CRASH

Pharmacology

elow.

Other Titles in the Crash Course Series

There are 23 books in the Crash Course series in two ranges: Basic Science and Clinical. Each book follows the same format, with concise text, clear illustrations, and helpful learning features, including access online USMLE test questions.

Basic Science titles
Pathology
Nervous System
Renal and Urinary Systems
Gastrointestinal System
Respiratory System
Endocrine and Reproductive Systems
Metabolism and Nutrition
Pharmacology
Immunology
Musculoskeletal System
Cardiovascular System

Forthcoming:
Cell Biology and Genetics
Anatomy

Clinical titles
Surgery
Cardiology
History and Examination
Internal Medicine
Neurology
Gastroenterology

Forthcoming:
OBGYN
Psychiatry
Imaging
Pediatrics

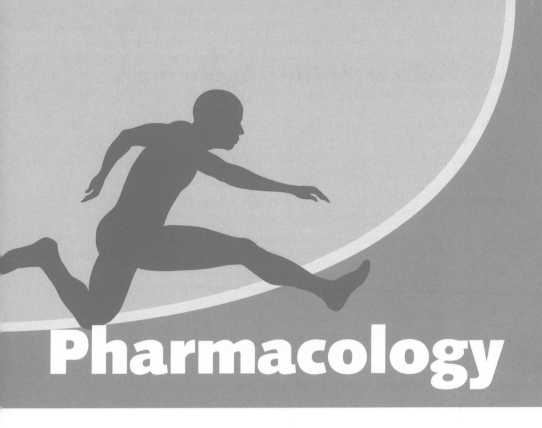

Pharmacology

Donald W. Barnes, PhD

Professor and Course Director, Medical Pharmacology
Department of Pharmacology and Toxicology
The Brody School of Medicine
East Carolina University
Greenville, North Carolina

UK edition authors
**James S. Dawson, Magali N.F. Taylor,
Peter J.W. Reide**

UK Series editor
Daniel Horton-Szar

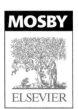

MOSBY

ELSEVIER

MOSBY
ELSEVIER

1600 John F. Kennedy Boulevard
Suite 1800
Philadelphia, PA 19103-2899

CRASH COURSE: PHARMACOLOGY ISBN-13: 978-1-4160-2959-5
Copyright © 2006 by Mosby, Inc., an affiliate of Elsevier Inc. ISBN-10: 1-4160-2959-1

Adapted from Crash Course Pharmacology 2e by James S. Dawson, ISBN 0-7234-3246-5.
© 2002, Elsevier Science Limited. All rights reserved.

The rights of James S. Dawson to be identified as the author of this work have been asserted by him in accordance with the Copyright Designs and Patents Act, 1988.

Library of Congress Cataloging-in-Publication Data

Barnes, Donald, MD.
  Crash course: pharmacology/Donald Barnes.—1st American ed.
    p. ; cm.—(Crash course)
  Includes index.
  ISBN 1-4160-2959-1
  1. Clinical pharmacology—Outlines, syllabi, etc. I. Title: Pharmacology. II. Title. III. Series.
  [DNLM: 1. Pharmacology, Clinical. QV 38 B261c 2006]
  RM301.28.B37 2006
  615'.1—dc22   2005056126

Commissioning Editor: Alex Stibbe
Developmental Editor: Stan Ward
Project Manager: David Saltzberg
Design: Andy Chapman
Cover Design: Antbits Illustration
Illustration Manager: Mick Ruddy

Printed in China.

Last digit is the print number:
9 8 7 6 5 4 3 2 1

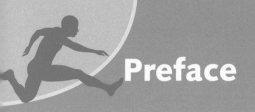

Preface

A major goal of *Crash Course Pharmacology* is to give a concise and clear presentation of basic pharmacologic concepts. The figures in this text are especially useful for grasping these major concepts. An additional goal is to provide a concise but sufficient description of drug information that can be read easily in a relatively short amount of time. However, unlike many review texts, explanations and information are discussed with enough detail to provide an essential understanding of important concepts rather than presented as simple statements for memorization.

Knowledge and practice in pharmacology and pharmacotherapeutics is highly dynamic. Drugs and their indications change almost daily with the frequent entry of newer drugs and withdrawal of other drugs. While no text can keep pace with all of these changes, the primary effort of *Crash Course Pharmacology* is to provide a timely and practical description of the drugs that are currently used in the United States.

Students should find that this book is an excellent supplement to their class notes and to more traditional texts.

Donald W. Barnes, PhD

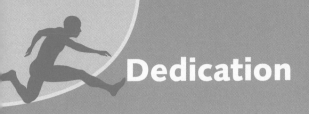

Dedication

*To
my most special
wife, children,
and grandchildren*

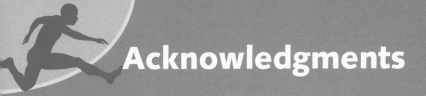

Acknowledgments

Figure credits

Figures 1.1–3, 1.12, 1.13, 6.1, 6.4, 6.11, 7.1–4, 8.3, 9.1, 9.3–5, 10.2, 11.1–5, 11.7, 11.11, 11.16, 11.18, 12.1–3, 12.6–8 redrawn from Integrated Pharmacology 2nd ed., edited by Professor C Page, Dr. M Curtis, Professor M Sutter, Professor M Walker and Professor B Hoffman, Mosby, 2002.

Contents

Preface v
Dedication. vii
Acknowledgments ix

Part I: Principles of Pharmacology 1

1. **Introduction to Pharmacology** 3
   Molecular basis of pharmacology 3
   Drugs and receptors. 8
   Pharmacokinetics. 10
   Drug interactions and adverse
   effects. 17
   Drug history and drug development 18

Part II: Clinical Pharmacology 21

2. **Cancer** 23
   Concepts of cancer chemotherapy 23

3. **Infectious Diseases** 31
   Antibacterial drugs. 31
   Antiviral drugs. 41
   Antifungal drugs 47
   Antiprotozoal drugs 49
   Antihelminthic drugs 53

4. **Inflammation, Pain, and
   Immunosuppression** 57
   Inflammation. 57
   Pain 63
   Immunosuppression 69

5. **Peripheral Nervous System** 73
   Basic concepts. 73
   Somatic nervous system. 76
   Autonomic nervous system 81
   Nitrergic nervous system 88

6. **Central Nervous System** 91
   Parkinsonism. 91
   Dementia 95
   Anxiety and sleep disorders 95
   Affective disorders. 99
   Psychotic disorders. 104

Nausea and vertigo 108
Epilepsy. 108
General anesthetics 113
Drug misuse 118

7. **Cardiovascular System.** **127**
   Heart 127
   Circulation. 138
   Hemostasis and thrombosis 148
   The blood and fluid replacement 153

8. **Respiratory System** **157**
   Reversible airways disease 157
   Respiratory stimulants and pulmonary
   surfactants 162
   Antitussives, mucolytics, and
   decongestants 162
   Allergic disorders and drug therapy. . . . 163

9. **Kidney and Urinary System** **167**
   Kidney 167
   Edema. 171
   Urinary system 172

10. **Gastrointestinal System.** **175**
    Stomach 175
    Nausea and vomiting. 179
    Intestines. 180
    Pancreas and gallbladder 185

11. **Endocrine and Reproductive
    Systems** **187**
    Thyroid gland 187
    Endocrine pancreas 190
    Adrenal cortex. 195
    Reproductive system 201
    Bone and calcium 207

12. **Eyes and Skin** **209**
    Eyes 209
    Skin 212

Index 219

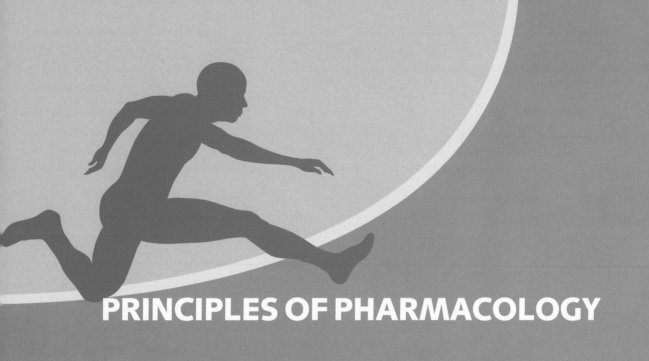

PRINCIPLES OF PHARMACOLOGY

1. Introduction to Pharmacology   3

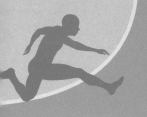

1. Introduction to Pharmacology

What is pharmacology?

The word "pharmacology" derives from the Greek word for drug, *pharmakon*.

Pharmacology is the study of the actions, mechanisms, uses, and adverse effects of drugs.

A drug is any natural or synthetic substance that alters the physiologic state of a living organism. Drugs can be divided into two groups:

- Medicinal drugs are substances used for the prevention, treatment, and diagnosis of disease.
- Nonmedicinal drugs, or social drugs, are substances used for recreational purposes. Nonmedicinal drugs include illegal mood-altering substances such as cannabis, heroin, and cocaine as well as everyday substances such as caffeine, nicotine, and alcohol.

Although drugs are intended to have a selective action, this is rarely achieved.

There is always a risk of adverse effects associated with the use of any drug, and each time a drug is used, the prescriber should be confident that the benefits of giving the drug outweigh potential drawbacks or adverse effects.

Drug names and classification

A single drug can have a variety of names and belong to many classes.

Factors used for classifying drugs include their:

- Pharmacotherapeutic actions.
- Pharmacologic actions.
- Molecular actions.
- Chemical nature.

The generic name of a drug is that which appears in official national pharmacopoeias. All drugs available on prescription or sold over the counter have a generic name that may vary from country to country. Newly patented drugs usually have one generic name (e.g., salmeterol) and one or more brand or proprietary names (e.g., Serevent®). However, once the patent expires, the marketing of the drug is open to any number of manufacturers, and, although the generic name is retained, the variety of brand names inevitably increases.

How do drugs work?

Drugs cause a change in physiologic function by interacting with the organism at the chemical level.

Certain drugs (e.g., general anesthetics, antacids) work by means of their physicochemical properties, and these are said to have a nonspecific mechanism of action. For this reason, these drugs must be given in much higher doses (mg–g) than the more specific drugs.

Most drugs produce their effects by targeting specific cellular macromolecules. This may involve modification of DNA or RNA function, inhibition of transport systems or enzymes, or, more commonly, action on receptors.

Detailed knowledge about the molecular structures of the cell is not required, though a simple understanding of them is useful in appreciating how drugs cause their effects and side effects.

Transport systems
Ion channels

Ion channels are pores located in the cell membrane that allow selective transfer of ions (charged species) in and out of the cell. Opening or closing of these channels, known as "gating," occurs as a result of the channel proteins undergoing a change in shape. Gating is controlled either by transmitter substances or by the membrane potential (voltage-operated channels).

Some drugs modulate ion channel function directly by binding to a part of the channel protein itself (e.g., the blocking action of local anesthetics on sodium channels). Other drugs interact with ion channels indirectly via a G-protein and other intermediates.

Carrier molecules

Transfer of ions and molecules against their concentration gradients is facilitated by carrier molecules located in the cell membrane. There are two types of carrier molecule:

- Energy-independent carriers are transporters (move one type of ion/molecule in one direction), symporters (move two or more ions/molecules), or antiporters (exchange one or more ions/molecules for one or more other ions/molecules).
- Energy-dependent carriers are termed pumps (e.g., the Na^+/K^+ ATPase pump).

Enzymes

Enzymes are protein catalysts that increase the rate of specific chemical reactions without undergoing any net change themselves during the reaction.

All enzymes are potential targets for drugs. Drugs either act as a false substrate for the enzyme, or they inhibit the enzyme's activity directly by binding to other sites on the enzyme protein.

Certain drugs may require enzymatic modification. This degradation converts a drug from its inactive form (prodrug) to its active form.

Receptors

Receptors are the means through which most drugs produce their effects.

A receptor is a specific protein molecule that is usually located in the cell membrane, though intracellular receptors and intranuclear receptors also exist. Agonist drugs mimic endogenous mediators and activate the receptor, while antagonist drugs bind to the receptor, preventing receptor activation by endogenous mediators.

Synaptic transmitter substances and hormones, the body's chemical messengers, are natural ligands (i.e., molecules that bind with a molecular target) for receptors, and they have the following modes of action:

- Neurotransmitters are chemicals that are released from nerve terminals, diffuse across the synaptic cleft, and bind to pre- or postsynaptic receptors.
- Hormones are chemicals that, after being released into the bloodstream from specialized cells, act at neighboring or distant cells.

Each cell expresses only certain receptors, depending on the function of the cell.

Receptor number and responsiveness to messengers can be modulated.

In many cases, there is more than one receptor for each messenger, so that the messenger often has different pharmacologic specificity and different functions according to where it binds (e.g., epinephrine). This may be a result of gene splicing and other processes that led to polypeptide diversity in evolution.

Using conventional molecular biology techniques, it is now possible to clone the genes' encoding receptors and express them in cultured cells, thus allowing their properties to be studied. In particular, substitutions of amino acid residues that may be caused by mutations can be reproduced, so that the relation between protein structure and function can be evaluated.

The four types of receptors for chemical messengers and growth factors are those:

- Linked directly to multimeric ion channels (inotropic).
- Linked via G-proteins to membrane enzymes and intracellular processes (metabotropic).
- Linked directly to tyrosine kinases.
- Linked to DNA interactions (steroid receptors).

Receptors directly linked to ion channels

Receptors that are directly linked to ion channels (Fig. 1.1) are mainly involved in fast synaptic neurotransmission, where the delay between ligand binding and channel opening lasts only a matter of milliseconds. A classic example of a receptor linked directly to an ion channel is the nicotinic

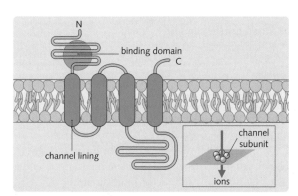

Fig. 1.1 General structure of the subunits of receptors directly linked to ion channels (N, N-terminal; C, C-terminal). (Redrawn from Page et al., 2002.)

acetylcholine receptor (nicAChR). The nicAChR consists of five subunits—two α, one β, one γ, and one δ—each of molecular weight 40–58 kDa and of great sequence identity.

The nicAChRs possess several characteristics:

- Acetylcholine (ACh) must bind to the N-termini of both α-subunits in order to activate the receptor.
- The whole receptor oligomer incorporates 20 transmembrane segments arranged around a central aqueous channel. One of the transmembrane helices (M_2) from each of the subunits is believed to form the lining of the channel.
- The receptor shows marked similarities with the two other receptors for fast transmission, namely the γ-aminobutyric acid ($GABA_A$) and glycine receptors.

G-protein-linked receptors

G-protein-linked receptors (Fig. 1.2) are involved in relatively rapid transduction, a response being generated in seconds. Muscarinic ACh, adrenergic, dopamine, serotonin, and opiate receptors are all examples of G-protein-linked receptors.

Molecular structure of the receptor

Most of the G-protein-linked receptors consist of a single polypeptide chain of 400–500 residues and have seven transmembrane α-helices. The third intracellular loop of the receptor is larger than the other loops, and this interacts with the G-protein.

The ligand-binding domain is buried within the membrane on one or more of the α-helical segments. This is unlike ion channel-coupled receptors, where the ligand binds to the extracellular N-terminal region—an area easily accessible to small hydrophobic molecules.

G-proteins

Fig. 1.3 describes the mechanism of G-protein-linked receptors:

- In the resting state, the G-protein exists as an unattached trimer consisting of α-, β-, and γ-subunits (Fig. 1.3A).
- The occupation of the receptor by an agonist produces a conformational change, causing its affinity for the trimer to increase. Subsequent association of the trimer with the receptor results in the dissociation of bound guanosine diphosphate (GDP) from the α-subunit. Guanosine triphosphate (GTP) replaces GDP in the cleft, thus activating the G-protein and causing the α-subunit to dissociate from the βγ-dimer (Fig. 1.3B).
- The α–GTP complex represents the active form of the G-protein (although this is not always the case: in the heart, potassium channels are activated by the βγ-dimer, and recent research has shown that the γ-subunit alone may play a role in activation). This component diffuses in the plane of the membrane, where it is free to interact with downstream effectors such as enzymes and ion channels. The βγ-dimer remains associated with the membrane, owing to its hydrophobicity (Fig. 1.3C).

The cycle is completed when the α-subunit, which has enzymic activity, hydrolyses the bound GTP to GDP. The GDP-bound α-subunit dissociates from the effector and recombines with the βγ-dimer (Fig. 1.3D).

This whole process results in an amplification effect because the binding of an agonist to the receptor can cause the activation of numerous G-proteins, which in turn can each, via their association with the effector, produce many molecules of product.

Targets for G-proteins

G-proteins interact with either ion channels or second messengers.

Ion channels

G-proteins may activate ion channels directly. For example, muscarinic receptors in the heart are linked

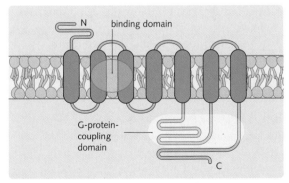

Fig. 1.2 General structure of the subunits of receptors linked to G-proteins (N, N-terminal; C, C-terminal). (Redrawn from Page *et al.*, 2002.)

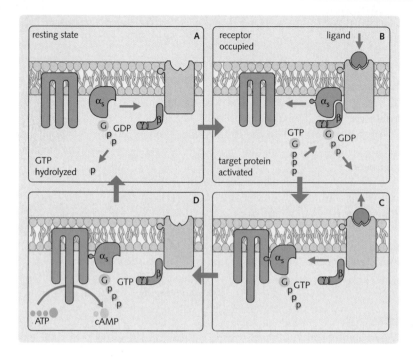

Fig. 1.3 Mechanism of G-protein-linked receptors (α, β, γ, subunits of G-protein; cAMP, cyclic adenosine monophosphate; ATP, adenosine triphosphate; G, guanosine; GDP, GTP, guanosine diphosphate and triphosphate; p, phosphate). (Redrawn from Page *et al.*, 2002.)

to potassium channels that open directly upon interaction with the G-protein, causing a slowing down of the heart rate.

Second messengers

Three second-messenger systems exist as targets of G-proteins (Fig. 1.4).

Adenylyl cyclase/cyclic AMP system

Many types of G-protein exist. This is probably attributable to the variability of the α-subunit. G_S and G_i/G_o cause stimulation and inhibition, respectively, of the target enzyme adenylyl cyclase. This explains why muscarinic ACh receptors and β-adrenoreceptors located in the heart produce opposite effects.

The bacterial toxins cholera and pertussis can be used in order to determine which G-protein is involved in a particular situation. Each has enzymic action on a conjugation reaction with the α-subunit, such that:

- Cholera affects G_S, causing continued activation of adenylyl cyclase. This explains why infection with cholera toxin results in uncontrolled fluid secretion from the gastrointestinal tract.
- Pertussis affects G_i and G_o, causing continued inactivation of adenylyl cyclase. This explains why infection with *Bordetella pertussis* causes a

"whooping" cough, characteristic of this infection, as the airways are constricted, and the larynx experiences muscular spasms.

Adenylyl cyclase catalyses the conversion of adenosine triphosphate (ATP) to cyclic adenosine monophosphate (cAMP) within cells. The cAMP produced in turn causes activation of certain protein kinases, enzymes that phosphorylate serine and threonine residues in various proteins, thereby producing either activation or inactivation of these proteins. This can lead to:

- Increased lipolysis through activation of hormone-sensitive lipase.
- Reduced glycogen synthesis through inactivation of glycogen synthase.
- Increased glycogen breakdown through the activation of phosphorylase kinase and, therefore, conversion of inactive phosphorylase b to active phosphorylase a.

Activation of $β_1$-adrenergic receptors found in cardiac muscle results in activation of cAMP-dependent protein kinase A, which phosphorylates and opens voltage-operated calcium channels. This increases calcium levels in the cell and results in an increased rate and force of contraction.

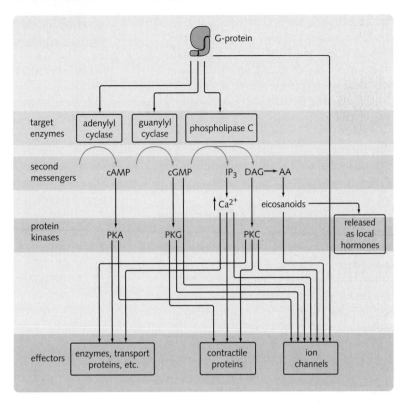

Fig. 1.4 Second-messenger targets of G-proteins and their effects (cAMP, cyclic adenosine monophosphate; cGMP, cyclic guanosine monophosphate; DAG, diacylglycerol; IP$_3$, inositol (1,4,5) triphosphate; PK, protein kinase; AA, arachidonic acid).

In contrast, activation of β$_2$-adrenergic receptors found in smooth muscle causes activation of protein kinase and, therefore, phosphorylation, but inactivation of another enzyme (myosin light-chain kinase) needed for contraction.

Receptors linked to G$_i$ inhibit adenylyl cyclase and reduce cAMP production. Examples of these receptors are the M$_2$ and M$_4$ muscarinic, the opioid, the 5-HT$_1$ (5-hydroxytryptamine), and the α$_2$-adrenoreceptors.

Phospholipase C/inositol phosphate system

Activation of M$_1$, M$_3$, 5-HT$_2$, peptide, and α$_1$-adrenoreceptors, via G$_q$, causes activation of phospholipase C, a membrane-bound enzyme, which increases the rate of degradation of phosphatidylinositol (4,5) bisphosphate into diacylglycerol (DAG) and inositol (1,4,5) triphosphate (IP$_3$). DAG and IP$_3$ act as second messengers.

IP$_3$ binds to the membrane of the endoplasmic reticulum, opening calcium channels and increasing the concentration of calcium within the cell by 10–100-fold. Increased calcium levels may result in smooth muscle contraction, increased secretion from exocrine glands, increased hormone or transmitter release, or increased force and rate of contraction of the heart.

DAG, which remains associated with the membrane owing to its hydrophobicity, causes protein kinase C to move from the cytosol to the membrane where DAG can regulate its activity. There are at least six types of protein kinase C, with 50 or more targets having effects such as:

- Release of hormones and neurotransmitters.
- Smooth muscle contraction.
- Inflammation.
- Ion transport.
- Tumor promotion.

Guanylyl cyclase system

Guanylyl cyclase catalyses the conversion of GTP to cGMP. This cGMP goes on to cause activation of protein kinase G, which in turn phosphorylates contractile proteins and ion channels.

Transmembrane guanylyl cyclase activity is exhibited by the atrial natriuretic peptide receptor upon the binding of atrial natriuretic peptide.

Cytoplasmic guanylyl cyclase activity is exhibited when bradykinin activates receptors on the membrane of endothelial cells to generate nitric oxide, which then acts as a second messenger to activate guanylyl cyclase within the cell.

Sodium nitroprusside is a nitrovasodilator that relaxes the smooth muscle of arteries and veins by increasing cGMP production. Because both central venous pressure and arterial pressure drop, there is little change in cardiac output. Sodium nitroprusside is used for angina and hypertension.

Tyrosine-kinase-linked receptors

Tyrosine-kinase-linked receptors are involved in the regulation of growth and differentiation, and the responses to metabolic signals.

The response time of enzyme-initiated transduction is slow (minutes). Examples include the receptors for insulin, platelet-derived growth factor, and epidermal growth factor.

Activation of tyrosine kinase receptors results in autophosphorylation of tyrosine residues, leading to the activation of pathways involving protein kinases.

DNA-linked receptors

Corticosteroids, thyroid hormone, retinoic acid, and vitamin D are all molecules with receptors that are linked so as to interact with DNA. The receptors are intracellular, and so agonists must pass through the cell membrane in order to reach the receptor. Receptor–agonist complexes are then transported to the nucleus. Once in the nucleus, the complex can bind to specific DNA sequences and so alter the expression of specific genes. As a result, secondary transduction involving an increase or decrease in the synthesis of various proteins occurs. The process is much slower than for other receptor–ligand interactions, and the effects usually last longer.

Drugs, like naturally occurring chemical mediators, act on receptors located in the cell membrane, in the cytoplasm of the cell, or in the cell nucleus, to bring about a cellular and, eventually, organ or tissue response.

Drugs and receptors

Drug–receptor interactions

Most drugs produce their effects by acting through specific protein molecules called receptors.

Receptors respond to endogenous chemicals in the body that are either synaptic transmitter substances (e.g., ACh, norepinephrine) or hormones (endocrine, e.g., insulin; or local mediators, e.g., histamine). These chemicals or drugs will do one of the following:
- Activate receptors and produce a subsequent response (agonists).
- Associate with receptors but not cause activation (antagonists). Antagonists reduce the chance of transmitters or agonists binding to the receptor and thereby oppose their action by effectively diluting or removing the receptors from the system.

Electrostatic forces initially attract a drug to a receptor. If the shape of the drug corresponds to that of the binding site of the receptor, then it will be held there temporarily by weak bonds or, in the case of irreversible antagonists, permanently by stronger covalent bonds. The number of bonds, and the level of perfection of fit, between drug and receptor determine the affinity of the drug for that receptor. The greater the number of bonds and the more perfect the fit, the higher the affinity.

The affinity is defined by the dissociation constant, which is given the symbol K_d. The lower the K_d, the higher the affinity. K_d values in the nanomolar range represent drugs (D) with a high affinity for their receptor (R):

$$D + R \underset{k_{-1}}{\overset{k_{+1}}{\rightleftharpoons}} DR$$

The rate at which the forward reaction occurs is dependent upon the drug concentration [D] and the receptor concentration [R]:

Forward rate = $k_{+1}[D][R]$

The rate at which the backward reaction occurs is mainly dependent upon the interaction between the drug and the receptor [DR]:

Backward rate = $k_{-1}[DR]$

$$K_d = \frac{k_{-1}}{k_{+1}}$$

K_a is the association constant and is used to quantify affinity. It can be defined as the concentration of drug that produces 50% of the maximum response at equilibrium, in the absence of receptor reserve:

$$K_a = \frac{1}{k_d}$$

Drugs with a high affinity stay bound to their receptor for a relatively long time and are said to have a slow off-rate. This means that at any time, the probability that any given receptor will be occupied by the drug is high.

The ability of a drug to combine with one type of receptor is termed specificity. Although no drug is truly specific, most exhibit relatively selective action on one type of receptor.

Agonists

An agonist (A) binds to the receptor (R), and the chemical energy released on binding induces a conformational change that sets off a chain of biochemical events within the cell, leading to a response (AR*). The equation for this is:

$$A + R \xrightarrow{(1)} AR \xrightarrow{(2)} AR^*$$

(1): affinity dependent   (2): efficacy dependent

Partial agonists cannot bring about the same maximum response as full agonists, even if their affinity for the receptor is the same (Figs. 1.5 and 1.6).

The ability of agonists, once bound, to activate receptors is termed efficacy. Full agonists have high efficacy, and they are able to produce a maximum response while occupying only a small percentage of the receptors available. Partial agonists have low efficacy, and they are unable to elicit the maximum response, even if they are occupying all the available receptors.

Antagonists

Antagonists bind to receptors, but they do not activate them; they do not induce a conformational change and so have no efficacy. However, because antagonists occupy the receptor, they prevent agonists from binding and, therefore, block their action.

Two types of antagonists exist, competitive and noncompetitive.

Competitive antagonists

These bind to receptors reversibly and effectively produce a dilution of the receptors, such that:

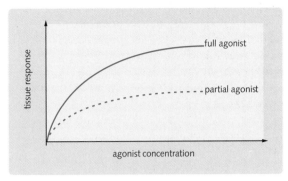

Fig. 1.5 Comparison of the dose–response curve for a partial agonist and a full agonist (From Medical Pharmacology at a Glance, 2nd ed., by MJ Neal. Courtesy of Blackwell Scientific Publications).

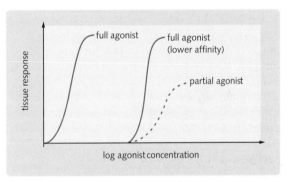

Fig. 1.6 Comparison of the log dose–response curve for a partial agonist and a full agonist (From Medical Pharmacology at a Glance, 2nd ed., by MJ Neal. Courtesy of Blackwell Scientific Publications).

- A parallel shift is produced to the right of the agonist dose–response curve (Fig. 1.7).
- The maximum response is not depressed. This reflects the fact that the antagonist's effect can be overcome by increasing the dose of agonist; that is, the block is surmountable. Increasing the concentration of agonist increases the probability of the agonist taking the place of an antagonist leaving the receptor.
- The size of the shift in the agonist dose–response curve produced by the antagonist reflects the affinity of the antagonist for the receptor. High-affinity antagonists stay bound to the receptor for a relatively long period of time, allowing the agonist little chance to take the antagonist's place.

This concept can be quantified in terms of the dose ratio. The dose ratio is the ratio of the concentration of agonist producing a given response in the presence

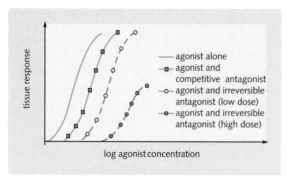

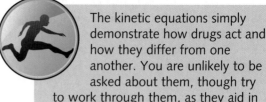

The kinetic equations simply demonstrate how drugs act and how they differ from one another. You are unlikely to be asked about them, though try to work through them, as they aid in the building of a good foundation in the subject.

Fig. 1.7 Comparison of the log dose–response curves for competitive and noncompetitive (irreversible) antagonists (From Medical Pharmacology at a Glance, 2nd ed., by MJ Neal. Courtesy of Blackwell Scientific Publications).

and absence of a certain concentration of antagonist (e.g., a dose ratio of 3 tells us that three times as much agonist was required to produce a given response in the presence of the antagonist than it did in its absence).

Noncompetitive antagonists

These are also known as irreversible antagonists. Like competitive antagonists, their presence also produces a parallel shift to the right of the agonist dose–response curve (see Fig. 1.7). However, noncompetitive antagonists also depress the maximum response, reflecting the fact that the antagonist's effect cannot be overcome by the addition of greater doses of agonist. At low concentrations of antagonist, however, a parallel shift may occur without a reduced maximum response. This tells us that not all of the receptors need be occupied by agonist in order to elicit a maximum response, since irreversible antagonists effectively remove receptors, and there must be a number of spare receptors.

Receptor reserve

Although on a log scale the relationship between the concentration of agonist and the response produces a symmetrical sigmoid curve, very rarely does a 50% response correspond to 50% receptor occupancy. This is due to the fact that there are spare receptors.

This excess of receptors is known as receptor reserve and serves to sharpen the sensitivity of the cell to small changes in agonist concentration.

The low efficacy of partial agonists can be overcome in tissues with a large receptor reserve, and in these circumstances partial agonists may act as full agonists.

Potency

Potency relates to the concentration of a drug needed to elicit a response.

The EC_{50}, where EC stands for effective concentration, is a number used to quantify potency. The EC_{50} is the concentration producing 50% of the maximum response. Therefore, the lower the EC_{50}, the more potent the drug.

Where agonists are concerned, potency is related to both the affinity and the efficacy.

Pharmacokinetic variables also affect potency. For example, the acidic pH of the stomach may break down a drug that has been found to be very potent in a test tube. This means that, if given as a tablet, it would have very little potency and would be ineffective.

Pharmacokinetics

Pharmacology can be divided into two disciplines:
- Pharmacokinetics, which considers drug disposition and the way the body affects the drug with time (i.e., the factors that determine its absorption, distribution, metabolism, and excretion).
- Pharmacodynamics, which deals with the effect of the drug on the body.

Compliance

Compliance on the patient's behalf is very important as far as taking drugs is concerned. In order for some drugs to be effective (e.g., antibiotics), they must be taken at regular intervals and for a certain period of time. For certain forms of treatment, patients may even need to come to the hospital, in which case transport, work, and having young children may be a problem.

Compliance tends to be more of a problem in pediatric practice since it involves both parents and the child: the parent must remember to give the medication and follow directions accurately; the child must cooperate and not spit out or spill the medicine.

Practical dosage forms are important in achieving compliance. Many tablets are now sugar coated, making them easier to take; and a large number of the drugs manufactured for children are in the form of elixirs or suspensions, which may be available in a variety of different flavors, making their administration less of a problem.

The route of administration of a drug may affect compliance. Taking a drug orally, for example, is simpler than having it injected.

The dosing schedule is also an important aspect of compliance. The easier this is to follow, and the less frequently a drug needs to be taken or administered, the more likely it is that compliance will occur.

Routes of administration
Topical
Topical drugs are placed where they are needed, giving them the advantage that they do not have to cross any barriers or membranes. Examples include skin ointments; ear, nose, or eye drops; and aerosols inhaled in the treatment of asthma.

Enteral
Enteral administration means that the drug reaches its target via the gut. It is the least predictable route of administration, owing to metabolism by the liver, chemical breakdown, and the possible binding to food. Drugs must cross several barriers, which may or may not be a problem according to their physicochemical properties such as charge and size. However, most drugs are administered orally unless the drug is unstable or is rapidly inactivated in the gastrointestinal tract, or if its efficacy of absorption from the gastrointestinal tract is uncertain owing to metabolism by the liver or the intestines, vomiting, or a disease that may affect drug absorption.

Absorption of drugs via the buccal or sublingual route avoids the portal circulation, and it is, therefore, valuable when administering drugs subject to a high degree of first-pass metabolism (which is unavoidable if taken orally). It is also useful for potent drugs with an agreeable taste, such as sublingual nitroglycerin given to relieve acute attacks of angina.

Administration of drugs rectally, such as in the form of suppositories, means that there is less first-pass metabolism by the liver because the venous return from the lower gastrointestinal tract is less than that from the upper gastrointestinal tract. It has the disadvantage, however, of being inconsistent.

Antacids have their effect in the stomach and may be considered as being topical.

Parenteral
Parenteral administration means that the drug is administered in a manner that avoids the gut. The protein drug insulin, for example, is destroyed by the acidity of the stomach and the digestive enzymes within the gut; therefore, it must be injected, usually subcutaneously.

Intravenous injection of drugs has several advantages:
- It is the most direct route of administration. The drug enters the bloodstream directly and bypasses absorption barriers.
- A drug is distributed in a large volume and acts rapidly.

For drugs that must be given continuously by infusion, or for drugs that damage tissues, this is an important method of administration.

Alternative parenteral routes of administration include subcutaneous, intramuscular, epidural, or intrathecal injections, and transdermal patches such as are used in angina.

The rate of drug absorption from the site of the injection can be decreased by binding the drug to a vehicle or coadministering a vasoconstrictor, such as epinephrine, to reduce blood flow to the site.

Drug absorption
Bioavailability takes into account both absorption and metabolism and describes the proportion of the drug that passes into the systemic circulation. This will, of course, be 100% after an intravenous injection; but following oral administration it will depend on the drug, the individual, and the circumstances under which the drug is given.

Since drugs must cross membranes in order to enter cells or to transfer between body compartments, drug absorption will be affected by both chemical and physiological factors.

Cell membranes
Cell membranes are composed of lipid bilayers, and thus absorption is usually proportional to the lipid solubility of the drug. Un-ionized molecules (B) are far more lipid soluble than those that are ionized

(BH^+) and surrounded by a "shell" of water.

$$B + H^+ \leftrightarrows BH^+$$

Size

Small size is another factor that favors absorption. Most drugs are small molecules (molecular weight <1000) that are able to diffuse across membranes in their uncharged state.

pH

Since most drugs are either weak bases, weak acids, or amphoteric, the pH of the environment in which they dissolve, as well as the pK_a value of the drug, will be important in determining the fraction in the un-ionized form that is in solution and able to diffuse across cell membranes. The pK_a of a drug is defined as the pH at which 50% of the molecules in solution are in the ionized form, and is characterized by the Henderson-Hasselbalch equation:

For acidic molecules: $HA \leftrightarrows H^+ + A^-$

$$pk_a = pH + \log\frac{[HA]}{[A^-]}$$

For basic molecules: $BH^+ \leftrightarrows B + H^+$

$$pk_a = pH + \log\frac{[BH^+]}{[B]}$$

Drugs will tend to exist in the ionized form when exposed to an environment with a pH opposite to their own state. Therefore, acids become increasingly ionized with increasing pH (i.e., basic).

It is useful to consider three important body compartments—plasma (pH = 7.4), stomach (pH = 2.0), and urine (pH = 8.0)—in relation to drugs:

- Aspirin is a weak acid (pK_a = 3.5), and its absorption will, therefore, be favored in the stomach, where it is uncharged, and not in the plasma or the urine, where it is highly charged. Aspirin in high doses may even damage the stomach.
- Morphine is a weak base (pK_a = 8.0) that is highly charged in the stomach, quite charged in the plasma, and half charged in the urine. Morphine is able to cross the blood–brain barrier, but it is poorly and erratically absorbed from the stomach and intestines, and metabolized by the liver. It must, therefore, be given by injection or delayed-release capsules. Some drugs, such as quaternary ammonium compounds (e.g., succinylcholine, tubocurarine), are always charged and must, therefore, be injected.

Drug distribution

Once drugs have reached the circulation, they are distributed around the body. As most drugs are of a very small molecular size, they are able to leave the circulation by capillary filtration to act on the tissues.

The half-life of a drug ($t_{1/2}$) is the time taken for the plasma concentration of that drug to fall to half of its original value.

Bulk transfer in the blood is very quick. Drugs exist either dissolved in blood or bound to plasma proteins such as albumin. Albumin is the most important circulating protein for binding many acidic drugs. Basic drugs tend to be bound to a globulin fraction that increases with age. A drug that is bound is confined to the vascular system, and it is unable to exert its actions; this becomes a problem if more than 80% of the drug is bound. Drugs also interact, and one drug may displace another. For example, aspirin can displace the benzodiazepine diazepam from albumin.

The apparent volume of distribution (V_d) is the calculated pharmacokinetic space into which a drug is distributed.

$$V_d = \frac{\text{dose administered}}{\text{initial apparent plasma concentration}}$$

V_d values that amount to less than a certain body compartment volume indicate that the drug is contained within that compartment. For example, when the volume of distribution is less than 5L, it is likely that the drug is restricted to the vasculature. If it is less than 15L, this implies that the drug is restricted to the extracellular fluid; if it is greater than 15L, this suggests distribution within the total body water. Some drugs (usually basic) have a volume of distribution that exceeds body weight, in which case tissue binding is occurring. These drugs tend to be contained outside the circulation and may accumulate in certain tissues. Very lipid-soluble substances, such as thiopental, can build up in fat; lead accumulates in bone; and quinacrine, an antimalarial drug, has a concentration in the liver 200 times that in the plasma because it binds to nucleic acids. Some drugs are even actively transported into certain organs.

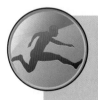

Highly lipid-soluble drugs such as thiopental will accumulate in fat, and as such, its half life will be much longer in obese than in thin patients.

Drug metabolism

Before being excreted from the body, most drugs are metabolized. A small number of drugs exist in their fully ionized form at physiological pH (7.4), and, because of this highly polar nature, they are metabolized to only a minor extent, if at all. The sequential metabolic reactions that occur have been categorized as phases 1 and 2.

Sites of metabolism

The liver is the major site of drug metabolism although most tissues are able to metabolize specific drugs. Other sites of metabolism include the kidney, the lung, and the gastrointestinal tract.

Orally administered drugs, which are usually absorbed in the small intestine, reach the liver via the portal circulation. At this stage, or within the small intestine, the drugs may be extensively metabolized; this is known as first-pass metabolism and means that considerably less drug reaches the systemic circulation than enters the portal vein. This causes problems because it means that higher doses of drug must be given, and, owing to individual variation in the degree of first-pass metabolism, the effects of the drug can be unpredictable. Drugs that are subject to a high degree of first-pass metabolism, such as the local anesthetic lidocaine (lignocaine), cannot be given orally and must be administered by some other route.

Phase 1 metabolic reactions

Phase 1 metabolic reactions include oxidations, reductions, and hydrolyses. These reactions introduce a functional group, such as $-OH$, $-NH_2$, $-SH$, or $COOH$, which increases the polarity of the drug molecule and provides a site for phase 2 reactions.

Oxidations

Oxidations are the most common type of phase 1 reactions and are catalyzed by an enzyme system known as the microsomal mixed function oxidase system, which is located on the smooth endoplasmic reticulum and consists of a number of enzymes known as the cytochromes P450.

The cytochromes P450 are the most important phase 1 enzymes, although other enzymes are involved in phase 1 metabolism. Cytochromes P450 are hemoproteins that require the presence of oxygen, reduced nicotinamide adenine dinucleotide phosphate (NADPH), and NADPH cytochrome P450 reductase in order to oxidize a drug.

There are over 50 isoforms of human cytochromes P450, some of which are constitutive, while others are synthesized (induced) in response to specific signals. The substrate specificities of the isoforms for drugs tend to be low and can overlap among different isoforms, meaning that a whole variety drugs can be oxidized by one or more isoforms (CYPs) of cytochromes P450.

The major human P450 families that are involved in phase 1 drug metabolism are CYP1A2, CYP2C9, CYP2D6, CYP2E, and CYP3A. CYP3A is responsible for the metabolism of the largest proportion of drugs.

Although oxidative reactions usually result in inactivation of the drug, sometimes a metabolite is produced that is pharmalogically active and may have a duration of action exceeding that of the original drug. In such cases, the drug is known as a prodrug (e.g., codeine, which is demethylated to morphine).

Reductions

Reduction reactions also involve microsomal enzymes but are much less common than oxidation reactions. Examples of drugs subject to reduction include prednisone, which is given as a prodrug and reduced to the active glucocorticoid prednisolone; and warfarin, an anticoagulant, which is inactivated by the transformation of a ketone group to a hydroxyl group.

Hydrolysis

Hydrolysis is not restricted to the liver and occurs in a variety of tissues. Aspirin is spontaneously hydrolyzed to salicylic acid in moisture.

Phase 2 metabolic reactions

Drug molecules that possess a suitable site that was either present before phase 1 or is the result of a phase 1 reaction are susceptible to phase 2 reactions. Phase 2 reactions involve conjugation—the attachment of a large chemical group to a functional group on the drug molecule. Conjugation results in the drug being more hydrophilic and thus more easily excreted from the body. In conjugation, it is mainly the liver that is involved, although conjugation can occur in a wide variety of tissues.

Chemical groups involved are endogenous activated moieties such as glucuronic acid, sulphate, methyl and acetyl groups, and glutathione. The conjugating enzymes exist in many isoforms, and they show relative substrate and metabolite specificity.

Unlike the products of phase 1 reactions, the conjugate is almost invariably inactive. An important exception is morphine, which is converted to morphine-6-glucuronide, which has an analgesic effect lasting longer than that of its parent molecule.

Factors affecting metabolism

Enzyme induction is the increased synthesis or decreased degradation of enzymes, and it occurs as a result of the presence of an exogenous substance. For example:

- Some drugs are able to increase the activity of certain isoenzyme forms of cytochrome P450 and thus increase their own metabolism as well as that of other drugs.
- Smokers can show increased metabolism of certain drugs because of the induction of cytochrome P448 (CYP 1A2) by a constituent in tobacco smoke.
- In contrast, some drugs inhibit microsomal enzyme activity and, therefore, increase their own activity as well as that of other drugs.
- Some dietary substances can increase or decrease cytochrome P450-mediated drug metabolism. Grapefruit juice is a potent inhibitor of CYP3A4.

Fig. 1.8 gives some examples of enzyme-inducing agents and the drugs whose metabolism is affected.

Competition for a metabolic enzyme may occur between two drugs, in which case there is a decreased metabolism of one or both drugs. This is known as inhibition.

Enzymes that metabolize drugs are affected by many aspects of diet, such as the ratio of protein to carbohydrate, flavonoids contained in vegetables, and polycyclic aromatic hydrocarbons found in barbecued foods.

Acetaminophen poisoning

Acetaminophen is a classic example of a drug that can be lethal at high doses (2–3 times the maximum therapeutic dose), owing to the accumulation of its metabolites.

In phase 2 of the metabolic process, acetaminophen is conjugated with glucuronic acid and sulphate. When high doses of acetaminophen are taken, these pathways become saturated, and the drug is metabolized by the mixed-function oxidases. This results in the formation of the toxic metabolite N-acetyl-p-benzoquinone, which is inactivated by glutathione. However, when glutathione is depleted, this toxic metabolite reacts with nucleophilic constituents in the cell, leading to necrosis in the liver and kidneys.

N-Acetylcysteine or methionine can be administered in cases of acetaminophen overdose, since they increase liver glutathione formation and the conjugation reactions, respectively.

Drug excretion

Drugs are excreted from the body in a variety of different ways. Excretion can occur by the kidneys into urine, by the gastrointestinal tract into bile and feces, and by the lungs into exhaled air. Drugs may also leave the body through breast milk and sweat. The most important routes for drug excretion are through the urine and feces.

The volume of plasma cleared of drug per unit time is known as the clearance rate.

Examples of drugs that induce or inhibit drug-metabolizing enzymes	
Drugs modifying enzyme action	**Drugs whose metabolism is affected**
Enzyme induction Phenobarbital and other barbiturates Rifampin Phenytoin Ethanol Carbamazepine	Warfarin Oral contraceptives Corticosteroids Cyclosporine
Enzyme inhibition Allopurinol Chloramphenicol Corticosteroids Cimetidine MAO inhibitors Erythromycin Ciprofloxacin	Azathioprine Phenytoin Various drugs- TCA, cyclophosphamide Many drugs-amiodarone, phenytoin meperidine Meperidine Cyclosporine Theophylline

Fig. 1.8 Examples of drugs that induce or inhibit drug-metabolizing enzymes (MAO, monoamine oxidase; TCA, tricyclic antidepressant). (Adapted from Pharmacology, by H Rang, M Dale and J Ritter, 4th ed., 2001, Churchill Livingstone.)

Renal excretion

Glomerular filtration, tubular reabsorption (passive and active), and tubular secretion all determine the extent to which a drug will be excreted by the kidneys.

Glomerular capillaries allow the passage of molecules with a molecular weight <20000. The glomerular filtrate thus contains most of the substances in plasma except proteins. In the glomerular capillaries:

- The negative charge of the corpuscular membrane also repels negatively charged molecules, including plasma proteins.
- Drugs that bind to plasma proteins such as albumin will not be filtered.

Most of the drug in the blood does not pass into the glomerular filtrate but passes into the peritubular capillaries of the proximal tubule, where it may be transported into the lumen of the tubule by either of two transport mechanisms. One transport mechanism deals with acidic molecules, the other with basic molecules. In the peritubular capillaries:

- Tubular secretion is responsible for most of the drug excretion carried out by the kidneys and, unlike glomerular filtration, allows the clearance of drugs bound to plasma proteins. Competition between drugs that share the same transport mechanism may occur, in which case the excretion of these drugs will be reduced. Probenecid is a drug that was designed to compete with penicillin for excretion and, therefore, increase the duration of action of penicillin.
- Reabsorption of a drug will depend upon the fraction of molecules in the ionized state, which is in turn dependent on the pH of the urine. Intoxification with aspirin (weak acid, $pK_a = 3.5$) can be treated by administering bicarbonate, which makes the urine more alkaline; this ionizes aspirin and renders it less prone to reabsorption.
- Renal disease will affect the excretion of certain drugs. The extent to which excretion is impaired can be deduced by measuring 24-hour creatinine clearance.

Gastrointestinal excretion

Some drug conjugates are excreted into the bile and subsequently released into the intestines, where they can be hydrolyzed back to the parent compound and reabsorbed. This "enterohepatic circulation" prolongs the effect of the drug.

Mathematical aspects of pharmacokinetics
Kinetic order

Two types of kinetics, related to the plasma concentration of a drug, describe the rate at which a drug leaves the body:

- Zero-order kinetics (Fig. 1.9) describes a decrease in drug levels in the body that is independent of the plasma concentration, and the rate is held constant by a limiting factor, such as availability of an enzyme cofactor. When the plasma concentration is plotted against time, the decrease is a straight line. Ethanol is an example of a drug that displays zero-order kinetics.
- First-order kinetics (Fig. 1.10) is displayed by most drugs. It describes a decrease in drug levels in the body that is dependent on the plasma concentration, as the concentration of the substrate (drug) is the rate-limiting factor. When the plasma concentration is plotted against time, the decrease is exponential.

One-compartment model

The one-compartment model considers the body to be a single compartment. Within this single compartment, a drug is absorbed, immediately distributed, and subsequently eliminated by metabolism and excretion.

If the volume of the compartment is V_d and the dose administered D, then the initial drug concentration, C_o, will be:

$$C_o = \frac{D}{V_d}$$

The time taken for the plasma drug concentration to fall to half of its original value is the half-life of that drug. The decline in concentration may be exponential, but this situation expresses itself

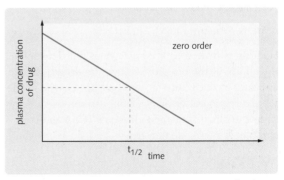

Fig. 1.9 Plasma drug concentration versus time plot for a drug displaying zero-order kinetics ($t_{1/2}$, half-life).

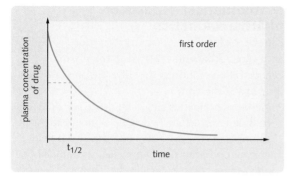

Fig. 1.10 Plasma drug concentration versus time plot for a drug displaying first-order kinetics ($t_{1/2}$, half-life).

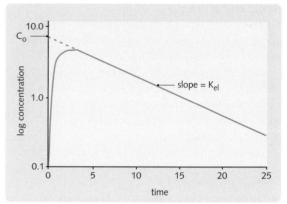

Fig. 1.12 Log plasma drug concentration versus time plot for a drug compatible with the one-compartment open pharmacokinetic model for drug disposition after an oral dose (Kel, elimination rate constant; C_0, initial drug concentration; $t_{1/2}$, half-life). (Redrawn from Page et al.,

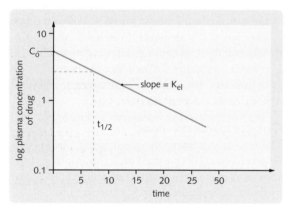

Fig. 1.11 Log plasma drug concentration versus time plot compatible with the one-compartment open pharmacokinetic model for drug disposition after a parenteral dose, assuming first-order kinetics (Kel, elimination rate constant; C_0, initial drug concentration; $t_{1/2}$, half-life).

graphically as a straight line when the log plasma concentration is plotted against the time after intravenous dose (Fig. 1.11).

Half-life is related to the elimination rate constant (K_{el}) by the following equation:

$$t_{1/2} \times K_{el} = \text{natural log 2 (ln 2)}$$

Half-life is related to V_d, but it does not determine the ability of the body to remove the drug from the circulation, since both V_d and half-life change in the same direction. The body's ability to remove a drug from the blood is termed clearance (Cl_p) and is constant for individual drugs:

$$Cl_p = V_d \times K_{el}$$

If the drug is not administered parenterally, plotting the log plasma drug concentration against

time will require the consideration of both absorption and elimination from the compartment (Fig. 1.12).

The one-compartment model is widely used to determine the dose of drug to be administered.

Two-compartment model

The distribution of drugs between the peripheral compartment (i.e., tissues) and the central compartment (i.e., plasma) occurs at rates varying from rapid to insignificant.

Some drugs distribute slowly or extensively, and in these cases a curvilinear relationship between the log of the plasma concentration and time is seen. Two phases can be observed (Fig. 1.13):

- An early, rapid α-phase, which represents the redistribution of the drug to the peripheral compartment and a modest component of elimination.
- A later, slower β-phase, which is a combination of elimination and return of the drug from the peripheral compartment to the central compartment, in which the drug then distributes rapidly.

The liver is the main site of drug inactivation, and the kidneys and gastrointestinal tract the main sites for drug excretion—disease of these organs will alter a drug's pharmacokinetics.

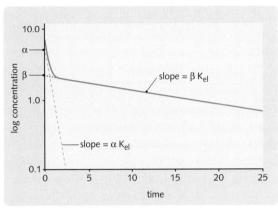

Fig. 1.13 Log plasma drug concentration versus time plot that requires a two-compartment open model to account for its disposition after a parenteral dose (K_{el}, elimination rate constant). (Redrawn from Page *et al.*, 2002.)

Model-independent approach

For drugs displaying first-order kinetics, the level of the drug in the body increases until it is equal to the level excreted, at which point steady-state is reached (Fig. 1.14), such that:

- The time to reach steady-state is usually equal to four to five half-lives.
- The amount of drug in the body at steady-state will depend on the frequency of drug administration—the greater the frequency, the greater the amount of drug and the less the variation between peak and trough plasma concentrations. If the frequency of administration is greater than the half-life, then accumulation of the drug will occur.

The loading dose can be calculated according to the desired plasma concentration at steady-state (CSS) and the volume of distribution (V_d) of the drug:

Loading dose $(mg/kg) = V_d(L/kg) \times C_{SS}(mg/L)$

Drug interactions and adverse effects

Drug interactions

Drugs interact in a number of ways that may produce unwanted effects. Two types of interactions exist, pharmacodynamic and pharmacokinetic.

Pharmacodynamic interactions

Pharmacodynamic interactions involve a direct conflict between the effects of drugs. This conflict results in the effect of one of the two drugs being enhanced or reduced. For example:

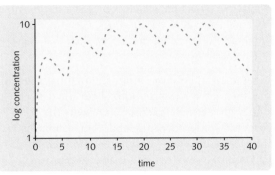

Fig. 1.14 Log plasma drug concentration versus time plot for a drug administered by mouth every 6 hours when its terminal disposition half-life is 6 hours.

- Propranolol, a β-adrenoceptor antagonist given for angina and hypertension, will reduce the effect of salmeterol, a β_2-adrenoceptor agonist given for the treatment of asthma. The administration of β-blockers to asthmatics should, therefore, be avoided, or undertaken with caution.
- Administration of monoamine oxidase inhibitors, which inhibit the metabolism of catecholamines, enhances the effects of drugs such as ephedrine. This enhancement causes the release of norepinephrine from stores in the nerve terminal and is known as "potentiation."

Pharmacokinetic interactions

Absorption, distribution, metabolism, and excretion all affect the pharmacokinetic properties of drugs. Therefore, any drug that interferes with these processes will be altering the effect of other drugs. For example:

- If administered with diuretics, nonsteroidal anti-inflammatory drugs (NSAIDs) will reduce the antihypertensive action of these drugs. NSAIDs bring about this effect by reducing prostaglandin synthesis in the kidney, thus impairing renal blood flow and consequently decreasing the excretion of waste and sodium. This results in an increased blood volume and a rise in blood pressure.

 Adverse reactions and allergy to a drug are different. Adverse reactions can be minor irritations or upset, though an allergic reaction can be life threatening.

- Enzyme induction, which occurs as a result of the administration of certain drugs, can affect the metabolism of other drugs served by that enzyme (see Fig. 1.8).

In some cases, however, drugs are used together so that their interaction can bring about the desired effect. For example, carbidopa prevents the conversion of levodopa (L-dopa) to dopamine and is therefore used with L-dopa in the treatment of Parkinson's disease. L-Dopa is able to cross the blood–brain barrier and enter the brain, where it is converted to dopamine. Carbidopa reduces the peripheral side effects of L-dopa, but it cannot cross the blood–brain barrier.

Adverse effects

As well as interacting with one another and with their target tissue, drugs will also interact with other tissues and organs and alter their function. No drug is without side effects, although the severity and frequency of these will vary from drug to drug and from person to person.

The liver and the kidneys are susceptible to the adverse effects of drugs, as these are the sites of drug metabolism and excretion. Some drugs cause hepatotoxicity or nephrotoxicity.

Those who are more prone to the adverse effects of drugs, include:

- Pregnant women, who must be careful about taking drugs, as certain drugs are teratogenic; that is, they cause fetal malformations (e.g., thalidomide taken in the 1960s for morning sickness).
- Breastfeeding women, who must also be careful about which drugs they take, as many drugs can be passed on in the breast milk and consumed by the developing infant.
- Patients with an underlying illness other than the one being treated, such as liver or kidney disease. These illnesses will result in decreased metabolism and excretion of the drug, and they will produce the side effects of an increased dose of the same drug.
- The elderly, who tend to take a large number of drugs, greatly increasing the risk of drug interactions and the associated side effects. In addition, elderly patients have a reduced renal clearance and a nervous system that is more sensitive to drugs. The dose of drug initially given is often less than 50% of the adult dose, and certain drugs are contraindicated.
- Patients with genetic enzyme defects, such as glucose-6-phosphate dehydrogenase deficiency.

This deficiency will result in hemolysis if an oxidant drug (e.g., aspirin) is taken.

Certain drugs are carcinogenic (i.e., induce cancer). Genotoxic carcinogens cause mutations, either directly (primary carcinogens) or through their metabolites (secondary carcinogens). Epigenetic carcinogens, such as phorbol esters, do not induce mutations themselves, but they increase the likelihood that a mutagen will do so.

Allergic reactions to certain drugs are common, occurring in 2–25% of cases. Most of these are not serious (e.g., skin reactions); however, rarely, reactions such as anaphylactic shock (type 1 hypersensitivity) occur, which may be lethal unless treated with parenteral epinephrine. The most common allergic reaction is to penicillin, which produces anaphylactic shock in approximately 1 in 50,000 people.

Some drugs (e.g., the vasodilator hydralazine) induce autoimmune reactions similar to systemic lupus erythematosus. Stopping the drug usually puts an end to this reaction, although in some cases glucocorticoid therapy may be needed.

Drug history and drug development

The drug history

A patient's drug history is a crucial component of the clerking process, as drug effects account for a significant proportion of hospital admissions, and foreseeing potential drug interactions and adverse events is crucial.

A complete list of the names and doses of prescribed drugs taken by patients (noting the proprietary or trade name and the generic or chemical name, such as Viagra® and sildenafil, respectively) and any other medications or supplements they may have bought themselves over the counter at the pharmacy should be documented. Women often forget the contraceptive pill and hormone replacement therapy, and they should be sensitively questioned about these. Nonsteroidal anti-inflammatory drugs and acetaminophen are often taken by the bucket load in patients with arthritis, and again these should be specifically asked about. Make sure to note how often the drugs are taken and at what times.

If presented with numerous bottles and packets of tablets, it is important to ensure that they all belong to the patient and not the partner of the patient or someone else; the effects could be devastating. Ask the patient if he or she was taking all his or her medicines as prescribed—it is not unusual for people to alter their dosages without consulting a doctor!

Occasionally, it is useful to know what drugs have been taken in the recent and distant past. For example, monoamine oxidase inhibitors should be stopped for at least 3 weeks prior to starting a different antidepressant therapy, and the cytotoxic drug bleomycin can cause lung fibrosis years later.

It is essential to ascertain previous adverse reaction to drugs and to nondrug products such as latex. Explore what happened to the patient and what was done about it. A simple upset stomach and loose stools just for one day after taking amoxicillin previously is an acceptable side effect, and it is not grounds for choosing another antibiotic when treating a penicillin-sensitive infection in the future. Widespread cutaneous rash and difficulty breathing, which required epinephrine and hospital admission, are genuinely worrying adverse effects of penicillin, and any such drug should be clearly avoided in the future, as this was an allergic drug reaction. Allergy to drugs should be clearly marked in the patient's notes and drug charts.

Family history of adverse drug reactions is usually confined to the anesthetic history, where the concern is largely in relation to the muscle-relaxing drugs, particularly succinylcholine.

Asking a patient about recreational or illicit drug use is occasionally important, though on the whole patients find it uncomfortable to talk about, and usually this adds little to the overall drug history.

Knowledge about any hepatic or renal disease, and general health problems, is important when it comes to management and prescribing, as are specific considerations, such as not prescribing aspirin in peptic ulcer disease, or estrogen to patients with estrogen-dependent cancers. These aspects are usually brought to light in the rest of the history-taking.

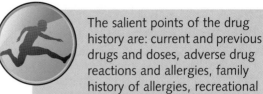

The salient points of the drug history are: current and previous drugs and doses, adverse drug reactions and allergies, family history of allergies, recreational drug use, and existing renal, hepatic, or general disease.

Drug development

Hundreds of thousands of substances have been produced by the pharmaceutical industry over the past 50 years, although few ever get past preclinical screening, and fewer than 10% of these survive clinical assessment.

Preclinical screening is performed using laboratory animals in order to evaluate the pharmacokinetic properties and adverse effects of the potential drug. The information gained from these studies is submitted to the Food and Drug Administration (FDA) as part of an "investigational new drug" (IND) application. FDA approval of the IND allows the clinical phases of drug development to begin.

A potential drug goes through four clinical stages (phases 1–4) as part of the assessment of pharmacokinetics, pharmacodynamics, efficacy, dose–response relationships, and safety in humans (Fig. 1.15). A "new drug application" (NDA) is submitted to the FDA based on the results of phase 1–3 studies.

Phase 4 occurs after the drug has been approved/licensed for use in humans and can be regarded as an ongoing phase during which drugs are monitored once they have been marketed for use in the general public. By this stage, the efficacy and dose–response relationship are known, although the side-effect profile is often incomplete. Information is gathered about any "adverse reactions" and "drug interactions" that are due to, or probably due to, new drugs. The reporting of this information is voluntary during phase 4.

The five stages of drug development and monitoring		
Phase	Main aims/means of investigation	Subjects
Preclinical	• Pharmacology • Toxicology	• *In vitro* • In laboratory animals
Phase 1	• Clinical pharmacology and toxicology • Drug metabolism and bioavailability • Evaluate safety	• Healthy individuals and/or patients
Phase 2	• Initial treatment studies • Evaluate efficacy	• Small numbers of patients
Phase 3	• Large randomized controlled trials • Comparing new to old treatments • Evaluate safety and efficacy	• Large numbers of patients
Phase 4	• Post-marketing surveillance • Long-term safety and rare events • Yellow card scheme	• All patients prescribed the drug

Fig. 1.15 The five stages of drug development and monitoring.

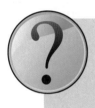

- What is meant by the term "drug"? How are drugs named?
- What are the specific and nonspecific actions of drugs?
- What is a cellular receptor? List the types of cellular receptors known.
- By what mechanisms does receptor activation bring about a cellular/physiologic response?
- Give an example of a receptor that interacts directly with DNA. How does this receptor bring about its cellular/physiologic action?
- What is meant by the terms agonist and antagonist?
- How does the presence of either a competitive or noncompetitive antagonist affect the action of an agonist?
- What is receptor reserve? How can it be measured?
- What is potency? What factors affect the potency of a drug?
- What are the differences between pharmacokinetics and pharmacodynamics?
- What is compliance? How can doctors increase compliance?
- What are the common routes by which drugs are administered? (Give an example of a drug for each and its indication.)
- What barriers must drugs cross in order to have their effects for each of the routes mentioned above?
- What are the principal steps and location of drug metabolism in the body?
- What is meant by the term enzyme induction? What effects does this have upon a drug's activity?
- By which route out of the body are drugs and their metabolites commonly excreted? What factors accelerate or hinder drug excretion?
- What are the differences between zero-order and first-order kinetics?
- What is a drug interaction? Give an example.
- What are the main areas of the drug history?

CLINICAL PHARMACOLOGY

2. Cancer   23

3. Infectious Diseases   31

4. Inflammation, Pain, and
   Immunosuppression   57

5. Peripheral Nervous System   73

6. Central Nervous System   91

7. Cardiovascular System   127

8. Respiratory System   157

9. Kidney and Urinary System   167

10. Gastrointestinal System   175

11. Endocrine and Reproductive
    Systems   187

12. Eyes and Skin   209

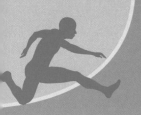

2. Cancer

Cancer

Cancers are malignant neoplasms ("new growths"). Despite their variability, cancers share the characteristics of:

- Uncontrolled proliferation.
- Local invasiveness.
- Tendency to spread (metastasis).
- Changes in some aspects of original cell morphology/retention of other characteristics.

Cancers account for a large proportion of deaths in the Western world. Attempts to cure or palliate cancer employ four principal methods: surgery, radiotherapy, immunotherapy, and chemotherapy. These methods are not mutually exclusive, often being used in combination (e.g., adjuvant chemotherapy after surgical removal of a tumor).

Chemotherapy

The aim of cancer chemotherapy is the use of drugs to inhibit the rate of growth of, or to kill, cancerous cells, while having minimal effects upon non-neoplastic host cells.

In a fashion similar to antimicrobial chemotherapy, the ideal anticancer drugs target malignant cells in preference to nonmalignant cells. This is achieved by exploiting the molecular differences between them.

The most striking difference between cancerous and noncancerous cells is their accelerated rate of cell division. Rapidly growing cancers, such as leukemia, are generally more responsive to chemotherapy than slower growing solid tumors. This difference remains the main target for therapeutic intervention at present, although newer drugs are being designed which recognize other molecular differences.

The chemotherapeutic techniques currently used include:
- Cytotoxic therapy, which is the main approach.
- Endocrine therapy.
- Immunotherapy.

Cancers differ in their sensitivity to chemotherapy, from the highly sensitive (e.g., lymphomas, testicular carcinomas), for which complete clinical cures can be achieved, to the resistant (generally solid tumors, such as colorectal carcinoma and squamous cell bronchial carcinoma).

A diagnosis of cancer carries a significant social stigma and also many myths. Hair loss and sickness are more often the initial concern for patients rather than other potentially serious side effects of chemotherapy. Nausea and vomiting should be taken seriously in cancer management, as these can have a devastating impact upon patients' quality of life. Antiemetic drugs are discussed in Chapter 10.

Cytotoxic chemotherapy
Mechanisms of action

Most cytotoxic drugs affect DNA synthesis. They can be classified according to their site of action on the process of DNA synthesis within the cancer cell (Fig. 2.1). Cytotoxic drugs are, therefore, most effective against actively cycling/proliferating cells, both normal and malignant, and least active against nondividing cells.

Some drugs are only effective at killing cycling cells during specific parts of the cell cycle. These are known as phase specific (Fig. 2.2). Other drugs are cytotoxic toward cycling cells throughout the cell cycle (e.g., alkylating agents), and these are known as cycle specific.

Selectivity

Cytotoxic drugs are not specifically toxic to cancer cells, and the selectivity they show is marginal at best. The side effects of cytotoxic drugs limit the amount and frequency of treatment as well as therapeutic effectiveness.

Cytotoxic drugs affect all dividing tissues, both normal and malignant; therefore, they are likely to have general toxic side effects (see Fig. 2.4). The side effects of cytotoxic drugs are most often related to the inhibition of division of noncancerous host cells, namely in the gut, in the bone marrow, and in the reproductive and immune systems.

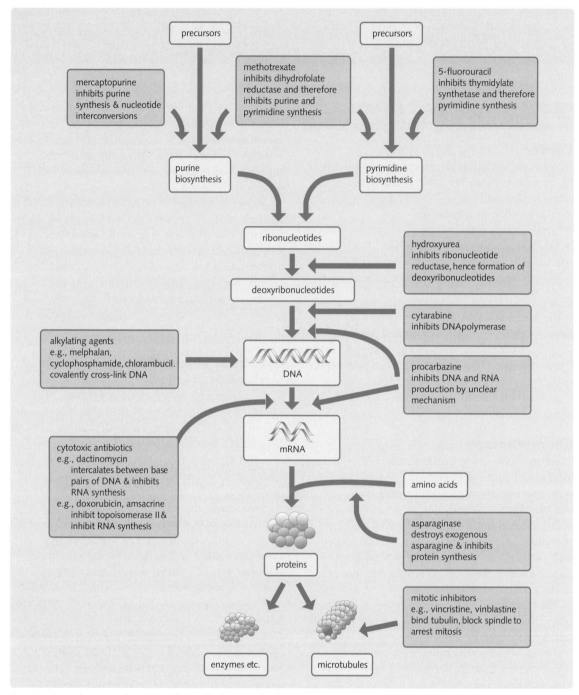

Fig. 2.1 Site of action of cytotoxic drugs that act on dividing cells.

Relative selectivity can occur with some cancers because:

- In malignant tumors, a higher proportion of cells are undergoing proliferation than in normal proliferating tissues.

- In some cases, normal cells seem to recover from chemotherapeutic inhibition faster than some cancer cells.

- Synchronized cell cycling may leave discrete periods of vulnerability to cytotoxic drugs.

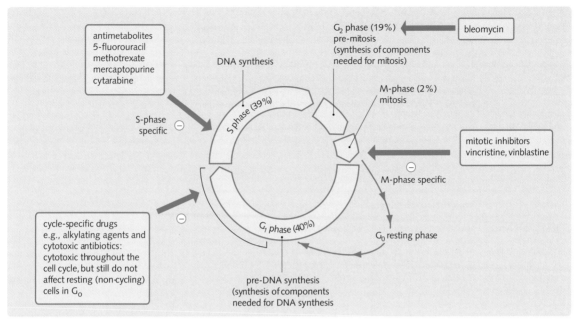

Fig. 2.2 Cell cycle and point of action of phase-specific drugs.

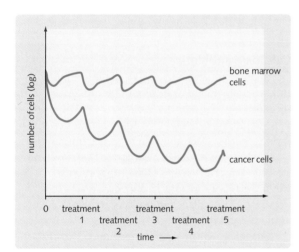

Fig. 2.3 Theoretical anticancer cytotoxic dosing schedule, allowing recovery of normal tissues.

Knowledge of these principles and knowing that cytotoxic drugs kill a constant fraction, not a constant number, of cells, lay down the foundation for chemotherapeutic dosing schedules (Fig. 2.3).

Resistance to cytotoxic drugs

Genetic resistance to cytotoxic drugs can be inherent to the cancer cell line or acquired during the course of chemotherapy as a result of selection imposed by the chemotherapeutic agent.

The mechanisms of genetic resistance to cytotoxic drugs include:

- Abnormal transport.
- Decreased cellular retention.
- Increased cellular inactivation (binding/ metabolism).
- Altered target protein.
- Enhanced repair of DNA.
- Altered processing.

Some tumors are relatively resistant to chemotherapy because they exist in so-called "pharmacologic sanctuaries." These occur when a tumor is in a privileged compartment (e.g., protected by the blood–brain barrier) or in large solid tumors when poor blood supply and diffusion limit the penetration of the drug.

In clinical practice, cancers may be treated more successfully with combinations of cytotoxic drugs simultaneously. An example is MOPP therapy (melphalan, Oncovin® [vincristine], procarbazine, and prednisolone) for Hodgkin's lymphoma. The theory is that multiple attacks with cytotoxic agents acting at different biochemical sites will increase efficacy while reducing the likelihood of resistance.

Cytotoxic agents

Cytotoxic agents, the major group of anticancer drugs, include:

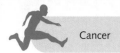

General adverse effects of cytotoxic drugs	
Site	**Effect**
Bone marrow	Myelosuppression can lead to leukopenia, thrombocytopenia and sometimes anaemia; this is often the close-limiting side effect; there is a high risk of hemorrhage, immunosuppression, and infection as a result.
Gastrointestinal tract	Inhibition fo mucosal cell division may produce anorexia, ulceration, or diarrhea; nausea and vomiting are comon, especially with alkylating agents and cisplatin.
Skin	Loss of hair (alopecia) may be partial or complete but is usually reversible.
Wounds	Impaired wound healing results from cell reproduction inhibition.
Reproductive system	Sterility, teratogenesis, and mutagenicity are all possible.
Secondary cancers	Many cytotoxic drugs are carcinogenic; additionally, the immunosuppression resulting from myelosuppression may reduce immune surveillance of emergin dysplastic cells, leading to an increased risk of development of some cancers after chemotherapy.

Fig. 2.4 General adverse effects of cytotoxic drugs.

- Alkylating agents.
- Antimetabolites.
- Cytotoxic antibiotics.
- Mitotic inhibitors.
- Miscellaneous agents.

Alkylating agents
Examples of alkylating agents include melphalan, cyclophosphamide, and chlorambucil.

Mechanism of action: Alkylating agents act via a reactive alkyl group that reacts to form covalent bonds with nucleic acids. There follows either cross-linking of the two strands of DNA, preventing replication, or DNA strand breakage (see Fig. 2.1).

Route of administration: Melphalan and cyclophosphamide orally and intravenously; chlorambucil orally.

Indications: Melphalan is used in myeloma and in some solid tumors. Cyclophosphamide is used to treat a variety of leukemias, lymphomas, and some solid tumors. Chlorambucil is used for leukemias, lymphomas, and ovarian cancers.

Adverse effects: Generalized cytotoxicity is common with alkylating agents (Fig. 2.4).

A urinary metabolite of cyclophosphamide, acrolein, may cause serious hemorrhagic cystitis.

Damage to gametogenesis and the development of secondary acute nonlymphocytic leukemias are particular problems with these alkylating agents.

Therapeutic notes: Extensive clinical experience is available with alkylating agents.

Cytotoxic antibiotics
Dactinomycin (actinomycin D), bleomycin, and doxorubicin are examples of cytotoxic antibiotics.

Mechanism of action: Cytotoxic antibiotics act by various means. Dactinomycin prevents transcription by interfering with RNA polymerase. Doxorubicin inhibits transcription and DNA replication by inhibiting topoisomerase II. Bleomycin acts to fragment DNA chains but appears to be more active in the G2 phase.

Route of administration: Intravenous. Doxorubicin can be given intravesically for bladder cancer.

Indications: Dactinomycin is principally used in pediatric cancers. Doxorubicin is used for acute leukemias, lymphomas, and a variety of solid tumors, including breast cancer. Bleomycin is used for lymphomas and certain solid tumors, including testicular cancer.

Adverse effects: Generalized cytotoxicity (see Fig. 2.4). Doxorubicin produces dose-dependent cardiotoxicity as a result of irreversible free radical damage to the myocardium. Bleomycin may cause pulmonary fibrosis but is associated with less myelosuppression than other cytotoxic antibiotics.

Mitotic inhibitors

Examples of mitotic inhibitors include the vinca alkaloids, vincristine, vinblastine, and vinorelbine.

Mechanism of action: Mitotic inhibitors act by binding tubulin and inhibiting the polymerization of microtubules, which is necessary to form the mitotic spindle. This prevents mitosis and arrests dividing cells at metaphase (see Fig. 2.1).

Route of administration: The vinca alkaloids are administered intravenously, and etoposide is administered orally or intravenously.

Indications: Mitotic inhibitors are used for acute leukemias, lymphomas, and some solid tumors.

Adverse effects: Side effects of mitotic inhibitors result from the fact that tubulin polymerization is relatively indiscriminate, inhibiting other cellular processes that involve microtubules, as well as cell division.

Generalized cytotoxicity occurs (see Fig. 2.4), except that vincristine is unusual in producing little or no bone marrow suppression.

Neurologic and neuromuscular effects occur, especially with vincristine, and include peripheral neuropathy leading to paraesthesia, loss of reflexes, and weakness. Recovery from these effects occurs, but it is slow.

Therapeutic notes: The intrathecal administration of vinca alkaloids is contraindicated, as it is usually fatal.

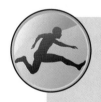

As with most drugs, understanding how anticancer agents work allows potential side effects and complications to be predicted.

Antimetabolites

Examples of antimetabolites include the folic acid antagonists (e.g., methotrexate), pyrimidine antagonists (e.g., fluorouracil and cytarabine), and purine antagonists (e.g., mercaptopurine).

Mechanism of action: Antimetabolites are analogs of normal metabolites and act by competition, replacing the natural metabolite and then subverting cellular processes (see Fig. 2.1).

Methotrexate competitively antagonizes dihydrofolate reductase and prevents the regeneration of intermediates (tetrahydrofolate) essential for the synthesis of purine and thymidylate, thus inhibiting the synthesis of DNA.

Fluorouracil is converted into a fraudulent pyrimidine nucleotide, fluorodeoxyuridine monophosphate, which inhibits thymidylate synthetase, impairing DNA synthesis.

Cytarabine is converted intracellularly to a triphosphate form that inhibits DNA polymerase.

Mercaptopurine is converted into a fraudulent purine nucleotide that impairs DNA synthesis.

Route of administration: Methotrexate is administered orally, intravenously, intramuscularly, and intrathecally. Fluorouracil is usually given intravenously, although it can be given orally and topically. Cytarabine is given subcutaneously, intravenously, and intrathecally. Mercaptopurine is given orally.

Indications: Methotrexate is used for acute lymphoblastic leukemia, and non-Hodgkin's lymphoma; fluorouracil for solid tumors and some malignant skin conditions; cytarabine for acute myeloblastic leukemia; and mercaptopurine as maintenance therapy for acute leukemias.

Adverse effects: Common side effects of antimetabolites are generalized cytotoxicity (see Fig. 2.4).

Therapeutic notes: Methotrexate should not be given to people with significant hepatic or renal impairment.

Miscellaneous agents

Several chemotherapeutic cytotoxic agents do not fall into any of the aforementioned groups.

Procarbazine

Mechanism of action: Procarbazine is a methylhydrazine derivative with monoamine oxidase inhibitor actions and cytotoxicity. It inhibits DNA and RNA synthesis by a mechanism that is unclear (see Fig. 2.1).

Route of administration: Oral.

Indications: Procarbazine is the first-line drug for lymphomas such as Hodgkin's.

Adverse effects: Generalized cytotoxicity (see Fig. 2.4). It causes an adverse reaction in combination with alcohol.

Therapeutic notes: Procarbazine forms part of MOPP therapy for Hodgkin's lymphoma.

Hydroxyurea

Mechanism of action: Hydroxyurea causes the inhibition of ribonucleotide reductase and hence the formation of deoxyribonucleotides (see Fig. 2.1).

Route of administration: Oral.

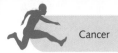

Indications: Hydroxyurea is used for chronic myeloid leukemia. Polycythemia rubra vera.

Adverse effects: Generalized cytotoxicity (see Fig. 2.4).

Asparaginase

Mechanism of action: Some tumor cells lose the ability to synthesize asparagine, requiring an exogenous source of the substance to grow. Normal host cells can synthesize their own. Asparaginase is an enzyme produced by bacteria that breaks down any circulating asparagine, hence inhibiting the growth of some cancers, namely acute lymphoblastic leukemia (ALL) (see Fig. 2.1).

Route of administration: Intramuscular, subcutaneous.

Indications: Asparaginase is used for ALL.

Adverse effects: The most serious side effects of asparaginase include severe toxicity to the liver and pancreas. Central nervous system (CNS) depression and anaphylaxis are also risks.

Therapeutic notes: Regular testing of patients given asparaginase is necessary to monitor organ functions.

Mitotane

Mechanism of action: Mitotane is related to the insecticide dichlorodiphenyltrichloroethane (DDT). It interferes with the formation of adrenocortical steroids and has a selective cytotoxic effect on the cells of the adrenal cortex (see Fig. 2.1).

Route of administration: Oral.

Indications: Mitotane is used for tumors of the adrenal cortex.

Adverse effects: Side effects of mitotane include adrenosuppression.

Amsacrine

Mechanism of action: Like doxorubicin, amsacrine works by intercalation between base pairs in the DNA double helix. This stabilizes the DNA structure and stops it from being an effective template for RNA synthesis.

Route of administration: Intravenous.

Indications: Amsacrine is used for acute myeloid leukemia.

Adverse effects: Bone marrow suppression. Cardiotoxicity due to hypokalemia has been reported.

Therapeutic notes: Electrolytes should be monitored in patients given amsacrine.

Many other anticancer agents are used in the management of malignant tumors, including altretamine, dacarbazine, pentostatin, platinum compounds, taxanes, thalidomide, topoisomerase I inhibitors, trastuzumab, and tretinoin.

Endocrine therapy

Hormones and hormone antagonists

The growth of some cancers is hormone dependent. Growth of such tumors can be inhibited by surgical removal of the source of the driving hormone, such as the gonads, adrenals, or pituitary. Increasingly, however, administration of hormones or hormone antagonists is preferred.

Endocrine therapy can cause side effects, the nature of which can normally be deduced from the physiologic effects of the hormone being given or antagonized. Endocrine therapy generally has the advantage that it carries far fewer serious adverse effects than do cytotoxic agents.

Hormones used in endocrine therapy include:

- Adrenocortical steroids (Chapter 11), such as prednisolone, which inhibit the growth of cancers of the lymphoid tissues and blood. In addition, they are used to treat some of the complications of the cancer (e.g., edema).
- Estrogen antagonists, such as tamoxifen, which are competitive inhibitors at estrogen receptors. Inhibition of the stimulatory effects of estrogen suppresses the division of breast cancer cells. Tamoxifen is indicated for use in postmenopausal women with metastatic disease, where it has definitely been shown to increase survival times.
- Estrogens (Chapter 11), such as diethylstilbestrol, which have an antiandrogenic effect and can be used to suppress androgen-dependent prostatic cancers.
- Progesterones (Chapter 11), which inhibit endometrial cancer and carcinomas of the prostate and breast.
- Androgen antagonists, such as flutamide, which inhibit androgen-dependent prostatic cancers. Gonadotrophin-releasing hormone (GnRH) analogs have a similar effect, as they inhibit GnRH release via negative feedback.

Immunotherapy

Immunotherapy of cancer is a recent advance derived from the nineteenth-century observation that bacterial infections sometimes provoked the regression of cancer (i.e., indirect immunostimulation).

Approaches of immunotherapy include:

- The use of tumor-specific monoclonal antibodies to target drugs specifically to cancerous cells, the so-called magic-bullet approach (e.g., trastuzumab, rituximab).
- The use of vaccines (e.g., BCG) to provide nonspecific immunostimulation.
- The use of specific vaccines prepared using tumor cells from similar cancers, in an attempt to raise an adaptive immune response against the cancer.
- Immunostimulation using drugs (e.g., levamisole).
- The use of cytokines to regulate the immune response so as to favorably target the cancer. Cytokines used include interferon-α, interleukin-2, and tumor necrosis factor.
- The use of recombinant colony-stimulating factors to reduce the extent and duration of neutropenia after cytotoxic chemotherapy.

Recombinant human granulocyte colony-stimulating factor (rh-G-CSF; filgrastim) and granulocyte-macrophage colony stimulating factor (GM-CSF; sargramostim) promote the development of their respective hematopoietic stem cells in the marrow. Their use to raise white blood cell counts after cytotoxic chemotherapy is effective, although this has not been shown to alter overall survival rates.

The future

There are many drugs which are potential candidates as anticancer agents, and numerous drugs are in ongoing trials across the world. The most promising areas appear to be the use of antisense oligonucleotides, inhibitors of enzymes responsible for cell invasiveness and metastasis, and agents which interfere with tumor angiogenesis (formation of new blood vessels).

Modulation of the host's immune system is believed to become part of cancer therapy in the future, in addition to novel methods of drug delivery, including liposomes and viral vectors.

- What is cancer, and how does it arise? How do malignant cells differ from normal cells?
- What is the definition of chemotherapy? What are the goals of chemotherapy?
- What are the principal targets for cytotoxic chemotherapeutic agents?
- What is resistance to cytotoxic drugs, and how does it arise?
- How do current cytotoxic agents target malignant cells and have minimal effect upon normal host cells?
- What is the basis of the cell cycle? Which cells of the normal human actively proliferate regularly?
- What are the common adverse effects of cytotoxic agents?
- What are the main classes of cytotoxic agents?
- What is the role of steroids in the management of malignant disease?
- What therapies might be used to treat cancer in the future? How are these proposed to work?

3. Infectious Diseases

Antibacterial drugs

Concepts of antibacterial chemotherapy

Bacteria belong to the kingdom of prokaryotic organisms. Some bacteria are pathogenic to humans and responsible for a number of medically important diseases.

The principal treatment of infections is chemotherapy, which in its simplest definition is the use of chemicals (drugs) to combat disease (Chapter 2).

The chemotherapy of infections aims to selectively target the invading bacteria while having minimal effect upon the host. This is achieved by exploiting differences that exist between the structure and physiology of the prokaryotic bacterial cells and the host eukaryotic cell (Figs. 3.1 and 3.2).

Antibacterial agents can be considered as bacteriostatic (i.e., they inhibit bacterial growth but do not kill the bacteria) or bactericidal (i.e., they kill bacteria).

Note that the distinction is not clear cut, as the ability of an antibacterial agent to inhibit or kill bacteria is partially dependent on its concentration. Also, the distinction is rarely of clinical significance, the exception being immunocompromised patients in whom bactericidal agents are necessary, as the host's immune system is not capable of final elimination of the bacteria.

Antibiotics: definition

The term "antibiotic" strictly refers to antimicrobial agents that are synthesized and released by microorganisms (e.g., penicillins from fungi). In practice, the term antibiotic has become

Differences between prokaryotic and eukaryotic cells		
Site	**Exploitable difference**	**Antibacterial drugs**
Peptidoglycan cell wall	Peptidoglycan cell walls are a uniquely prokaryotic feature not shared by eukaryotic (mammalian) cells. Drugs that act here are therefore very selective.	Penicillins Cephalosporins Vancomycin Carbapenems Aztreonam Bacitracin
Cytoplasmic membrane	Bacteria possess a plasma membrane within the cell wall which is a phospholipid bilayer, as in eukaryotes. However, in bacteria the plasma membrane does not contain any sterols, and this results in differential chemical behavior that can be exploited.	Polymixins
Protein synthesis	The bacterial ribosome (50S+30S subunits) is sufficiently different from the mammalian ribosome (60S+40S subunits) that sites on the bacterial ribosome are good targets for drug action.	Aminoglycosides Tetracyclines Chloramphenicol Macrolides/ketolides Quinupristin/dalfopristin Linezolid
Nucleic acids	The bacterial genome is in the form of a single circular strand of DNA plus ancillary plasmids unenclosed by a nuclear envelope, in contrast to the eukaryotic chromosomal arrangement within the nucleus. Drugs may interfere directly or indirectly with microbial DNA and RNA metabolism, replication, and transcription.	Antifolates Quinolones/ fluoroquinolones Rifampin

Fig. 3.1 Site of action of cytotoxic drugs that act on dividing cells.

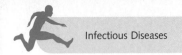
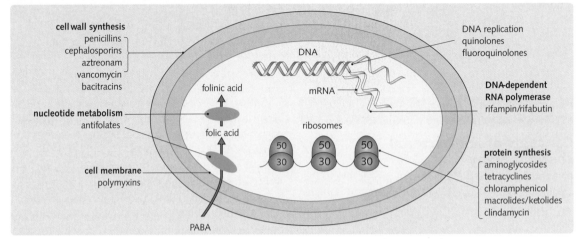

Fig. 3.2 Sites of action of different types of antibiotic agent (PABA, para-aminobenzoic acid).

synonymous with all antibacterial agents, whether natural or synthetic, and it is used as such in this chapter.

Spectrum of activity: definition

Antibiotics have a narrow or broad spectrum of activity. Broad-spectrum antibiotics are active against many bacterial species, whereas narrow-spectrum antibiotics are active against only a few species.

Classification of antibiotics

There are three main ways of classifying antibiotics:
- Whether they are bactericidal or bacteriostatic.
- By their site and mechanism of action.
- By their chemical structure.

Antibiotics will be described according to their site of action in this chapter.

Antibiotic resistance

When an antibiotic is ineffective against a bacterium, that bacterium is said to be resistant. Resistance to antibiotics can be acquired or innate.

Innate resistance

Innate resistance is a long-standing characteristic of a particular species of bacteria. For instance, *Pseudomonas aeruginosa* has always been resistant to treatment with several antibiotics, including penicillin G and vancomycin.

Acquired resistance

Acquired resistance occurs when bacteria that were sensitive to an antibiotic become resistant.

Biochemical mechanisms responsible for resistance to an antibiotic include:
- Production of enzymes that inactivate the drug (e.g., β-lactamases produced by many bacteria, which inactivate penicillin).
- Alteration of drug binding site (e.g., aminoglycosides and erythromycin bind to the bacterial ribosome and inhibit protein synthesis). Resistant organisms have modified the sites of drug binding so that they no longer have affinity for the drugs.
- Reduction in drug uptake and accumulation (e.g., some bacteria are resistant to tetracycline because they have altered their cell membrane to make it impermeable to the drug). Other bacteria may use active transport mechanisms to pump a drug out of the cell before it accumulates to an effective level.
- Development of altered metabolic pathways (e.g., bacteria can become resistant to trimethoprim because of acquired changes in their dihydrofolate reductase enzyme that gives it very little affinity for the drug).

The major stimulus for the development of acquired resistance is the use of antibiotics themselves. Antibiotic use exerts selective pressure on bacteria to "acquire" resistance in order to survive.

Acquired resistance to antibiotics can develop in bacterial populations in many ways, although all involve genes that code for the resistance mechanism located either on the bacterial chromosome or on plasmids.

The "acquisition" of resistance by a bacterium can either be achieved *de novo* by spontaneous mutation or by being transferred from another bacterium.

The development of clinical antibiotic drug resistance is a major problem imposing serious constraints on the medical treatment of many bacterial infections. Methicillin-resistant *Staphylococcus aureus* (MRSA) and some strains of *Mycobacteria tuberculosis* are real examples of multiple drug-resistant bacteria that are not uncommon in hospitals across the world.

Prescribing antibiotics

Like most drugs, many antibiotics have side effects, some more serious than others (Chapter 1). When prescribing antibiotics, there are many considerations to take into account that determine which antibiotic to use, by which route, for how many days, etc. These include:

- Organism responsible for, or likely to be responsible for, the symptoms (e.g., *Staphylococcus* infection of a pierced belly-button).
- Severity of illness (e.g., oral or parenteral antibiotics).
- Previous antibiotic therapy (e.g., symptoms have not responded to a 7-day course of a penicillin).
- Previous adverse/allergic response to antibiotics (e.g., penicillin rash).
- Other medications being taken (e.g., warfarin, phenytoin, oral contraceptive drugs [OCDs]).
- Ongoing medical considerations (e.g., pregnancy, breastfeeding, renal failure).

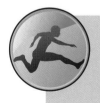

Always try to get a sample for microbial culture prior to starting antibiotics unless there is a threat to life by withholding antibiotics.

Antibacterial drugs that inhibit cell-wall synthesis

Examples of antibacterial drugs that inhibit bacterial cell-wall synthesis include the penicillins and the cephalosporins (the β-lactam antibiotics), and the glycopeptides (see Fig. 3.2).

Penicillins

Examples of penicillins include benzylpenicillin, phenoxymethylpenicillin, amoxicillin, ampicillin, ticarcillin, and piperacillin.

Mechanism of action: Penicillins are bactericidal. Structurally, they possess a thiazolidine ring connected to a β-lactam ring. The side chain from the β-lactam ring determines the unique pharmacologic properties of the different penicillins.

Penicillins bind to penicillin-binding proteins on susceptible microorganisms. This interaction results in inhibition of peptide cross-linking within the microbial cell wall and indirect activation of autolytic enzymes. The combined result is lysis (see Fig. 3.2).

Spectrum of activity: Penicillins exhibit considerable diversity in their spectrum of activity (Fig. 3.3).

Penicillin G is active against aerobic gram-positive and gram-negative cocci and many anaerobic organisms (excluding *Bacteroides* sp.). Most staphylococci are now resistant to penicillin G (and most other penicillins). The isoxazolyl penicillins (e.g., dicloxacillin and nafcillin) can be used against penicillinase-producing staphylococci because they are not inactivated by staphylococcal β-lactamases. Some staphylococci ("methicillin-resistant") are resistant to all penicillins and most other antibiotics. Penicillin V has a similar antibacterial spectrum to penicillin G but may be less active against some organisms. Amoxicillin and ampicillin are also active against some aerobic gram-negative bacilli such as *H. influenzae*, *E. coli*, and *Proteus mirabilis*. Ticarcillin and piperacillin are parenteral drugs that have extended activity against several gram-negative aerobes, especially *Pseudomonas aeruginosa*.

Route of administration: Penicillin G, nafcillin, ticarcillin, and piperacillin must be administered parenterally, as they are inactivated when given orally. Penicillin V, dicloxacillin, amoxicillin, and ampicillin are active when given orally. Ampicillin can be administered intravenously.

Contraindications: Known hypersensitivity to penicillins, cephalosporins, or other beta-lactam antibiotics.

Adverse effects: Generally highly specific and safe antibiotics. Hypersensitivity reactions are the main adverse effect, including rashes (common) and anaphylaxis (rare). Neurotoxicity occurs at excessively high cerebrospinal fluid (CSF)

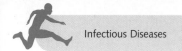

concentrations. Diarrhea is common, owing to disturbance of normal colonic flora.

Therapeutic notes: Resistance to penicillins is often due to production of β-lactamases by some microorganisms, which hydrolyses the β-lactam ring. This type of resistance may be constitutive or inducible and is transferable via plasmids. Some organisms, especially staphylococci and streptococci, develop resistance through changes in "penicillin-binding proteins" with decreased affinity for penicillins. Other organisms produce changes in membrane porins which render the bacterial cell membrane less permeable to the penicillins.

Cephalosporins

The cephalosporins comprise a large group of drugs which, for convenience, are divided into three general subgroups:

- First-generation (G1) cephalosporins, such as cephalexin (oral) and cefazolin (parenteral).
- Second-generation (G2) cephalosporins, such as cefuroxime (oral and parenteral) and cefoxitin (parenteral).
- Third-generation (G3) cephalosporins, such as cefixime (oral) and ceftriaxone (parenteral).
- Fourth-generation (G4) cephalosporins, such as cefepime (parenteral).

Drugs of choice and alternatives for selected common bacterial pathogens			
Bacterium	**Drug(s) of Choice**	**Alternatives**	**Comments**
Streptococcus species	Penicillin G/V	G1 cephalosporins Erythromycin Clindamycin Vancomycin	Erythromycin for mild infections Vancomycin for serious infections Some strains of *Strep. pneumoniae (Pneumococcus)* are resistant; "intermediate-resistant" strains are susceptible to G3 cephalosporins; Vancomycin is used for "highly resistant" strains.
Enterococcus species	Penicillin or ampicillin plus an aminoglycoside	Vancomycin plus aminoglycoside	Some strains are resistant to synergy with an aminoglycoside.
Staphylococcus species	Penicillinase-resistant penicillin e.g., dicloxacillin, (oral) nafcillin, (i.v.)	G1 cephalosporin Vancomycin	Vancomycin is required for "methicillin-resistant" strains. Rifampin is occasionally used to eradicate the nasal carrier state.
Neisseria meningitidis	Penicillin G	G3 cephalosporin Fluoroquinolone	Rare strains are pencicillin resistant.
Neisseria gonorrhoeae	Cefixime, (oral) Ceftriaxone, (i.m.)	Fluoroquinolone	Some strains are fluoroquinolone resistant.
Bordetella pertussis	Erythromycin Clarithromycin	Trimethoprim-sulfamethoxazole	
Haemophilus influenzae	Trimethoprim-sulfamethoxazole Amoxicillin/clavulanate	Amoxicillin/ampicillin G2 or G3 cephalosporin, Azithromycin Fluoroquinolone	At least 30% are resistant to aminopenicillins; amoxicillin or ampicillin should not be used empirically in serious infections until susceptibility results are available.
Enterobacteria in urine	Trimethoprim-sulfamethoxazole Fluoroquinolone	Aminoglycoside Nitrofurantoin	β-lactams are less effective than Trimethoprim-sulfamethoxazole or fluoroquinolones.
Enterobacteria in cerebrospinal fluid	G3 cephalosporin	Trimethoprim-sulfamethoxazole Aminoglycoside	Aminoglycosides have poor CSF penetration and must be administered by intrathecal route.

Fig. 3.3A Drugs of choice and alternatives for selected common bacterial pathogens.

	Drugs of choice and alternatives for selected common bacterial pathogens—cont'd		
Bacterium	Drugs(s) of Choice	Alternatives	Comments
Enterobacteria elsewhere (blood, lung, etc.)	Aminoglycoside G3 or G4 cephalosporin Ciprofloxacin	Carbapenem Ticarcillin/clavulanate Piperacillin/tazobactam Trimethoprim-sulfamethoxazole	Combination therapy is sometimes used in serious infections.
Pseudomonas aeruginosa	Ticarcillin/clavulanate or Piperacillin/tazobactam plus an Aminoglycoside	Ceftazidime Cefepime Ciprofloxacin Carbapenem Aztreonam	Combination therapy is recommended, except for urinary tract infection.
Bacteroides fragilis	Metronidazole or Clindamycin	Carbapenem Cefoxitin Ticarcillin/clavulanate Piperacillin/tazobactam	*Bacteroides fragilis* is involved in polymicrobial infections; therefore, another antibiotic against Enterobacteriaceae is often required.
Mycoplasma pneumoniae	Macrolide Doxycycline	Doxyciciline G2 fluoroquinolone	Although tetracyclines are as effective as macrolides, macrolides are recommended because of better activity against *Pneumococcus*, which can mimic this infection.
Chlamydia trachomatis	Doxycycline Azithromycin	Erythromycin Fluoroquinolone	Azithromycin is the only therapy effective in a single dose. Erythromycin is used in pregnancy.
Rickettsial species	Doxycycline	Chloramphenicol	
Listeria monocytogenes	Ampicillin with or without an aminoglycoside	Trimethoprim-sulfamethoxazole	
Legionella species	Azithromycin Fluoroquinolone	Doxycycline Trimethoprim-sulfamethoxazole	Rifampin is used as a second agent in severe cases.
Clostridium difficile	Metronidazole (oral)	Vancomycin (oral) Bacitracin (oral)	
Mycobacterium tuberculosis	Isoniazid plus rifampin plus ethambutol plus pyrazinamide	Aminoglycoside Fluoroquinolone Clarithromycin Cycoserine Capreomycin	Drug combinations will vary depending on resistance. Direct observation of therapy is recommended. Isoniazid is used alone for prophylaxis.
Mycobacterium leprae	Dapsone plus rifampin ± cofazimine	Clarithromycin	Thalidomide is useful for erythema nodosum leprosum.

Fig. 3.3B—cont'd

Mechanism of action: Cephalosporins are bactericidal. They are β-lactam antibiotics and inhibit bacterial cell-wall synthesis in a manner similar to the penicillins. Structurally, cephalosporins possess a dihydrothiazine ring connected to the β-lactam ring that makes them more resistant to hydrolysis by β-lactamases than are the penicillins. In general, G2 cephalosporins are less susceptible to gram-negative β-lactamases than G1 cephalosporins; the G3 and G4 cephalosporins are least susceptible to these β-lactamases.

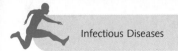

Spectrum of activity: The cephalosporins are broad-spectrum antibiotics used to treat many infections (see Fig. 3.3).

Route of administration: Oral, intravenous, or intramuscular. Varies among individual cephalosporins.

Contraindications: Known severe hypersensitivity to penicillins, cephalosporins, or other beta-lactam antibiotics.

Adverse effects: Hypersensitivity reactions occur in a similar and cross-reacting fashion to the penicillins. Approximately 10% of patients allergic to penicillins experience allergic reactions to cephalosporins. Diarrhea is common, especially with oral G3 cephalosporins, owing to disturbance of normal colonic flora. Nausea and vomiting may also occur. A few cephalosporins (e.g., cefotetan) contain a side chain (MTT) that can cause bleeding via the inhibition of vitamin K activation. In addition, these drugs can inhibit aldehyde oxidase ("disulfiram effect") in some patients who have consumed ethanol.

Therapeutic notes: The primary cause of resistance to the cephalosporins is production of β-lactamase enzymes, although the later generation drugs are more resistant to hydrolysis.

Glycopeptides

Vancomycin is the classic glycopeptide.

Mechanism of action: Vancomycin is bactericidal and inhibits peptidoglycan synthesis in the cell wall, with possible effects on RNA synthesis (see Fig. 3.2).

Spectrum of activity: Vancomycin is active only against aerobic and anaerobic gram-positive bacteria and is used to treat resistant staphylococcal and enterococcal infections. It is also an alternate to metronidazole in the treatment of *Clostridium difficile* in antibiotic-associated pseudomembranous colitis (see Fig. 3.3). Vancomycin is the current drug of choice for "methicillin-resistant" staphylococci.

Route of administration: Poor oral absorption requires parenteral administration (slow intravenous infusion). Oral administration is reserved for cases when a local gastrointestinal tract effect is required (e.g., in colitis).

Adverse effects: Side effects include ototoxicity and nephrotoxicity at high plasma levels; blood levels and renal function should be monitored. Other side effects include fever, rashes, and local phlebitis at the site of infection. Too rapid administration can result in vasodilation and hypotension due to histamine release ("red man" syndrome).

Therapeutic notes: Acquired resistance to vancomycin has been rare, but vancomycin-resistant enterococci are becoming more common.

Aztreonam and carbapenems

Aztreonam is a monobactam antibiotic and is active against gram-negative aerobic bacilli only. It is associated with a lower frequency of allergic reactions than other beta-lactam antibiotics. The carbapenems include imipenem, meropenem, and ertapenem. They are broad-spectrum β-lactam antibiotics that are resistant hydrolysis by bacterial beta-lactamases.

Inhibitors of beta-lactamase

Clavulanate, sulbactam, and tazobactam are beta-lactam antibiotics with minimal inherent antibacterial activity, but they produce antibacterial synergy when combined with penicillins such as amoxicillin, ampicillin, ticarcillin, and piperacillin.

Antibacterial drugs that inhibit bacterial nucleic acids

Antibacterial drugs that inhibit bacterial nucleic acids (see Fig. 3.2) include:

- The antimetabolites (antifolates), which affect synthesis of methionine and purines.
- The quinolones/fluoroquinolones, which inhibit bacterial DNA gyrase and topoisomerase IV, thus affecting DNA replication and unpackaging.
- Rifampin/rifabutin, which inhibit DNA-dependent RNA polymerase, thus affecting transcription.
- Metronidazole, which causes breaks in DNA strands.

Antifolates

Examples include the sulfonamides, sulfones, and trimethoprim.

Mechanism of action: Folate is an essential cofactor in the synthesis of purines and hence of DNA. Bacteria, unlike mammals, must synthesize their own folate from para-aminobenzoic acid (see Fig. 3.2). This pathway can be inhibited at two points: the sulfonamides inhibit the synthesis of dihydrofolate, while trimethoprim inhibits dihydrofolate reductase. These drugs are bacteriostatic.

Spectrum of activity: The primary indication for sulfonamides as single agents is treatment of uncomplicated urinary tract infections (UTIs). Trimethoprim and co-trimoxazole (trimethoprim-sulfamethoxazole) are used for UTIs and respiratory tract infections (see Fig. 3.3).

Route of administration: Oral, intravenous.

Contraindications: Pregnant women, because of theoretical teratogenic risk with antifolates. Neonates: avoid at term, as bilirubin displacement can damage the neonatal brain (kernicterus).

Adverse effects: Nausea, vomiting, and hypersensitivity reactions (e.g., rashes, fever, Stevens–Johnson syndrome). The sulfonamides are relatively insoluble and can cause crystalluria, while trimethoprim can cause myelosuppression/ agranulocytosis (more common in HIV-infected patients).

Therapeutic notes: Antifolates are often used in combined preparations, as they have synergistic effects. Resistance is common, and it is due to the production of enzymes that have reduced affinity for the drugs. Resistance can be acquired on plasmids in gram-negative bacteria.

Quinolones/fluoroquinolones

Ciprofloxacin is the prototype of the fluoroquinolones.

Mechanism of action: Quinolones/fluoroquinolones are bactericidal. They act by inhibiting prokaryotic DNA gyrase and Topisomerase IV. These enzymes package DNA into supercoils and is essential for DNA replication and repair (see Fig. 3.2).

Spectrum of activity: Ciprofloxacin has a broad spectrum of activity. Newer, second-generation (G2) fluoroquinolones, such as moxifloxacin, have enhanced activity against *Streptococcus pneumoniae*, mycoplasma, and enterococci (see Fig. 3.3).

Route of administration: Oral, intravenous. Ciprofloxacin is so well absorbed orally that intravenous administration is rarely required unless the patient is unable to tolerate oral medication.

Contraindications: Some fluoroquinolones (e.g., ciprofloxacin) should not be given with theophylline, as theophylline-toxicity may be precipitated. These drugs are not recommended for use in pregnant women and children.

Adverse effects: Gastrointestinal upset. Rarely, hypersensitivity and CNS disturbances occur.

Antibacterial drugs that inhibit protein synthesis

Antibacterial drugs that inhibit protein synthesis are summarized in Fig. 3.4 and include:

- Aminoglycosides.
- Tetracyclines.
- Chloramphenicol.
- Macrolides/ketolides.
- Clindamycin.
- Quinupristin/dalfopristin.

Aminoglycosides

Examples of aminoglycosides include gentamicin, streptomycin, tobramycin, and amikacin.

Mechanism of action: Aminoglycosides are bactericidal. They bind irreversibly to the bacterial 30S ribosomal subunit. This inhibits the translation of mRNA to protein and causes more frequent misreading of the prokaryotic genetic code (see Fig. 3.4).

Spectrum of activity: Aminoglycosides have a broad spectrum of activity but with low activity against anaerobes, streptococci, and pneumococci (see Fig. 3.3). Streptomycin is used against *Mycobacterium tuberculosis*.

Route of administration: Parenteral only.

Contraindications: Acute neuromuscular blockade can occur if an aminoglycoside is used in combination with anesthesia or other neuromuscular blockers.

Adverse effects: Dose-related ototoxicity and nephrotoxicity at high plasma levels.

Therapeutic notes: Resistance to aminoglycosides is increasing and is primarily due to plasmid-borne genes encoding degradative enzymes. Amikacin is the most effective aminoglycoside against these organisms.

Tetracyclines

Examples of tetracyclines include tetracycline, minocycline, and doxycycline.

Mechanism of action: Tetracyclines are bacteriostatic. They work as a result of selective uptake into bacterial cells by active bacterial transport systems not possessed by mammalian cells. The tetracycline then binds reversibly to the bacterial 30S ribosomal subunit, interfering with the attachment of tRNA to the mRNA ribosome complex (see Fig. 3.4).

Spectrum of activity: Tetracyclines have broad-spectrum activity against gram-positive and gram-negative bacteria as well as intracellular pathogens (see Fig. 3.3).

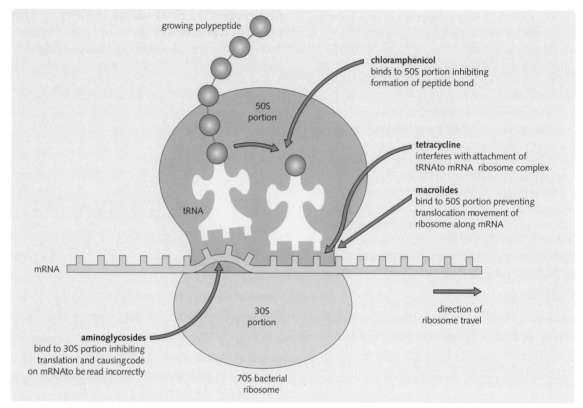

growing polypeptide

chloramphenicol
binds to 50S portion inhibiting
formation of peptide bond

50S
portion

tetracycline
interferes with attachment of
tRNA to mRNA ribosome complex

macrolides
bind to 50S portion preventing
translocation movement of
ribosome along mRNA

tRNA

mRNA

30S
portion

direction of
ribosome travel

aminoglycosides
bind to 30S portion inhibiting
translation and causing code
on mRNA to be read incorrectly

70S bacterial
ribosome

Fig. 3.4 Site of action of the antibiotics which inhibit bacterial protein synthesis.

Route of administration: Oral, intravenous. Oral absorption is incomplete and can be impaired by calcium (e.g., milk) and magnesium or aluminium salts (e.g., antacids).

Contraindications: Tetracyclines should not be given to children or pregnant women.

Adverse effects: Gastrointestinal disturbances are common after oral administration. In children, tetracyclines depress bone growth and produce permanent discoloration of teeth. Fatal hepatotoxicity has occurred in pregnant women.

Therapeutic notes: Resistance to tetracyclines is slow to develop, but it is now widespread. In the majority of cases, resistance is due to increased efflux of the drug and is plasmid mediated. Remember that tetracyclines are contraindicated in pregnant women and children.

Chloramphenicol

Mechanism of action: Chloramphenicol is both bactericidal and bacteriostatic, depending on the bacterial species. It reversibly binds to the bacterial ribosome, inhibiting the formation of peptide bonds (see Fig. 3.4).

Spectrum of activity: Chloramphenicol has a broad spectrum of activity against many gram-positive cocci and gram-negative organisms (see Fig. 3.3). Because of its toxicity, it is reserved for life-threatening infections, especially typhoid fever and meningitis.

Route of administration: Oral, intravenous.

Contraindications: Chloramphenicol is not recommended for use in pregnant women or neonates.

Adverse effects: Myelosuppression and reversible anemia. Neutropenia and thrombocytopenia may occur during chronic administration. Aplastic anemia, although rare, is often fatal.

Neonates cannot metabolize chloramphenicol; and "gray baby syndrome" may develop, which consists of pallor, abdominal distention, vomiting, and collapse.

Therapeutic notes: Resistance to chloramphenicol is due to a plasmid-borne gene encoding an enzyme that inactivates the drug by acetylation. Blood monitoring is necessary.

Macrolides/ketolides

Erythromycin, clarithromycin, and azithromycin are examples of macrolides. Telithromycin is a ketolide.

Mechanism of action: Macrolides are bacteriostatic/bactericidal. They reversibly bind to the bacterial ribosome, preventing the translocation movement of the ribosome along mRNA (see Fig. 3.3).

Spectrum of activity: Erythromycin is effective against most gram-positive bacteria and spirochetes. Clarithromycin is active against *Haemophilus influenzae, Mycobacterium avium cellulare,* and *Helicobacter pylori.*

Route of administration: Oral, intravenous.

Adverse effects: Side effects of erythromycin include gastrointestinal disturbance, which is common after oral administration. Liver damage and jaundice can occur after chronic administration.

Therapeutic notes: Resistance to erythromycin results from a mutation of the binding site on the ribosome. Erythromycin has a similar spectrum of activity to penicillin, and it is an effective alternative in penicillin-sensitive patients. Azithromycin can be given for uncomplicated chlamydial infections of the genital tract. Telithromycin is active against respiratory pathogens resistant to the macrolides.

Clindamycin

Clindamycin is a lincosamide.

Mechanism of action: Similar to the macrolides.

Spectrum of activity: Clindamycin is active against gram-positive cocci, including penicillin-resistant staphylococci, and many anaerobes.

Route of administration: Oral, parenteral.

Adverse effects: Antibiotic-associated (pseudomembranous) colitis; greater risk than for other antibiotics.

Therapeutic notes: Clindamycin is used for staphylococcal joint and bone infections.

Miscellaneous antibacterials

Miscellaneous antibacterials include:
- Metronidazole.
- Nitrofurantoin.
- Bacitracin.
- Polymyxins.

Metronidazole and tinidazole

Mechanism of action: Metronidazole is bactericidal. It is metabolized to an intermediate that inhibits bacterial DNA synthesis and degrades existing DNA. Its selectivity is due to the fact that the intermediate toxic metabolite is not produced in mammalian cells.

Spectrum of activity: Metronidazole is antiprotozoal, and it has antibacterial activity against anaerobic bacteria (see Fig. 3.3).

Route of administration: Oral, rectal, intravenous, and topical.

Contraindications: If possible, metronidazole should not be used in pregnant women.

Adverse effects: Mild headache and gastrointestinal disturbance. Adverse drug reactions occur with alcohol.

Therapeutic notes: Acquired resistance to metronidazole is rare. Tinidazole is similar to metronidazole but has a longer duration of action.

Nitrofurantoin

Mechanism of action: The mechanism of action of nitrofurantoin is uncertain, although it possibly interferes with bacterial DNA metabolism.

Spectrum of activity: Nitrofurantoin is active against gram-positive bacteria (including some enterococci resistant to vancomycin) and *Escherichia coli* (see Fig. 3.3).

Route of administration: Oral; it reaches high therapeutic concentrations in the urine.

Adverse effects: Gastrointestinal disturbance. Pulmonary complications can occur with chronic therapy.

Therapeutic notes: Rarely, chromosomal resistance to nitrofurantoin can occur.

Bacitracin

Mechanism of action: Bacitracin is a natural antibiotic, isolated from *Bacillus subtilis,* that inhibits bacterial cell-wall formation.

Spectrum of activity: Bacitracin is similar in its spectrum of activity to penicillin (see Fig. 3.3).

Route of administration: Topical. Oral for *Clostridium difficile* enterocolitis.

Adverse effects: Well tolerated when used topically. Serious nephrotoxicity can occur if it is used systemically.

Therapeutic notes: Bacitracin is much less likely to cause hypersensitivity reactions than penicillin. Acquired resistance is rare.

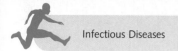

Polymyxins

Colistin is an example of a polymyxin, though this class is seldom prescribed, due to its toxicity.

Mechanism of action: Polymyxins are bactericidal. They are peptides that interact with phospholipids on the outer plasma cell membranes of gram-negative bacteria, disrupting their structure. This disruption destroys the bacteria's osmotic barrier, leading to lysis (see Fig. 3.2).

Spectrum of activity: Polymyxins are active only against gram-negative bacteria, including *Pseudomonas aeruginosa* (see Fig. 3.3).

Route of administration: Intravenous, intramuscular, inhalation. Oral polymyxins are given to sterilize the bowel in neutropenic patients.

Adverse effects: Perioral and peripheral, paraesthesia, vertigo, nephrotoxicity, and neurotoxicity.

Therapeutic notes: Resistance to polymyxins is rare. Clinical use of polymyxins is re-emerging because of increasing resistance of gram-negative bacteria to currently available antibiotics.

Antimycobacterial drugs

The mycobacteria are slow-growing intracellular bacilli that cause tuberculosis (*Mycobacterium tuberculosis*) and leprosy (*Mycobacterium leprae*) in humans.

Mycobacteria differ in their structure and lifestyle from gram-positive and gram-negative bacteria, and they are treated with different drugs.

Antituberculosis therapy

The first-line drugs used in the treatment of tuberculosis are:

- Isoniazid, which inhibits the production of mycolic acid, a component of the cell wall unique to mycobacteria, and is bactericidal against growing organisms. Taken orally, it penetrates tuberculous lesions well. Adverse effects occur in about 5% of patients and include peripheral neuropathy, hepatotoxicity, and autoimmune phenomena. Resistance is rare in developed countries, but not in less-developed areas.
- Rifampin, which inhibits DNA-dependent RNA polymerase, causing a bactericidal effect. It is a potent drug, active orally. Adverse effects are infrequent, but they can be serious (e.g., hepatotoxicity and "toxic syndromes"). Rifampin

is a potent inducer of cytochrome P450 enzymes and is associated with many DDIs. Orange discoloration of the urine, tears, and other secretions is a common side effect. There are many drug interactions, and resistance can develop rapidly.

- Ethambutol, which is bacteriostatic. The mechanism of action is uncertain, involving impaired synthesis of the mycobacterial cell wall. Ethambutol is administered orally. Adverse effects are uncommon, but reversible optic neuritis may occur. Resistance often develops.
- Pyrazinamide, the mechanism of action of which is uncertain but may involve metabolism of drug within *Mycobacterium tuberculosis* to produce a toxic product, pyrazinoic acid, which works as a bacteriostatic agent in the low pH environment of the phagolysosome. It is active orally. Adverse effects are hepatotoxicity and raised plasma urate levels that can lead to gout. Resistance can develop rapidly.
- Streptomycin, which is now rarely used for tuberculosis.

Other aminoglycosides and macrolides are used to treat mycobacteria.

The second-line drugs used for tuberculosis infections when first-line drugs have been discontinued owing to resistance or adverse effects are:

- Capreomycin, which is a peptide drug given intramuscularly. It can cause ototoxicity and kidney damage.
- Cycloserine, which is a broad-spectrum drug that inhibits peptidoglycan synthesis. This drug is administered orally and can cause CNS toxicity.
- New macrolides (e.g., azithromycin and clarithromycin).
- Fluoroquinolones (e.g., ciprofloxacin).

To reduce the emergence of resistant organisms, a compound drug therapy is used to treat tuberculosis, involving:

- An initial phase of about 2 months, consisting of three drugs: isoniazid, rifampicin, and pyrazinamide.
- Continuation phase of 4 months, consisting of two drugs: isoniazid and rifampin.
  Longer treatment regimens may be needed for patients with meningitis or bone/joint involvement.

Antileprosy therapy

Tuberculoid leprosy is treated with dapsone and rifampicin for 6 months.

Lepromatous leprosy is treated with dapsone, rifampin, and clofazimine for up to 2 years.

Dapsone resembles sulfonamides chemically, and it may inhibit folate synthesis in a similar way. It is active orally. Adverse effects are numerous, and some are fatal.

Clofazimine is a chemically complex dye that accumulates in macrophages, possibly acting on mycobacterial DNA. As a dye, clofazimine can discolor the skin and turn urine red. Other adverse effects are numerous. It is active orally.

Grouping of antibacterial drugs by their mechanism of action rather than chemical structure is easier, more important, and more relevant to your understanding.

Concepts of viral infection

Viruses are obligate intracellular parasites that lack independent metabolism and can only replicate within the host cells they enter and infect. A virus particle, or virion, consists essentially of DNA or RNA enclosed in a protein coat (capsid). In addition, certain viruses may possess a lipoprotein envelope and replicative enzymes (Fig. 3.5).

Viruses are classified largely according to the architecture of the virion and the nature of their genetic material. Viral nucleic acid may be single stranded (ss) or double stranded (ds) (Fig. 3.6).

Antiviral agents

Because viruses have an intracellular replication cycle and they share many of the metabolic processes of the host cell, it has proved extremely difficult to find drugs that are selectively toxic to them. Additionally, by the time a viral infection becomes detectable clinically, the viral replication process tends to be very far advanced, making chemotherapeutic intervention difficult. All current antiviral agents are virustatic rather than virucidal, and, therefore, they

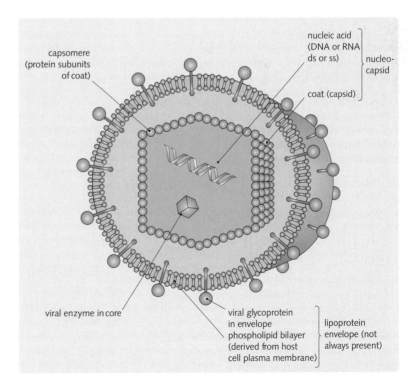

Fig. 3.5 Diagrammatic representation of the components of a virion.

Classification of medically important viruses and the diseases they cause

Family	ss/ds	Viruses	Diseases
DNA viruses Herpes viruses	ds	Herpes simplex (HSV)* Varicella-zoster (VZV)* Cytomegalovirus (CMV)* Epstein–Barr virus (EBV)*	Cold sores, genital herpes Chickenpox, shingles Cytomegalic disease Infectious mononucleosis
Poxviruses	ds	Variola	Smallpox
Adenoviruses	ds	Adenoviruses	Acute respiratory disease
Hepadnaviruses	ds	Hepatitis B	Hepatitis
Papovaviruses	ds	Papilloma	Warts
Parvoviruses	ss	B19	Erythema infectiosum
RNA viruses Orthomyxoviruses	ss	Influenza A* and B*	Influenza
Paramyxoviruses	ss	Measles virus Mumps virus Parainfluenza Respiratory syncytial*	Measles Mumps Respiratory infection Respiratory infection
Coronaviruses	ss	Coronavirus	Respiratory infection
Rhabdoviruses	ss	Rabies virus	Rabies
Picornaviruses	ss	Enteroviruses Rhinoviruses Hepatitis A	Meningitis Colds Hepatitis
Calciviruses	ss	Norwalk virus	Gastroenteritis
Togaviruses	ss	Alphaviruses Rubivirus	Encephalitis, haemorrhagic fevers Rubella
Reoviruses	ds	Rotavirus	Gastroenteritis
Arenavirus	ss	Lymphocytic choriomeningitis Lassavirus*	Meningitis Lassa fever
Retroviruses	ss	HIV I, II*	AIDS

Fig. 3.6 Classification of selected medically important viruses and the diseases they cause (*, viruses for which effective chemotherapy exists; ds, double-stranded; ss, single-stranded).

rely upon host immunocompetence for a complete clinical cure.

Nevertheless, antiviral chemotherapy is clinically effective against some viral diseases (identified with an asterisk in Fig. 3.6). The viruses include:

- Herpesviruses (herpes simplex virus, HSV; varicella zoster virus, VZV; cytomegalovirus, CMV).
- Influenza viruses A and, more recently, B.
- Respiratory syncytial virus, arenaviruses.
- Human immunodeficiency virus 1 (HIV–1).

The selective inhibition of these viruses by drugs depends on either:

- Inhibition of unique steps in the viral replication pathways, such as adsorption of the virion to the cell receptor, penetration, uncoating, assembly, and release.
- Preferential inhibition of steps shared with the host cell, which include transcription and translation.

In addition to chemotherapy, immune-based therapies, such as the use of immunoglobulins and cytokines in viral infection, are also mentioned below.

Inhibition of attachment to or penetration of host cells
Amantadine and Rimantidine
Mechanism of action: These drugs block a primitive ion channel in the viral membrane (named M_2), preventing fusion of a virion to host cell membranes, and they inhibit the release of newly synthesized viruses from the host cell (Fig. 3.7).

Route of administration: Oral.

Indications: Amantadine is used for the prophylaxis and treatment of acute influenza A in groups at risk. It is not effective against influenza B.

Adverse effects: Some patients (5–10%) report nonserious dizziness, slurred speech, and insomnia. Neurologic side effects and renal failure can occur at high concentrations.

Therapeutic notes: Emergence of resistance to amantadine associated with clinical failure has been reported in 25–50% of patients. Amantadine is not used widely because of problems with resistance, its narrow spectrum of activity, and because influenza vaccines are often preferred.

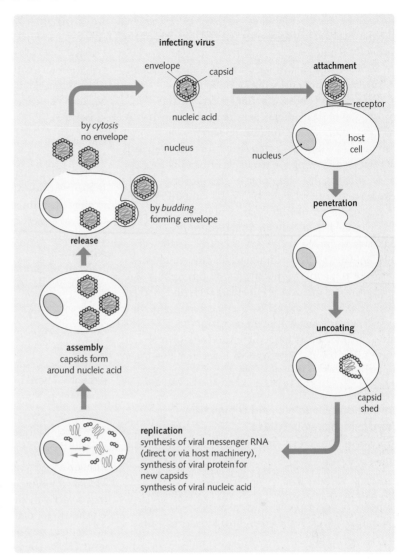

Fig. 3.7 Stages in the infection of a host's cell and replication of a virus. Several thousand virus particles may be formed from each cell (redrawn from *Medical Microbiology*, 2nd ed., by Mims *et al.* Mosby, 1998).

Neuraminidase inhibitors

Zanamivir and oseltamivir belong to the neuraminidase inhibitor class of drugs.

Mechanism of action: These drugs inhibit the release of newly synthesized viruses from the host cell by inhibiting the enzyme—neuraminidase—that is responsible for cleaving the peptide links between virus and host.

Route of administration: Zanamivir is delivered by inhalation, but its sister drug oseltamivir may be given orally.

Indications: Treatment of influenza A or B virus within 48 hours after onset of symptoms when influenza is endemic in the community.

Contraindications: Breastfeeding.

Adverse effects: Gastrointestinal disturbances.

Immunoglobulins

Examples of immunoglobulins include human normal immunoglobulin (HNIG/γ-globulin) and specific immunoglobulins, including hepatitis B (HBIG), rabies (RIG), varicella zoster (VZIG), and cytomegalovirus (CMVIG) immunoglobulins.

Mechanism of action: Immunoglobulins bind specifically to antigenic determinants on the outside of virions. By specifically binding to a virus, the immunoglobulins may neutralize it by coating the virus and preventing its attachment and entry into host cells.

HNIG is prepared from pooled plasma of ~1000 donors and contains antibodies to measles, mumps, varicella, and hepatitis A.

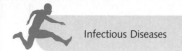

Specific immunoglobulins are prepared by pooling the plasma of selected donors with high levels of the antibody required.

Route of administration: Intramuscular, although intravenous immunoglobulins can be given.

Indications: HNIG is administered for the protection of susceptible contacts against hepatitis A, measles, mumps, and rubella. Specific immunoglobulins may attenuate or prevent hepatitis and rabies following known exposure and before the onset of signs and symptoms (e.g., following exposure to a rabid animal). VZIG and CMVIG are indicated for prophylactic use to prevent chickenpox and cytomegalic disease in immunosuppressed patients at risk.

Contraindications: Immunoglobulins should not be given to people with known antibody against IgA.

Adverse effects: Malaise, chills, fever, and (rarely) anaphylaxis.

Therapeutic notes: Protection with immunoglobulins is immediate and lasts several weeks. HNIG may interfere with vaccinations for 3 months.

Inhibition of nucleic acid replication
Acyclovir and related drugs
Acyclovir, famciclovir, and valacyclovir are all closely related antiviral drugs.

Mechanism of action: Acyclovir and related drugs are characterized by their selective phosphorylation in herpes-infected cells. This takes place by a viral thymidine kinase rather than host kinase, as a first step.

Phosphorylation yields a triphosphate nucleotide that inhibits viral DNA polymerase and viral DNA synthesis.

These drugs are selectively toxic to infected cells because, in the absence of viral thymidine kinase, the host kinase activates only a small amount of the drug. In addition, the DNA polymerase of herpes virus has a much higher affinity for the activated drug than has cellular DNA polymerase (see Fig. 3.7).

Route of administration: Topical, oral, parenteral.

Indications: Acyclovir and related drugs are used for the prophylaxis and treatment of herpes simplex virus (HSV) and varicella zoster virus (VZV) infections, superficial and systemic, particularly in the immunocompromised.

Adverse effects: Side effects are minimal. Rarely, renal impairment and encephalopathy occur.

Therapeutic notes: The herpes genome in latent (nonreplicating) cells is not affected by acyclovir therapy, and so recurrence of infection after cessation of treatment is to be expected.

Cytomegalovirus (CMV) is resistant to acyclovir because its genome does not encode thymidine kinase.

Ganciclovir
Mechanism of action: Ganciclovir is a synthetic nucleoside analog, structurally related to acyclovir. It also requires conversion to the triphosphate nucleotide form, though by a different kinase. Ganciclovir acts as a substrate for viral DNA polymerase and as a chain terminator, aborting virus replication.

Route of administration: Oral, intravenous.

Indications: While as active as acyclovir against HSV and VZV, ganciclovir is reserved for the treatment of severe CMV infections in immunocompromised people, owing to its side effects.

Adverse effects: Reversible neutropenia in 40% of patients. There is occasional rash, nausea, and encephalopathy.

Therapeutic notes: Maintenance therapy with ganciclovir at a reduced dose may be necessary to prevent recurrence of CMV.

Ribavirin
Mechanism of action: Ribavirin is a nucleoside analog that selectively interferes with viral nucleic acid synthesis in a manner similar to acyclovir.

Route of administration: For respiratory syncytial virus (RSV), by inhalation; for Lassa virus, intravenously.

Indications: Severe respiratory syncytial virus bronchiolitis in infants. Lassa fever.

Adverse effects: Reticulocytosis; respiratory depression.

Therapeutic notes: The necessity of aerosol administration for RSV limits the usefulness of this effective drug.

Nucleoside analog reverse transcriptase inhibitors
Examples of nucleoside reverse transcriptase inhibitors include zidovudine (AZT) and the newer drugs: abacavir, didanosine (ddI), lamivudine (3TC), stavudine (d4T), and zalcitabine (ddC).

Mechanism of action: These nucleotide analogs all require intracellular conversion to the corresponding triphosphate nucleotide for activation. The active triphosphates competitively inhibit reverse transcriptase, and they cause termination of DNA chain elongation once incorporated. Affinity for viral reverse transcriptase is 100 times that for host DNA polymerase (Fig. 3.8, site 3).

Route of administration: Oral.

Indications: Nucleoside reverse transcriptase inhibitors are used for the management of asymptomatic and symptomatic HIV infections, and the prevention of maternal–fetal HIV transmission.

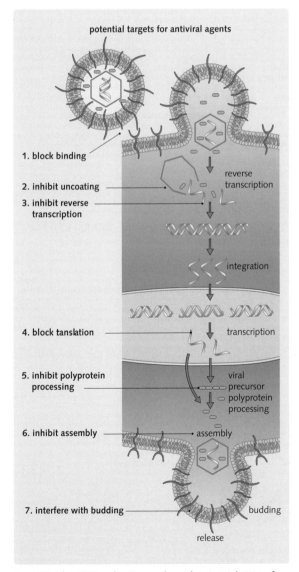

potential targets for antiviral agents

1. block binding

reverse transcription

2. inhibit uncoating

3. inhibit reverse transcription

integration

4. block tanslation

transcription

5. inhibit polyprotein processing

viral precursor polyprotein processing

6. inhibit assembly

assembly

7. interfere with budding

budding

release

Fig. 3.8 The HIV replicative cycle and potential sites of antiviral drug action.

Adverse effects: Side effects of AZT are uncommon at the recommended low dosage in patients with asymptomatic or mild HIV infections, but more common in AIDS patients on higher dosage regimens.

Toxicity to human myeloid and erythroid progenitor cells commonly causes anemia and neutropenia (i.e., bone-marrow suppression). Other common side effects include nausea, insomnia, headaches, and myalgia.

The major dose-limiting effects of ddI are pancreatitis and peripheral neuropathy; of ddC and d4T, peripheral neuropathy.

Therapeutic notes: Drug resistance evolves to all the current nucleoside reverse transcriptase inhibitors by the development of mutations in reverse transcriptase, although the kinetics of resistance development varies for the different drugs (e.g., 6–18 months for AZT). Combined therapies may have a place in increasing efficacy synergistically and reducing emergence of resistant strains.

Nonnucleoside reverse transcriptase inhibitors

Efavirenz and nevirapine are examples of drugs within this class.

Mechanism of action: Efavirenz and nevirapine both bind to reverse transcriptase near the catalytic site, leading to a conformational change that inactivates this enzyme.

Route of administration: Oral.

Contraindications: Breastfeeding, pregnancy.

Adverse effects: Generally well tolerated. Rash, dizziness, and headache may occur.

Therapeutic notes: Resistance can develop quickly when subtherapeutic doses are employed.

Inhibition of post-translational events
Protease inhibitors

Examples of protease inhibitors include saquinavir and the newer drugs: ritonavir, indinavir, nelfinavir, and amprenavir.

Mechanism of action: Protease inhibitors prevent the virus-specific protease of HIV cleaving the inert polyprotein product of translation into various structural and functional proteins (Fig. 3.8, site 5).

Route of administration: Oral.

Indications: Protease inhibitors are used for the management of asymptomatic and symptomatic HIV infections, in combination with nucleoside reverse transcriptase inhibitors.

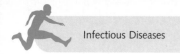
Adverse effects: Protease inhibitors are well tolerated. Nausea, vomiting, and diarrhea are common. In addition, indinavir and ritonavir may cause taste disturbances, and saquinavir may cause buccal and mucosal ulceration.

Therapeutic notes: Combination treatment between protease inhibitors and nucleoside reverse transcriptase inhibitors produces additive antiviral effects and reduces the incidence of resistance. Such combination therapy is termed highly active antiretroviral therapy (HAART).

Immunomodulators
Interferons

Mechanism of action: Interferons (IFNs) are endogenous cytokines with antiviral activity, which are normally produced by leukocytes and other cells in response to viral infection. Three major classes have been identified (α, β, and γ), and they have been shown to have immunoregulatory and antiproliferative effects.

The mechanism of the antiviral effect of IFN varies for different viruses and cells. IFNs have been shown to bind to cell-surface receptors and signal a cascade of events that interfere with viral penetration, uncoating, synthesis, or methylation of mRNA, translation of viral protein, viral assembly, and viral release (see Fig. 3.7).

Probably the most important effect of IFNs is the induction of enzymes in the host cell that inhibit the translation of viral mRNA.

The relatively recent production of IFNs in large quantities by cell culture and recombinant DNA technology has allowed their evaluation and prescription as antiviral agents.

Route of administration: Intravenous, intramuscular.

Indications: The exact role of interferons (IFNs) in the treatment of viral infections remains unclear. They have a wide spectrum of activity and have been shown to be effective in the treatmentof chronic hepatitis (B and C), among others.

Adverse effects: Influenza-like syndrome with fatigue, fever, myalgia, nausea, and diarrhea is the most common side effect. Chronic administration can cause bone-marrow depression and neurologic effects.

Therapeutic notes: The role of IFNs remains to be clearly established. Their usefulness has been limited by the need for repeated injections and by dose-limiting adverse effects.

Drugs used in HIV infection

Infection with the human immunodeficiency virus (HIV) ultimately results in progression to the acquired immunodeficiency syndrome (AIDS). There are currently no drugs which can prevent this progression, though there are numerous agents on the market and in clinical trials which delay the rate of progression.

The optimal treatment of HIV infection requires combination therapy with two or more drugs. This combination therapy is known as highly active antiretroviral therapy (HAART).

There are a variety of potential sites for antiviral drug action in the HIV–1 replicative cycle (see Fig. 3.8).

The three main classes of drug used in the treatment of HIV have already been discussed:
- Nucleoside reverse transcriptase inhibitors (Fig. 3.8, site 3).
- Nonnucleoside reverse transcriptase inhibitors (Fig. 3.8, site 3).
- Protease inhibitors (Fig. 3.8, site 5).

Future anti-HIV drug therapy

A number of strategies are being pursued in research laboratories across the world in the quest for effective drugs to treat HIV infection. These strategies include:
- Drugs which interrupt HIV binding to host cells, notably the gp120 envelope protein.
- Drugs designed specifically to "smother" and prevent its entry into cells.
- Antisense oligonucleotides to complement specific portions of the viral genome and inhibit transcription and replication.

The development of antiviral drugs is a rapidly moving field and, with HIV especially, one that is currently topical. Keep up to date, as knowledge of recent developments in this area should impress examiners.

Antifungal drugs

Concepts of fungal infection

Fungi are members of a kingdom of eukaryotic organisms that live as saprophytes or parasites. A few species of fungi are pathogenic to humans.

Fungal infections are termed mycoses, and they may be superficial, affecting the skin, nails, hair, mucous membranes; or systemic, affecting deep tissues and organs.

Three main groups of fungi cause disease in humans (Fig. 3.9).

Fungal pathogenicity results from mycotoxin production, allergenicity/inflammatory reactions, and tissue invasion. Opportunistic fungal infections are important causes of disease in the immunosuppressed.

Antifungal drugs

There are four main classes of antifungal drugs:
- Polyene macrolides.
- Imidazole antifungals.
- Triazole antifungals.
- Other antifungals.

The sites of action of the antifungal drugs are summarized in Fig. 3.10.

Polyene macrolides

Examples of polyene macrolides include amphotericin B and nystatin.

Mechanism of action: Polyene macrolides bind to ergosterol in the fungal cell membrane, forming pores through which cell constituents are lost. This results in fatal damage (Fig. 3.11). These drugs are selectively toxic because in human cells the major sterol is cholesterol, not ergosterol.

Route of administration: Amphotericin B is administered topically and intravenously. Nystatin is too toxic for intravenous use. It is not absorbed orally at all, and so it is applied topically as a cream, vaginal pessaries, or tablets sucked so as to deliver the drug via the oral membranes.

Indications: Amphotericin is a broad-spectrum antifungal used in potentially fatal systemic infections. Nystatin is used to suppress candidiasis (thrush) on the skin and mucous membranes (oral and vaginal).

Adverse effects: Fever, chills, and nausea. Long-term therapy invariably causes renal damage. Nystatin may cause oral sensitization.

Therapeutic notes: Creatinine clearance must be monitored during amphotericin therapy to exclude renal damage. Resistance can develop *in vivo* to amphotericin but not to nystatin.

Imidazoles

Examples of imidazoles include clotrimazole, miconazole, and ketoconazole.

Mechanism of action: Imidazoles have a broad spectrum of activity. They inhibit fungal lipid (especially ergosterol) synthesis in cell membranes. Interference with fungal oxidative *N*-demethylases results in the accumulation of 14α-methyl sterols, which may disrupt the packing of acyl chains of phospholipids, inhibiting growth and interfering with membrane-bound enzyme systems.

Route of administration: Intravenous, topical. Ketoconazole is given orally as, unlike the other imidazoles, it is well absorbed by this route.

Fungi causing disease in humans			
Fungal class	Form	Example	Disease caused
Molds	Filamentous branching mycelia	Dermatophytes e.g., *Tinea spp.* *Aspergillus furnigatus*	Athlete's foot, ringworm, and other superficial mycoses Pulmonary or disseminated aspergillosis
True yeasts	Unicellular (round or oval)	*Cryptococcus neoformans*	Cryptococcal meningitis and lung infections in the immunocompromised
Yeast-like fungi	Similar to yeasts but can also form long (non-branching) filaments	*Candida albicans*	Oral and vaginal thrush, endocarditis, and septicemias

Fig. 3.9 Main groups of fungi causing disease in humans.

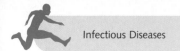

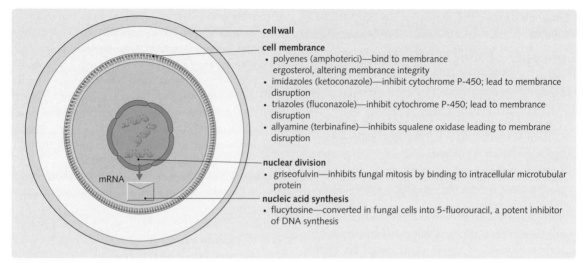

Fig. 3.10 Sites of action of antifungal drugs.

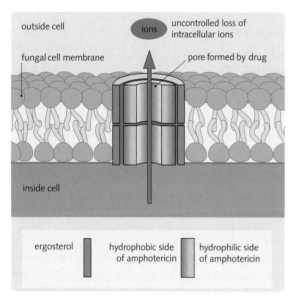

Fig. 3.11 Mechanism of action of polyene antifungal agents.

Indications: Candidiasis and dermatophyte mycoses. Miconazole can also be used intravenously as an alternative to amphotericin in disseminated mycoses. Because ketoconazole is active orally, it can be used for systemic mycoses.

Adverse effects: Topical use of imidazoles tends to be unproblematic. Intravenous miconazole is often limited by side effects of nausea, faintness, and hematologic disorders. Oral ketoconazole can cause serious hepatotoxicity and adreno-suppression. Ketoconazole also inhibits cytochrome P450 isozymes responsible for metabolism of many drugs.

Therapeutic notes: Resistance rarely develops to imidazoles.

Triazoles

Examples of triazoles include fluconazole and itraconazole.

Mechanism of action: Triazoles are similar to imidazoles (see above), although they have greater selectivity against fungi, and they cause fewer endocrinologic problems.

Route of administration: Oral.

Indications: Fluconazole can be used for a wide range of systemic and superficial infections, including cryptococcal meningitis, as it reaches the CSF in high concentrations. Itraconazole is similarly indicated, although unlike fluconazole, it can be used against *Aspergillus* sp.

Adverse effects: Nausea, diarrhea, and rashes. Itraconazole is well tolerated, although nausea, headaches, and abdominal pain can occur, but it should not be given to patients with liver damage. Itraconazole and, to a lesser extent, fluconazole inhibit P450 isozymes.

Therapeutic notes: Resistance rarely develops to the triazoles.

Other antifungals
Allylamines

Terbinafine is an example of an allylamine.

Mechanism of action: Terbinafine prevents ergosterol synthesis by inhibiting the enzyme squalene epoxidase, resulting in squalene accumulation, which leads to membrane disruption and cell death. It is lipophilic and penetrates superficial tissues well, including the nails.

Route of administration: Oral, topical.

Indications: Terbinafine has been recently introduced against dermatophyte infections including ringworm, where oral therapy is appropriate because of the site and severity of extent of infection.

Adverse effects: Mild nausea, abdominal pain, and skin reactions. Loss of taste has been reported.

Therapeutic notes: Resistance rarely develops. Initial trials with terbinafine show impressive clinical and mycologic cure rates.

Flucytosine

Mechanism of action: Flucytosine is imported into fungal, but not human, cells, where it is converted into 5-fluorouracil, a potent inhibitor of DNA synthesis.

Route of administration: Intravenous.

Indications: Flucytosine is most active against yeasts, and it is indicated for use in systemic candidiasis and as an adjunct to amphotericin in cryptococcal meningitis.

Adverse effects: Nausea and vomiting are common. Rare side effects include hepatotoxicity, hair loss, and bone-marrow suppression.

Therapeutic notes: Weekly blood counts of patients on flucytosine are necessary to monitor bone-marrow suppression.

Griseofulvin

Mechanism of action: The action of griseofulvin is not fully established, but it probably interferes with microtubule formation or nucleic acid synthesis and polymerization. It is selectively concentrated in keratin, and, therefore, it is suitable for treating dermatophyte mycoses.

Route of administration: Oral.

Indications: Griseofulvin is the drug of choice for widespread or intractable dermatophyte infections, where topical therapy has failed.

Adverse reactions: Hypersensitivity reactions, headaches, rashes, and photosensitivity.

Therapeutic notes: Because griseofulvin is fungistatic rather than fungicidal, treatment regimes are long, amounting to several weeks or months. Griseofulvin is more effective for skin than nail infections.

Superficial mycoses (e.g., "athlete's foot," "thrush") are common and usually easily treated with topical drugs that have few adverse effects. Deep mycoses are rare (except in the immunocompromised), serious, and may be fatal despite therapy with systemic drugs, which often have adverse effects.

Antiprotozoal drugs

Concepts of protozoal infection

Protozoa are members of a phylum of unicellular organisms, some of which are parasitic pathogens in humans causing several diseases of medical and global importance. Parasitic protozoa replicate within the host's body; they are usually divided into four subphyla according to their type of locomotion (Fig. 3.12).

Malaria

Malaria is the most important protozoan disease in tropical medicine. It is responsible for two million deaths per year and much morbidity in the 200 million people worldwide who are infected.

Malaria is caused by four species of plasmodial parasites (see below) that are transmitted by female anopheline mosquitoes.

Antimalarial drugs target different phases of the malarial life cycle (Fig. 3.13). This life cycle proceeds as follows:

- When an infected mosquito feeds on a human, it injects sporozoites into the bloodstream from its salivary glands.
- The sporozoites rapidly penetrate the liver, where they transform and grow into tissue schizonts containing large numbers of merozoites. In the case of *Plasmodium vivax* and *P. ovale*, some schizonts remain dormant in the liver for years (hypnozoites) before rupturing to cause a relapse.
- The large tissue schizonts rupture after 5–20 days, releasing thousands of merozoites that invade circulating red blood cells (RBCs), and multiply inside the cell.
- The host's RBCs rupture, leading to the release of more merozoites. These then invade and destroy

Classification of medically important protozoan species causing disease in humans			
Sub-phyla	Defining characteristics	Medically important species	Disease
Amebae (sarcodina)	Ameboid movement with pseudopods	*Entamoeba histolytica*	Amebiasis (amoebic dysentery)
Flagellates (mastigophora)	Flagella that produces a whip-like movement	*Giardia lamblia* *Trichomonas vaginalis* *Leishmania spp.* *Trypanosoma spp.*	Giardiasis Trichomonal vaginitis Leishmaniasis Trypanosomiasis (sleeping sickness and Chagas' disease)
Ciliates (ciliophora)	Cilia beat to produce movement	–	–
Sporozoans (sporozoa)	No locomotor organs in adult stage	*Plasmodium spp.*	Malaria

Fig. 3.12 Classification of medically important protozoan species causing disease in humans.

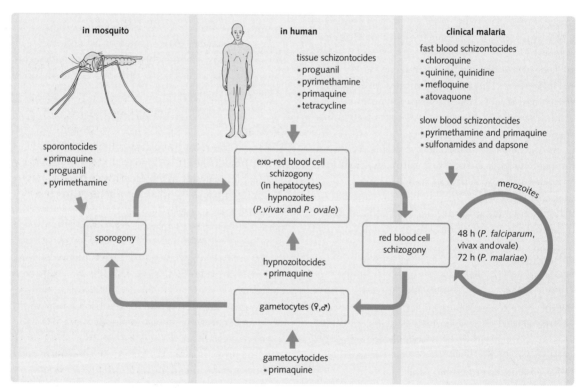

Fig. 3.13 Malarial life cycle and point of action of chemotherapeutic agents.

more RBCs. This cycle of invasion and destruction causes the episodic chills and fever that characterize malaria.

• Some merozoites develop into gametocytes. If these are taken up by a feeding mosquito, the insect becomes infected, thus completing the cycle.

The clinical features and severity of malaria depend upon the species of parasite and the immunologic status of the person infected. Clinically significant malaria is less common in adults who have always lived in endemic areas, as partial immunity develops.

The four types of plasmodium causing malaria are:
- *P. falciparum*, which is widespread and causes malignant tertian (fever every third day) malaria. There is no exo-erythrocytic stage, so that, if the erythrocytic forms are eradicated, relapses do not occur.
- *P. vivax*, which is widespread and causes benign, tertian relapsing malaria. Exo-erythrocytic forms may persist in the liver for years and cause relapses.
- *P. malariae*, which is rare and causes benign quartan (fever every fourth day) malaria. There is no exo-erythrocytic stage, so that, if the erythrocytic forms are eradicated, relapses do not occur.
- *P. ovale*, which is mainly African and causes a rare form of benign relapsing malaria. Exo-erythrocytic forms may persist in the liver for years and cause relapses.

Approaches to antimalarial chemotherapy

Antimalarial drugs are usually classified in terms of their action against different stages of the parasite (see Fig. 3.13). They are used to protect against or cure malaria or to prevent transmission.

Prophylactic use

The aim of prophylactic use is to prevent the occurrence of infection in a previously healthy individual who is at potential exposure risk.

Suppressive prophylaxis involves the use of blood schizonticides to prevent acute attacks; causal prophylaxis involves the use of tissue schizonticides or drugs against the sporozoite to prevent the parasite becoming established in the liver.

Curative (therapeutic use)

Antimalarial drugs can be used curatively (therapeutically) against an established infection.

Suppressive treatment aims to control acute attacks, usually with blood schizonticides; radical treatment aims to kill dormant liver forms, usually with a hypnozonticide, to prevent relapsing malaria.

Antimalarial drugs

4-aminoquinolines

Chloroquine is an example of a 4-aminoquinoline.

Mechanism of action: Chloroquine is a rapidly acting blood schizonticide (see Fig. 3.13). It is concentrated 100-fold in erythrocytes that contain plasmodial parasites; this occurs because ferriprotoporphyrin IX, a degradation product of

hemoglobin digestion by the parasites, acts as a chloroquine receptor. It is unclear how the high chloroquine concentrations kill the parasites; possibly, the digestion of hemoglobin is inhibited.

Route of administration: Oral. In severe falciparum malaria infections, injections or infusions can be used.

Indications: Suppressive chemoprophylaxis and treatment of susceptible strains of plasmodium.

Adverse effects: Nausea, vomiting, headache, rashes, and, rarely, neurologic effects.

Therapeutic effects: Chloroquine is considered safe for use in pregnant women. It rapidly controls fever (24–48 hours), but it cannot produce a lasting radical cure in *P. vivax* and *P. ovale* infections, as it does not affect hypnozoites.

In most areas, *P. falciparum* is resistant to chloroquine, necessitating combination chemoprophylaxis with antifolates (see later).

Quinoline–methanols

Examples of quinoline–methanols include quinine and mefloquine.

Mechanism of action: Quinoline–methanols are rapidly acting blood schizonticides (see Fig. 3.13). It is not precisely known how the quinoline–methanols work but, like chloroquine, they are known to bind to a product of hemoglobin digestion.

Route of administration: Quinine is administered orally or by rate-controlled infusion in severe cases. Mefloquine is only given orally.

Indications: Quinine is the drug of choice for treating the acute clinical attack of falciparum malaria resistant to chloroquine. Mefloquine is effective against all malarial species, including multidrug-resistant *P. falciparum*, and it can also be used for chemoprophylaxis.

Adverse effects: Quinine: tinnitus, headache, nausea, blurring of vision, hypoglycemia, and, rarely, blood disorders. Overdose results in profound hypotension due to peripheral vasodilatation and myocardial depression (see Chapter 7). Quinine is safe in pregnancy.

Mefloquine: nausea, vomiting, gastrointestinal disturbance, and postural hypotension. Rarely, acute neuropathic conditions may occur. Mefloquine may cause fetal abnormalities.

Therapeutic effects: The quinoline–methanols are used in combination therapy with other agents such as the sulfonamides or tetracyclines.

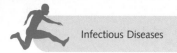

Antifolates

Examples of antifolates include type 1 drugs (e.g., sulfonamides and dapsone) and type 2 drugs (e.g., pyrimethamine and proguanil).

Mechanism of action: Antifolates are slow-acting (in comparison with chloroquine, quinine, and mefloquine) blood schizonticides, tissue schizonticides, and sporonticides. These drugs inhibit the formation of folate compounds and thus inhibit DNA synthesis and cell division. All growing stages of the malarial parasite are affected.

The sulfonamides and dapsone are known as type 1 antifolate drugs. They compete with *p*-aminobenzoic acid (PABA) for the enzyme dihydropteroate synthetase. These drugs selectively inhibit parasitic DHPA synthetase.

Proguanil and pyrimethamine are known as type 2 antifolate drugs. They selectively inhibit malarial dihydrofolate reductase.

These two groups of drug act on the same pathway but at different points; they are used in combination, as their synergistic blockade is more powerful than any one drug acting alone.

Route of administration: Oral.

Indications: Antifolates are used in combination for the causal chemoprophylaxis of malaria or in combination with quinine for the treatment of acute chloroquine-resistant malaria.

Adverse effects: In toxic doses, type 2 antifolates can inhibit mammalian dihydrofolate reductase and cause a megaloblastic anemia. Skin rashes occasionally occur.

Therapeutic notes: Common chemoprophylactic combinations include chloroquine plus pyrimethamine with a sulfonamide or dapsone.

8-Aminoquinolines

Primaquine is an example of an 8-aminoquinoline.

Mechanism of action: Primaquine is a hypnozonicide and gametocide. It is unclear how the drug works, but it may cause oxidative damage to the parasite. It is effective against the nongrowing stages of malaria (i.e., hypnozoites and gametocytes) (see Fig. 3.13).

Route of administration: Oral.

Indications: Primaquine is used for the radical cure of relapsing malarias (*P. ovale* and *P. vivax*) and prevention of transmission of *P. falciparum*.

Contraindications: Pregnancy.

Adverse effects: Nausea, vomiting, and bone-marrow depression. Acute hemolytic anemia can occur in people with glucose–6-phosphate deficiency.

Therapeutic notes: Primaquine is usually used in combination with chloroquine. Resistance is rare.

Treatment of other protozoal infections
Amebiasis

Amebic dysentery is caused by infection with *Entamoeba histolytica*, which is ingested in a cystic form. Dysentery results from invasion of the intestinal wall by the parasite. Occasionally, the organism encysts in the liver, forming abscesses.

Metronidazole is the drug of choice for acute invasive amebic dysentery; it kills the trophozoites but has no activity against the cyst forms. Diloxanide and tinidazole are also used to treat amebiasis.

Giardiasis

Giardiasis is a bowel infection caused by the flagellate *Giardia lamblia*. Infection follows ingestion of contaminated water or food and involves flatulence and diarrhea.

Metronidazole is the drug of choice for giardiasis.

Trichomonas vaginitis

Trichomonas vaginitis is caused by the flagellate *Trichomonas vaginalis*. It is a sexually transmitted inflammatory condition of the female vagina and, occasionally, male urethra.

Metronidazole is the drug of choice for trichomonas vaginitis.

Trypanosomiasis and leishmaniasis
Trypanosomiasis

African sleeping sickness and South American Chagas' disease are caused by species of flagellate trypanosome.

Insect vectors introduce the parasites into the human host, where they reproduce, causing bouts of parasitemia and fever. Toxins released cause damage to organs—the CNS in the case of sleeping sickness and the heart, liver, spleen, bone, and intestine in Chagas' disease.

Leishmaniasis

Leishmania species are flagellated parasites that are transmitted by a sandfly vector, assuming a nonflagellated intracellular form that resides within macrophages on infecting humans.

Clinical infections range from simple, resolving cutaneous infections to systemic "visceral" forms with hepatomegaly, splenomegaly, anemia, and fever.

The prophylaxis and treatment of trypanosomiasis and leishmaniasis are difficult and of variable efficacy. The drugs used are generally toxic and dangerous, making specialized knowledge essential.

Pneumocystis pneumonia

Pneumocystis pneumonia is most often associated with HIV infection and is now considered an AIDS-defining illness. The infective agent *Pneumocystis jiroveci* is not truly a protozoa; it has similarities with both protozoa and fungi and remains difficult to classify.

Signs and symptoms of *Pneumocystis jiroveci* pneumonia (PCP) are similar to other pneumonias, but culture is not possible, and the microorganism must be visualized by direct microscopy.

High-dose oral or parenteral trimethoprim/sulfamethoxazole is the drug of choice, with parenteral pentamidine as an alternative.

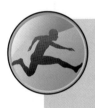

A decent knowledge of the plasmodial life cycle is a prerequisite to understanding the mechanism and site of action of antimalarial drugs.

Anthelminthic drugs

Concepts of helminthic infection

Helminth is derived from the Greek *helmins*, meaning worm. Anthelminthic drugs are, therefore, medicines acting against parasitic worms.

The three groups of helminths parasitize humans are:

- Cestoda (tapeworms).
- Nematoda (roundworms).
- Trematoda (flukes).

Fig. 3.14 lists medically important helminth infections and the main drugs used in their treatment.

Anthelminthic drugs

To be effective, an anthelminthic drug must be able to penetrate the cuticle of the worm or gain access to its alimentary tract, so that it may exert its pharmacologic effect on the physiology of the worm.

Anthelminthic drugs act on parasitic worms by a number of mechanisms:

- Damaging or killing the worm directly.
- Paralyzing the worm.
- Damaging the cuticle of the worm so that host defense mechanisms, such as digestion and immune rejection, can affect the worm.
- Interfering with worm metabolism.

Because there is great diversity across the different helminth classes, drugs highly effective against one species of worm are often ineffectual against another species.

Niclosamide

Mechanism of action: Before the introduction of praziquantel, niclosamide, a salicylamide derivative, was the most frequently used drug for tapeworm infestations. It blocks glucose uptake at high concentrations, irreversibly damaging the scolex (attachment end) of the tapeworm, leading to the release and expulsion of the tapeworm. It is a safe, selective drug since very little is absorbed from the gastrointestinal tract.

Route of administration: Oral.

Indications: Tapeworm infestation (see Fig. 3.14).

Adverse effects: Mild gastrointestinal disturbance.

Therapeutic notes: Patients are fasted before treatment with niclosamide. Purgatives to expel the dead worm segments (proglottides) can be used, but these are probably unnecessary, since the worm may be digested after the effects of the drug.

Praziquantel

Mechanism of action: Praziquantel increases the permeability of the helminth plasma membrane to calcium. At low concentrations, this causes contraction and spastic paralysis; higher concentrations cause vesiculation and vacuolization damage to the tegument of the worm.

Route of administration: Oral.

Indications: Praziquantel is the drug of choice for all schistosome infections (see Fig. 3.14) and for cysticercosis (a rare cestode condition caused by encystation of larvae of the tapeworm *Taenia solium* in human organs).

Adverse effects: Mild gastrointestinal disturbance, headache, and dizziness may occur shortly after administration.

53

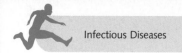

Classification of medically important helminth infections and the main drugs in their treatment		
	Helminth species	Drugs used in treatment
Cestodes		
Beef tapeworm	*Taenia saginata*	Niclosamide, praziquantel
Pork tapeworm	*Taenia solium*	Niclosamide, praziquantel
Fish tapeworm	*Diphyllobothrium latum*	Niclosamide, praziquantel
Hydatid tapeworm	*Echinococcus granulosus*	Albendazole
Nematodes		
Intestinal species		
Ascaris	*Ascaria lumbricoides*	Albendazole, mebendazole, ivermectin
Pinworm	*Enterobus vermicularis*	Mebendazole, albendazole, pyrantel pamoate
Threadworm	*Strongyloides stercoralis*	Thiabendazole, albendazole, ivermectin
Threadworm (US)	*Trichuris trichuria*	Mebendazole, ivermectin
Whipworm	*Necator americanus*	Mebendazole, albendazole, ivermectin
Hookworm	*Ankylostoma duodenale*	Mebendazole, albendazole, pyrantel pamoate
Tissue species		
Trichinella	*Trichinella spiralis*	Mebendazole, albendazole
Guinea worm	*Dracunculus medinesis*	Metronidazole
Filariaroidea	*Wucheria bancrofti*	Diethylcarbamazine
	Loa loa	Diethylcarbamazine
	Brugia malayi	Diethylcarbamazine
	Onchocerca volvulus	Ivermectin
Trematodes		
Blood flukes/schistosomes	*Schistosoma japonicum*	Praziquantel
	Schistosoma mansoni	Praziquantel
	Schistosoma haematobium	Praziquantel

Fig. 3.14 Classification of medically important helminth infections and the main drugs used in their treatment.

Therapeutic notes: Praziquantel should be taken after meals three times a day for 2 days only.

Piperazine

Mechanism of action: Piperazine is a reversible neuromuscular blocker that causes a flaccid paralysis in worms, leading to their expulsion by gastrointestinal peristalsis. It has very little effect on the host.

Route of administration: Oral.

Indications: Piperazine is used for roundworm and threadworm gastrointestinal infestation.

Adverse effects: Gastrointestinal disturbance and neurotoxic effects (dizziness) may occur.

Therapeutic notes: A single dose of piperazine is usually effective for treating roundworm infection; threadworm infestation may require a longer course (7 days).

Benzimidazoles

Examples of benzimidazoles include mebendazole, thiabendazole, and albendazole.

Mechanism of action: Benzimidazoles bind with high affinity to a site on tubulin dimers, thus preventing the polymerization of microtubules. Subsequent depolymerization leads to complete breakdown of the microtubule.

The selectivity of benzimidazoles arises because they are 250–400 times more potent in helminth than in mammalian tissue. The process takes time to have effect, and the worm may not be expelled for days.

Route of administration: Oral.

Indications: Benzimidazoles are used in the treatment of hydatid disease and many nematode infestations (see Fig. 3.14).

Contraindications: Benzimidazoles should not be given to pregnant women because they are teratogenic and embryotoxic.

Adverse effects: Occasional gastrointestinal disturbance. Thiabendazole causes more frequent gastrointestinal disturbance, headache, and dizziness. Serious hepatotoxicity rarely occurs.

Therapeutic notes: Dosage regimens of benzimidazoles range from a single dose for pinworm infestation to multiple doses for up to 5 days for trichinosis.

Diethylcarbamazine

Mechanism of action: It is not clear exactly how diethylcarbamazine exerts its filaricidal effect. It has been suggested that it damages or modifies the parasites in such a way as to make them more susceptible to host immune defenses.

Diethylcarbamazine kills both microfilariae in the peripheral circulation and adult worms in the lymphatics.

Route of administration: Oral.

Indications: Diethylcarbamazine is the drug of choice for lymphatic filariasis caused by *Wucheria bancrofti*, *Loa loa*, and *Brugia malayi* (see Fig. 3.14).

Adverse effects: Gastrointestinal disturbance, headache, and lassitude.

Material from the damaged and dead worms causes allergic side effects, including skin reactions, lymph gland enlargement, dizziness, and tachycardia, lasting from 3 to 7 days.

Therapeutic notes: To minimize the dangerous sudden release of dead worm material, the initial dose of diethylcarbamazine is started low and then increased and maintained for 21 days.

Ivermectin

Mechanism of action: Ivermectin immobilizes the tapeworm *Onchocerca volvulus* by causing tonic paralysis of the peripheral muscle system. It does this by potentiating the effect of γ-amino butyric acid (GABA) at the worm's neuromuscular junction.

Route of administration: Oral.

Indications: Ivermectin is the drug of choice for *Onchocerca volvulus*, which causes river blindness (see Fig. 3.14).

Adverse effects: Ocular irritation, transient electrocardiographic changes, and somnolence. An immediate immune reaction to dead microfilariae (Mazzotti reaction) can be severe.

All the anthelminthic drugs described in this chapter are administered orally.

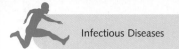

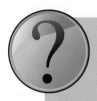

- What are the differences between bacterial (prokaryotic) and mammalian (eukaryotic) cells? How are these differences exploited by selective antibacterial agents?
- What are the differences between innate and acquired antibiotic resistance, the biochemical mechanisms of resistance, and the genetic mechanisms by which it is acquired?
- What are the classifications of mycobacterial diseases and the drugs used in their treatment?
- What are some of the more common side effects of antibiotic drugs and the likely mechanisms responsible for these?
- What are the main routes of administration for antibiotic drugs? (Give an example of an antibiotic drug that would be administered by this route, the microbial organism responsible for the disease, and the clinical features of the disease.)
- What are the peculiar features of viruses as infective pathogens? How does their life cycle make selective chemotherapy difficult?
- What is the broad classification of viruses? What are the major human diseases caused by viruses?
- What is the mechanism of action of the different classes of antiviral drugs and the point in the viral replication cycle they act upon?
- What are the drugs currently used in the treatment of HIV infection?
- By what routes can antiviral drugs be administered? What would be the indications for each route?
- What are the classifications of fungi and the types of infections that fungi can cause in humans?
- What are the main classes of antifungal drugs? (Describe their mechanism and site of action.)
- What is an opportunistic infection, and who is susceptible to this type of disease? (Name some of the more common opportunistic infections.)
- What are the three protozoan subphyla and the medically important diseases they cause?
- Draw a simple diagram illustrating the life cycle of the malaria parasite.
- Add the site of action of the antimalarial drugs to this life cycle.
- What is the classification of the helminths that parasitize humans?
- What are the medically important helminths in each group, the disease they cause, and the drugs used in their treatment?
- What are the mechanisms of action of the drugs used in the treatment of helminth infections?
- What are the more common infections that present to the health profession, the likely infective agents, and the most suitable drugs to treat these infections, considering all microbiologic and viral species?

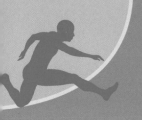

4. Inflammation, Pain, and Immunosuppression

Inflammation and pain go hand-in-hand and probably result in the majority of doctor–patient consultations.

In practice, the holistic approach allows the doctor to assess which therapeutics should be employed when a patient presents with pain or inflammation, but for the purpose of this chapter the two are described individually for simplicity. Arthritis provides an excellent example of where pain and inflammation are intimately married; therefore, the antirheumatic drugs are also described in this chapter.

Inflammation

Inflammation describes the changes seen in response to tissue injury or insult, as originally defined by the Latin words *dolor*, *rubor*, *calor*, and *tumor*, meaning pain, redness, heat, and swelling.

These changes result from alterations in local blood vessels. This leads to dilation of the blood vessels, their increased permeability, and increased receptiveness for leukocytes, resulting in the accumulation of inflammatory cells at the site of injury. The main cells seen in an acute inflammatory response are polymorphonuclear neutrophil leukocytes and macrophages. Lymphocytes, as well as basophils and eosinophils, also accumulate, especially in certain types of inflammation.

Inflammatory responses are produced and controlled by the interaction of a wide range of inflammatory mediators, some derived from leukocytes, some from the damaged tissues. Examples include histamine, kinins (bradykinin), neuropeptides (substance-P, calcitonin gene-related peptide), cytokines (e.g., interleukins), and the arachidonic acid metabolites (eicosanoids).

Arachidonic acid metabolites: the eicosanoids

Of the inflammatory mediators mentioned above, the eicosanoids are of special importance because:
- They are involved in the majority of inflammatory reactions.

- Most anti-inflammatory therapy is based on the manipulation of their biosynthesis—i.e., nonsteroidal anti-inflammatory drugs (NSAIDs) and steroidal anti-inflammatory drugs (glucocorticoids).

The eicosanoids are a family of polyunsaturated fatty acids formed from arachidonic acid. The biosynthetic pathway is shown in Fig. 4.1.

Arachidonic acid is derived mainly from phospholipids of cell membranes, from which it is mobilized by the action of the enzyme phospholipase A_2.

Arachidonic acid is then further metabolized:
- By cyclooxygenase to produce the "classic prostaglandins," thromboxane and prostacyclin, collectively known as the prostanoids.
- By lipoxygenase to produce the leukotrienes.

The actions of eicosanoids in inflammatory reactions are listed in Fig. 4.2.

Anti-inflammatory drugs

The main drugs used for their broad-spectrum anti-inflammatory effects are:
- Nonsteroidal anti-inflammatory drugs (NSAIDs).
- Steroidal anti-inflammatory drugs (glucocorticoids) (Chapter 11).

Both these classes of anti-inflammatory drug exert their effect by inhibiting the formation of eicosanoids (see Fig. 4.1).

In addition, a number of other drug classes, used clinically under certain circumstances, have more restricted anti-inflammatory actions:
- Disease-modifying antirheumatic drugs (DMARDs).
- Drugs used to treat gout.
- Antihistamines.

Nonsteroidal anti-inflammatory drugs

NSAIDs are a chemically diverse group of drugs that all possess the ability to inhibit both forms of the enzyme cyclooxygenase (see Fig. 4.1), an action that is responsible for their pharmacologic effects (see Fig. 4.4).

The first drugs of this type were the salicylates (e.g., aspirin) extracted from the

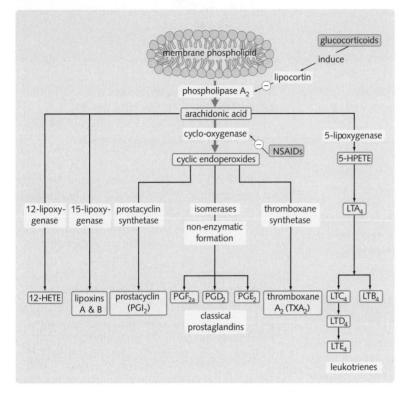

Fig. 4.1 Biosynthetic pathway of the eicosanoids (LT, leukotrienes; HETE, hydroxyeicosatetraenoic acid; PG, prostaglandin; HPETE, hydroperoxyeicosatetraenoic acid; NSAID, nonsteroidal anti-inflammatory drug).

Actions of the eicosanoids in the inflammatory reaction	
Eicosanoid	Actions in inflammation
• Prostanoids	
"Classical prostaglandins" e.g. PGD_2, PGE_2, PGF_2	Produce increased vasodilatation, vascular permeability, and edema in an inflammatory reaction; prostaglandins also sensitize nociceptive fibers to stimulation by other inflammatory mediators
Thromboxane A_2 (TXA_2)	Platelet aggregation and vasoconstriction
Prostacyclin (PGI_2)	Inhibition of platelet aggregation and vasodilatation
• Leukotrienes	
e.g. LTB_4, LTC_4	Increase vascular permeability, promote leucocyte chemotaxis (and cause contraction of bronchial smooth muscle)

Fig. 4.2 Actions of the eicosanoids in the inflammatory reaction.

bark of the willow tree. Subsequently, many synthetic and semisynthetic NSAIDs have been created by pharmacologists. Chemically and structurally heterogeneous, they are related through their common mechanism of action (Fig. 4.3).

Mechanism of action: The main action of all the NSAIDs is inhibition of the enzyme cyclooxygenase. This enzyme is involved in the metabolism of arachidonic acid to form the prostanoids (i.e., the "classic prostaglandins," prostacyclin and thromboxane A_2).

Inhibition of cyclooxygenase can occur by several mechanisms:

- Irreversible inhibition—e.g., aspirin causes acetylation of the active site.
- Competitive inhibition—e.g., ibuprofen acts as a competitive substrate.
- Reversible, noncompetitive inhibition—e.g., acetaminophen has a free-radical trapping action that interferes with the production of hydroperoxidases, which are believed to have an essential role in cyclooxygenase activity.

Non-steroidal anti-inflammatory drugs				
Chemical class	Examples	Analgesic	Antipyretic	Anti-inflammatory
Salicylic acids	Aspirin	+	+	+
Propionic acids	Ibuprofen	+	+	+
Acetic acids	Indomethacin	+	+	++
Oxicams	Piroxicam	+	+	++
Pyrazolones	Phenylbutazone	+/−	+	++
Fenemates	Mefenamic acid	+	+	+/−
para-Aminophenols	Acetaminophen	+	+	−

Fig. 4.3 Classes of nonsteroidal anti-inflammatory drugs and comparison of their main actions.

Cyclooxygenase exists in two enzyme isoforms:
- COX-1, which is expressed in most tissues, especially platelets, gastric mucosa, and renal vasculature; it is involved in physiological cell signaling. Most adverse effects of NSAIDs are caused by inhibition of COX-1.
- COX-2, which is induced at sites of inflammation and produces the prostanoids involved in inflammatory responses. Analgesic and anti-inflammatory effects of NSAIDs are largely a result of inhibition of COX-2.

COX-2–specific inhibitors were licensed for use in several countries for symptomatic relief in osteoarthritis and rheumatoid arthritis; evaluation of their therapeutic effects and reduced side-effect profile remains under scrutiny. Recently, rofecoxib and valdecoxib were withdrawn because of adverse cardiovascular events.

> Remember the reasons behind the conflict over NSAIDs. The cardiologist will want every patient on aspirin—for its antiplatelet action. The gastroenterologist and the nephrologist will want to stop aspirin—because it causes GI upset and ulceration and potentially worsens renal blood flow.

Clinical effects: NSAIDs work by the inhibition of cyclooxygenase and resulting inhibition of prostaglandin synthesis, producing three major clinical actions of potential therapeutic benefit: analgesia, an anti-inflammatory action, and an antipyretic (fever reducing) action (Fig. 4.4).

Not all NSAIDs possess these three actions to exactly the same extent, an example being the lack of anti-inflammatory activity possessed by acetaminophen (see Fig. 4.3).

In addition to these three main categories of effect, aspirin has a pronounced effect on inhibiting platelet aggregation, due to reduced thromboxane synthesis. This has led to its successful use in primary and secondary prevention of cardiovascular and cerebrovascular events (Chapter 7).

Indications: NSAIDs are widely used for a variety of complaints. They are available on prescription and over the counter. Their use includes musculoskeletal and joint diseases (e.g., strains, sprains, rheumatic problems, arthritis, gout), analgesia for mild to moderate pain relief (including headaches and dysmenorrhea), and symptomatic relief in fever.

Contraindications: NSAIDs should not be given to people with gastrointestinal ulceration or bleeding or a previous hypersensitivity to any NSAID. Caution should be used in asthma and when renal function is impaired.

Adverse effects: Generalized adverse effects of NSAIDs are common, especially in the elderly and in chronic users, and these mostly arise from the nonselective inhibition of COX-1 and COX-2 (Fig. 4.5).

Less commonly, liver disorders and bone marrow depression are seen.

Major clinical effects of NSAIDs	
Clinical action	Mechanism of action
Analgesic action	• The analgesic effect is largely a peripheral effect that is due to the inhibition of prostaglandin synthesis at the site of pain and inflammation. • Prostaglandins do not produce pain directly, but sensitize nociceptive fibre nerve endings to other inflammatory mediators (bradykinin, histamine, 5-HT) , amplifying the basic pain message; prostaglandins of the E and F series are implicated in this sensitizing action. • Thus NSAIDs are most effective against pain where there is an inflammatory component. • A small component of the analgesic action of NSAIDs is a consequence of a central effect in reducing prostaglandin synthesis in the CNS; acetaminophen especially works in this manner.
Anti-inflammatory action	• Prostaglandins produce increased vasodilatation, vascular permeability, and edema in an inflammatory reaction. • Inhibition of prostaglandin synthesis therefore reduces this part of the inflammatory reaction. • NSAIDs do not inhibit the numerous other mediators involved in an inflammatory reaction; thus, inflammatory cell accumulation, for example, is not inhibited.
Antipyretic action	• During a fever, leucocytes release inflammatory pyrogens (e.g. interleukin-1) as part of the immune response; these act on the thermoregulatory center in the hypothalamus to cause an increase in body temperature. • This effect is believed to be mediated by an increase in hypothalamic prostaglandins (PGEs), the generation of which is inhibited by NSAIDs. • NSAIDs do not affect temperature under normal circumstances or in heat stroke.

Fig. 4.4 Three major clinical actions of nonsteroidal anti-inflammatory drugs (NSAIDs).

General adverse effects of NSAIDs		
System	Adverse effect	Cause
GI	Dyspepsia, nausea, vomiting Ulcer formation and potential hemorrhage risk in chronic users	Inhibition of the normal protective actions of prostaglandins on the gastric mucosa PGE_2 and PGI_2 normally inhibit gastric acid secretion, increase mucosal blood flow, and have a cytoprotective action.
Renal	Renal damage/nephroxicity Renal failure can occur after years of chronic abuse.	Inhibition of PGE_2- and PGI_2-mediated vasodilatation in the renal medulla and glomeruli
Other	Bronchospasm, skin rashes, other allergic-type reactions	Hypersensitivity reaction/allergy to drug

Fig. 4.5 General adverse effects of nonsteroidal anti-inflammatory drugs (NSAIDs) (GI, gastrointestinal; PG, prostaglandin).

Other unwanted effects that are relatively specific to individual compounds are also seen (see below).

Therapeutic notes on individual NSAIDs
Salicylic acid (e.g., aspirin) is cheap and is still the drug of choice for many sorts of mild pain, despite a relatively high incidence of gastrointestinal side effects. It is also used for its antiplatelet action. However, it produces tinnitus in toxic doses.

Propionic acid (e.g., ibuprofen) is effective and well tolerated. It is the drug of choice for inflammatory joint disease, owing to its low incidence of side effects.

Acetic acid (e.g., indomethacin) is a highly potent inhibitor of COX that is effective but associated with a high incidence of side effects. It commonly causes neurologic effects such as dizziness and confusion as well as gastrointestinal upsets.

Oxicams—piroxicam is a potent drug widely used for chronic inflammatory conditions. It is given only once daily but causes a relatively high incidence of gastrointestinal problems.

Pyrazolones—phenylbutazone is an extremely potent agent but can produce a fatal bone marrow aplasia. For this reason, it is reserved for the treatment of intractable pain in ankylosing spondylitis.

Fenemates—mefenamic acid is a moderately potent drug, but it commonly causes gastrointestinal upsets and occasionally skin rashes.

para-Aminophenols—acetaminophen is used as an analgesic only and not as an anti-inflammatory drug. It is effective for pain, especially headaches, and fever. This is probably due to its mechanism of action in trapping free radicals and interfering with the production of hydroperoxidases, which are believed to have an essential role in cyclooxygenase activity. In areas of inflammation, phagocytic cells produce high levels of peroxide that swamp this effect.

Acetaminophen causes a serious, potentially fatal, hepatotoxicity in toxic doses (2–3 times therapeutic) that saturate the normal liver conjugation systems, leading to the formation of a toxic metabolite, N-acetyl-p-benzoquinone (Chapter 1).

COX-2-specific inhibitors (e.g., celecoxib) preferentially inhibit the inducible COX-2 enzyme, limiting COX-1-mediated side effects observed with other, nonspecific NSAIDs.

The COX-2 inhibitor, celecoxib, is licensed for symptomatic relief in osteoarthritis and rheumatoid arthritis but contraindicated in inflammatory bowel disease.

Steroidal anti-inflammatory drugs (glucocorticoids)

Glucocorticoids possess powerful anti-inflammatory actions that make them useful in several diseases (e.g., rheumatoid arthritis, inflammatory bowel conditions, bronchial asthma, and inflammatory conditions of the skin).

Their profound generalized inhibitory effects on inflammatory responses result from the effects of corticosteroids in altering the activity of certain corticosteroid-responsive genes. The anti-inflammatory action results from:

- Reduced production of acute inflammatory mediators, especially the eicosanoids (see Fig. 4.1). Corticosteroids prevent the formation of arachidonic acid from membrane phospholipids by inducing the synthesis of a polypeptide called lipocortin. Lipocortin inhibits phospholipase A_2, the enzyme normally responsible for mobilizing arachidonic acid from cell membrane phospholipids, and thus inhibits the subsequent formation of both prostaglandins and leukotrienes.
- Reduced numbers and activity of circulating immunocompetent cells, neutrophils, and macrophages.
- Decreased activity of macrophages and fibroblasts involved in the chronic stages of inflammation, leading to decreased inflammation and decreased healing.

Glucocorticoids are discussed in detail in Chapter 11.

Disease-modifying antirheumatic drugs

DMARDs are a diverse group of agents that are mainly used in the treatment of rheumatoid arthritis, which is a chronic, progressive, and destructive inflammatory disease of the joints (Fig. 4.6).

The mechanism of action of the DMARDs is often unclear—they appear to have a long-term depressive effect upon the inflammatory response as well as possibly modulating other aspects of the immune system.

Disease-modifying anti-rheumatic drugs (DMARDs)	
Class	Example
Gold salts	Sodium aurothimalate, auronofin
Penicillamine	Penicillamine
Antimalarials	Hydroxychloroguine
Sulfasalazine	Sulfasalazine
Immunosuppressants	Cytotoxic drugs: methotrexate, azathioprine, cyclosporine

Fig. 4.6 Disease-modifying antirheumatic drugs.

All DMARDs have a slow onset of action, with clinical improvement not becoming apparent until 4–6 months after the initiation of treatment. DMARDs have been shown to improve symptoms and reduce disease activity. Whether they alter the long-term outcome of the disease is controversial.

DMARDs are generally indicated for use in severe, active, progressive rheumatoid arthritis when NSAIDs alone have proved inadequate. DMARDs are frequently used in combination with an NSAID and/or low dose glucocorticoids.

Gold salts

Examples of gold salts include sodium aurothiomalate and auranofin.

Mechanism of action: The mechanism of action of gold salts is unknown—they may be taken up by, and inhibit, mononuclear macrophages; or they may affect the production of free radicals.

Route of administration: Sodium aurothiomalate is given by intramuscular injection, and auranofin is given orally.

Adverse effects: Rashes, proteinuria, ulceration, diarrhea, and bone marrow suppression.

Therapeutic notes: When administering gold salts, careful patient monitoring, including blood counts and urine analysis, is necessary. If any serious adverse effects develop, treatment must be stopped.

Penicillamine

Mechanism of action: The mechanism of action of penicillamine is unknown. It chelates metals, and it has immunomodulatory effects, including suppression of immunoglobulin production and effects on immune complexes. Penicillamine may also decrease interleukin 1 (IL-1) synthesis.

Route of administration: Oral.

Adverse effects: Rashes, proteinuria, ulceration, gastrointestinal upsets, fever, transient loss of taste, and bone marrow suppression.

Therapeutic notes: When administering penicillamine, careful patient monitoring, including blood counts and urine analysis, is necessary. If any serious adverse effects develop, treatment must be stopped.

Antimalarials

Examples of antimalarials include chloroquine and hydroxychloroquine (Chapter 3).

Mechanism of action: The mechanism of antimalarials is unclear. They interfere with a wide variety of leucocyte functions, including IL-1 production by macrophages, lymphoproliferative responses, and T-cell cytotoxic responses.

Route of administration: Oral.

Adverse effects: At the low doses currently recommended for antimalarials, toxicity is rare. The major adverse effect is retinal toxicity.

Therapeutic notes: People on antimalarials should have their vision monitored.

Sulfasalazine

Mechanism of action: Sulfasalazine is broken down in the gut into its two component molecules, 5-aminosalicylate (5-ASA) and sulfapyridine. The 5-ASA moiety is believed to be a free radical scavenger and responsible for most of this drugs antirheumatic effects.

Route of administration: Oral.

Adverse effects: Side effects of sulfasalazine are mainly due to sulfapyridine; they are common but rarely serious. These include nausea, vomiting, headache, and rashes. Rarely, blood disorders and oligospermia are reported.

Therapeutic notes: People on sulfasalazine should have their blood counts monitored.

Immunosuppressants

Certain drugs with immunosuppressive actions have been shown to be effective in rheumatoid arthritis. These include azathioprine, cyclosporine (cyclosporin A), and corticosteroids, which may work by suppressing the autoimmune component of rheumatoid arthritis.

The DMARDs are usually prescribed by a specialist. Their mechanisms of action are largely unknown, but remember that most patients taking these agents require regular blood tests to assess renal and liver function, and to monitor red and white blood cell counts.

Drugs used in gout

Gout is a condition in which uric acid (monosodium urate) crystals are deposited in tissues, especially in the joints, provoking an inflammatory response that

Drugs used in the treatment of gout	
• **Treatment of an acute attack**	**Example**
NSAIDs	Indomethacin
Immunosuppressive	Colchicine
• **Prophylaxis against recurrent attacks** (reduction of plasma uric acid concentration)	
Agents that reduce uric acid synthesis	Allopurinol
Agents that increase uric acid excretion (uricosurics	Sulfinpyrazone, probenecid

Fig. 4.7 Drugs used in the treatment of gout.

manifests as an extremely painful acute arthritis. Uric acid crystallizes in the tissues when plasma urate levels are high, as a result of either excessive production or reduced renal excretion.

There are two treatment strategies for gout—treatment of an acute attack and prophylaxis against further attacks (Fig. 4.7).

Treatment of an acute attack
Nonsteroidal anti-inflammatory drugs
At the onset of an acute attack of gout, NSAIDs are used for their general anti-inflammatory and analgesic effects.

Aspirin and other salicylates are not used in gout, as they inhibit uric acid excretion in the urine, exacerbating serum concentrations.

Colchicine
Mechanism of action: Colchicine helps in gouty arthritis by inhibiting the migration of leucocytes such as neutrophils into the inflamed joint. This effect is achieved as a result of the action of colchicine binding to tubulin, the protein monomer of microtubules, resulting in their depolymerization. The end result is that cytoskeletal movements and cell motility are severely inhibited.

The inhibition of microtubular function inhibits mitotic spindle formation, giving colchicine a cytotoxic effect on dividing cells. This cytotoxic effect is responsible for side effects of colchicine.

Route of administration: Oral, rarely intravenously.

Adverse effects: Side effects of colchicine include gastrointestinal toxicity, with nausea, vomiting, and diarrhea, occurring in 80% of people. Rarely, bone marrow suppression and renal failure occur.

Therapeutic notes: Colchicine is rapidly effective. It is given for the first 24 hours of an attack and then no further for 7 days. Nausea and vomiting are extremely common side effects.

Prophylaxis against recurrent attacks
Preventative management of gout includes diet and lifestyle changes as well as the use of drugs that reduce plasma uric acid concentration. These drugs should not be used during an acute attack, as they will initially worsen symptoms. NSAIDs or colchicine should be coadministered for the first 3 months of treatment, as initiation of prophylactic treatment may precipitate an acute attack.

Agents that reduce uric acid synthesis
Allopurinol is an example of a drug that reduces uric acid synthesis.

Mechanism of action: Allopurinol inhibits the enzyme xanthine oxidase, which converts purines (from DNA breakdown) into uric acid, thus reducing uric acid production.

Route of administration: Oral.

Adverse effects: Headaches, dyspepsia, diarrhea, rash, drug interactions, and acute exacerbation of gout initially. Rarely, life-threatening hypersensitivity occurs.

Agents that increase uric acid excretion
Uricosurics are drugs that increase uric acid excretion. Examples of uricosurics include sulfinpyrazone and probenecid.

Mechanism of action: Uricosurics compete with uric acid for reabsorption in the proximal tubules, preventing uric acid reabsorption and resulting in uricosuria.

Route of administration: Oral.

Adverse effects: Gastrointestinal upset, deposition of uric acid crystals in the kidney, interference with excretion of certain drugs, and acute exacerbation of gout initially.

Therapeutic notes: Uricosurics should not be used during an acute attack of gout. NSAIDs or colchicine should be coadministered for the first 3 months of treatment, as initiation of treatment may precipitate an acute attack.

Pain

Pain is a common everyday experience that performs an essential defensive function. However,

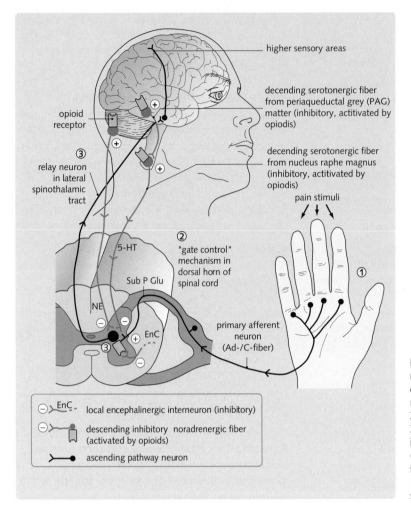

Fig. 4.8 Diagram showing nociceptive pathways and sites of opioid action. 1. Activation of nociceptors in the peripheral tissues; 2. Transmission of pain information; 3. Onward passage of pain information to higher centers (Glu, glutamate; 5-HT, 5-hydroxytryptamine [serotonin]; NE, norepinephrine; Sub P, substance P).

uncontrolled pain can severely diminish quality of life, and it may then be amenable to pharmacotherapy.

Pain, which may be acute or chronic, is defined as an unpleasant sensory and emotional experience associated with actual or potential tissue damage. Pain is a subjective experience, as there are currently no means of accurately and objectively assessing the degree of pain a patient is experiencing.

An analgesic drug is one that effectively removes (or at least lessens) the sensation of pain.

Pain perception

Pain perception is best viewed as a three-stage process—activation of nociceptors, followed by the transmission and onward passage of pain information.

Activation of nociceptors in the peripheral tissues

Noxious thermal, chemical, or mechanical stimuli can trigger the firing of primary afferent fibers (type C/Aδ), through the activation of nociceptors (pain-specific receptors) in the peripheral tissues (Fig. 4.8).

Transmission of pain information

Transmission of pain information from the periphery to the dorsal horn of the spinal cord is inhibited or amplified by a combination of local (spinal) neuronal circuits and descending tracts from higher brain centers. This constitutes the "gate-control mechanism."

In the gate-control mechanism:
• The primary afferent fibers synapse in lamina I and II of the dorsal horn of the spinal cord.

Receptor subtypes			
Action	μ/δ	κ	σ
Analgesia	Supraspinal and spinal	Spinal	–
Respiratory depression	Marked	Slight	–
Pupil	Constricts	–	Dilates
GIT motility	Reduced (constipating)	–	–
Mood/effect	Euphoria inducing but also sedating	Dysphoria inducing mildly sedating	Marked dysphoric and psychomimetic actions
Physical dependence	+++	+	–

Fig. 4.9 Actions mediated by opioid receptor subtypes (GIT, gastrointestinal tract).

- Transmitter peptides (substance P, calcitonin gene-related peptide, bradykinin, glutamate) and nitric oxide (NO) are involved in the ascending pain pathways, although the interactions are complex and have not yet been fully defined.
- The activity of the dorsal horn relay neurons is modulated by several inhibitory inputs. These include local inhibitory interneurons, which release opioid peptides; descending inhibitory noradrenergic fibers from the locus ceruleus area of the brainstem, which are activated by opioid peptides; and descending inhibitory serotonergic fibers from the nucleus raphe magnus and periaqueductal gray areas of the brainstem, which are also activated by opioid peptides (see Fig. 4.8).

Onward passage of pain information

The onward passage of pain information is via the spinothalamic tract, to the higher centers of the brain. The higher centers of the brain coordinate the cognitive and emotional aspects of pain and control appropriate reactions. Opioid peptide release in both the spinal cord and the brainstem can reduce the activity of the dorsal horn relay neurons and cause analgesia, known as "shutting the gate" (see Fig. 4.8).

Opioid receptors

All opioids, whether endogenous peptides, naturally occurring drugs, or chemically synthesized drugs, interact with specific opioid receptors to produce their pharmacologic effects.

Drugs interact with opioid receptors as either full agonists, partial agonists, mixed agonists/antagonists (full agonists on one opioid receptor, but partial agonists on another), or as antagonists. Opioid analgesics are agonists.

There are three major opioid receptor subtypes—μ, δ, and κ. The existence of a fourth receptor (σ) remains controversial.

The distinctions between the actions associated with μ- and δ-receptors are relatively unclear, because selective agonists and antagonists have only recently been discovered. However:

- μ-receptors are thought to be responsible for most of the analgesic effects of opioids and for some major adverse effects (e.g., respiratory depression). Most of the analgesic opioids in use are μ-receptor agonists.
- δ-receptors are probably more important in the periphery, but they may also contribute to analgesia.
- κ-receptors contribute to analgesia at the spinal level and may elicit sedation and dysphoria, but they produce relatively few adverse effects and do not contribute to physical dependence.
- σ-receptors are not selective opioid receptors, but they are the site of action of psychomimetic drugs, such as PCP. They may account for the dysphoria produced by some opioids.

Opioid receptor activation has an inhibitory effect on synapses in the CNS and in the gut (Fig. 4.9).

Secondary-messenger systems associated with opioid receptor activity include:

- μ/δ-receptors, the activation of which causes hyperpolarization of a neuron by opening potassium channels and inhibiting calcium channels.

Endogenous opioid peptides		
Precursor molecules	**Products**	**Relative opioid receptor affinity**
pro-opiomelanocortin (POMC)	Endorphins (e.g., β-endorphin) and other non-opioid peptides (e.g., ACTH)	μ
Proenkephalin	Enkephalins (e.g., Leu^5 enkephalin, Met^5 enkephalin, extended Met^5 enkephalins)	δ μ μ
Prodynorphin	Dynorphins (e.g., dynorphin A)	κ

Fig. 4.10 Endogenous opioid peptides.

Opioid analgesics	
Weak opioid analgesics	**Strong opioid analgesics**
Pentazocine	Morphine
Codeine	Oxymorphone
Dihydrocodeine	Oxycodone
Dextropropoxyphene	Meperidine
	Buprenorphine
	Nalbuphine

Fig. 4.11 Opioid analgesics.

- κ-receptors, the activation of which inhibits calcium channels.

Activation of all opioid receptors causes a decrease in cAMP production, the functional significance of which is not clear.

Endogenous opioids

Physiologically, the CNS has its own "endogenous opioids" that are the natural ligands for opioid receptors.

There are three main families of endogenous opioid peptides occurring naturally in the CNS:
- Endorphins.
- Dynorphins.
- Enkephalins.

They are derived from three separate gene products (precursor molecules), but all possess homology at their amino end.

The expression and anatomical distribution of the products of these three precursor molecules within the CNS are varied, and each has a distinct range of affinities for the different types of opioid receptor (Fig. 4.10).

Although it is known that the endogenous opioids possess analgesic activity, their precise function in the CNS and elsewhere is poorly defined. They are not used therapeutically.

Opioid analgesic drugs

Opioid analgesics are drugs, either naturally occurring (e.g., morphine) or chemically synthesized, that interact with specific opioid receptors to produce the pharmacologic effect of analgesia.

The first opioid drug was opium, the crude exudate of the seed head of the opium poppy *Papaver somniferum*; simple extraction yields morphine. Subsequently, many synthetic and semisynthetic opioids have been created by pharmacologists.

Examples of opioid analgesics are given in Fig. 4.11.

Mechanism of action: Opioid analgesic drugs work by agonist action at opioid receptors (see above).

Note that the sense of euphoria produced by strong opioids undoubtedly contributes to their analgesic activity by helping to reduce the anxiety and stress associated with pain. This effect also accounts for the illicit use of these drugs.

Route of administration: Oral, rectal, intravenous, or intramuscular.

Oral absorption is irregular and incomplete, necessitating larger doses; 70% is removed by first-pass hepatic metabolism.

Indications: Strong opioids are used in moderate to severe pain, particularly visceral, postoperative, or cancer related; in myocardial infarction and acute pulmonary edema; and in perioperative analgesia.

Weak opioids are used in the relief of mild to moderate pain, as antitussives (Chapter 8), and as antidiarrheal agents (Chapter 10), taking advantage of these "side effects" of opioid analgesics.

Contraindications: Opioid analgesics should not be given to people in acute respiratory depression, with acute alcoholism, at risk of paralytic ileus, or with head injuries prior to neurologic assessment (interferes with assessment of the level of consciousness).

Adverse effects: Opioid analgesics share many side effects, although qualitative and quantitative differences exist. These can be subdivided into central adverse actions and peripheral adverse actions.

Central adverse actions include the following:
- Drowsiness and sedation, in which initial excitement is followed by sedation and finally coma (on overdose).
- Reduction in sensitivity of the respiratory center to CO_2, leading to shallow and slow respiration.
- Tolerance and dependence (Chapter 6).
- Suppression of cough, an effect exploited clinically in antitussives (Chapter 8).
- Vomiting due to stimulation of the chemoreceptor trigger zone (CTZ).
- Pupillary constriction due to stimulation of the parasympathetic third cranial nerve nucleus.
- Hypotension and reduced cardiac output, which are partly due to reduced hypothalamic sympathetic outflow.

Peripheral adverse actions include the following:
- Constipation, which is partly due to stimulation of cholinergic activity in gut wall ganglia that results in smooth-wall spasm.
- Contraction of smooth muscle in the sphincter of Oddi and in the ureters, which results in an increase in blood amylase and lipase due to pancreatic stasis.
- Histamine release, which produces bronchospasm, flushing, and arteriolar dilatation.
- Lowered sympathetic discharge and direct arteriolar dilatation, which results in lowered cardiac output and hypotension.

Adverse effects of opioids tend to limit the dose that can be given and the level of analgesia that can be maintained. The most serious of all these effects is respiratory depression, which is the most common cause of death from opioid overdose.

Constipation and nausea are also common problems, and clinically it is common to coadminister laxatives and an antiemetic (Chapter 10). Tolerance to opioid analgesics can be detected within 24–48 hours from the onset of administration, and it results in larger and larger doses of the drug being needed to achieve the same clinical effect. Dependence

involves μ-receptors and is both physical and psychological in nature (Chapter 6).

If physical dependence develops, it is characterized by a definite withdrawal syndrome following cessation of drug treatment. This syndrome comprises a complex mixture of irritable and sometimes aggressive behavior combined with extremely unpleasant autonomic symptoms such as fever, sweating, yawning, and pupillary dilatation. The withdrawal syndrome is relieved by the administration of μ-receptor agonists and worsened by the administration of μ-receptor antagonists.

Psychological dependence on opioid analgesics is based on the positive reinforcement provided by euphoria.

In the clinical context, especially in terminal care, where tolerance and dependence can be monitored, they are not inevitably problematic. However, the fear of tolerance and dependence often leads to over-caution in the use of opioid analgesics and inadequate pain control in some patients. It is not uncommon for palliative care patients to take over 1000 mg of morphine sulphate twice daily and remain alert and active.

Therapeutic notes: Strong opioid analgesics include morphine, hydromorphone, oxymorphone, oxycodone, meperidine, buprenorphine, and nalbuphine:
- Morphine remains the most valuable drug for severe pain relief, though it frequently causes nausea and vomiting. It is the drug of choice for severe pain in terminal care. Morphine is the standard against which other opioid analgesics are compared.
- Meperidine is more lipid soluble than morphine, and it has a rapid onset and short duration of action, making it useful in labor. Meperidine is equianalgesic compared with morphine, but it produces less constipation. Interaction with MAOIs is serious, causing fever, delirium, and convulsions or respiratory depression.
- Buprenorphine has both agonist and antagonist actions at opioid receptors, and it may precipitate withdrawal symptoms in patients dependent on other opioids. It has a longer duration of action than morphine, and its lipid solubility allows sublingual administration. Vomiting may be a problem. Unlike most opioid analgesics, the effects of buprenorphine are only partially antagonized by naloxone, owing to its high-affinity attraction to opioid receptors.

- Nalbuphine is an agonist at κ-receptors and an antagonist at μ-receptors. It is equianalgesic compared with morphine, but it produces less nausea and vomiting. High doses cause dysphoria.

Weak opioid analgesics include pentazocine, codeine, dihydrocodeine, and dextropropoxyphene:

- Pentazocine has both κ/σ-receptor agonist and μ-antagonist actions, and it may precipitate withdrawal symptoms in patients dependent on other opioids. Pentazocine is weak orally, but by injection it has a potency between that of morphine and codeine. It is not recommended because of the side effects of thought disturbances and hallucinations, which probably are due to its action on σ-receptors.
- Codeine has about one twelfth of the analgesic potency of morphine. The incidence of nausea and constipation limits the dose and duration that can be used. Codeine is also used for its antitussive and antidiarrheal effects.
- Dihydrocodeine has an analgesic efficacy similar to that of codeine. It may cause dizziness and constipation.
- Dextropropoxyphene has an analgesic efficacy about half that of codeine (i.e., very mild), and so it is often combined with aspirin or acetaminophen. Such mixtures can be dangerous in overdose, with dextropropoxyphene causing respiratory depression and acute heart failure, while the acetaminophen is hepatotoxic.

Opioid antagonists

Examples of opioid antagonists include naloxone and naltrexone.

Mechanism of action: These drugs act by specific antagonism at opioid receptors: μ-, δ-, and κ-receptors are blocked more or less equally. They block the actions of endogenous opioids as well as those of morphine-like drugs.

Naloxone is short acting (half-life: 2–4 hours) while naltrexone is long acting (half-life: 10 hours).

Route of administration: Intravenous.

Indications: Opioid antagonists are given to reverse opioid-induced analgesia and respiratory depression rapidly, mainly after overdose, or to improve breathing in newborn babies that have been affected by the opioids given to their mother. Naltrexone is used to treat ethanol withdrawal.

Adverse effects: Precipitation of withdrawal in those with physical dependence on opioids. Reversal of analgesic effects of opiate agonist.

> When treating pain, remember the analgesic ladder. Start with nonopioid drugs such as acetaminophen or other NSAIDs; if these are ineffective, move up a step to weak opioid drugs such as codeine with acetaminophen. If these agents do not control the pain, then move up the final step to the strong opioid drugs such as morphine and oxycodone.

Headache and neuralgic pain
Headache

Headache is a very common presenting symptom, yet one which can be difficult to manage. The most common causes of headache include:

- Tension-type headache.
- Migraine.
- Headache associated with eye or sinus disease.

More sinister causes of headache (including meningitis and neoplasia) are less common, and these can often be confidently excluded by the history and by examination.

The pathophysiology underlying headache is unclear, although symptomatic relief is often obtained from NSAIDs and acetaminophen (see above). Some headaches are related to stress and anxiety, and these patients may benefit from antidepressant drugs (Chapter 6).

The management of migraine can address the acute attacks or attempt to prevent migraine episodes (prophylaxis) in those who experience frequent attacks.

Drugs used for acute migrainous attacks:

- NSAIDs and acetaminophen (see above).
- Antiemetics (Chapter 10).
- Serotonin (5-HT$_1$) agonists.

Drugs used in migraine prophylaxis:

- Antihistamine/serotonin (5-HT) antagonists.
- Beta antagonists (Chapter 7).
- Tricyclic antidepressants (Chapter 6).

Serotonin (5-HT₁) agonists

Sumatriptan and rizatriptan are serotonin agonists.

Mechanism of action: Serotonin agonists are believed to reverse the dilatation of cerebral blood vessels in the acute attack, which may be responsible for some of the symptoms of migraine.

Route of administration: Oral, intranasal, subcutaneous.

Indications: Acute migraine attacks.

Contraindications: Caution in coronary artery disease (may cause vasoconstriction or coronary vessels), hepatic impairment, pregnancy, and breastfeeding.

Adverse effects: Sensations of tingling, heat, chest tightness.

> Headache is a common complaint and, more often than not, does not represent a sinister pathology. Analgesics will simply help to control the symptoms. If a patient frequently returns with pain, be sure to look for a treatable underlying cause.

Neuralgic pain

Neuralgic pain is classically nerve pain, in the distribution of a particular nerve or nerve root. The more common pathologies, which come into this category, include sciatica and trigeminal neuralgia.

Neuralgia commonly occurs because of compression or entrapment of the nerve or nerve root, and definitive management relies on surgical release of the nerve.

Pharmacologic options can be employed when surgery is ill advised or ineffective or as an adjunct. NSAIDs are not particularly effective for neuralgic pain, and they have usually been self-prescribed prior to the patient consulting a professional opinion.

Antidepressants, in particular amitriptyline, often have an "analgesic" effect in neuralgic pain, often at a dose lower than their antidepressant effect (Chapter 6).

The other main class of drug used orally in neuralgic pain are the antiepileptics, notably carbamazepine, phenytoin, and, more recently, lamotrigine (Chapter 6). These potentially stabilize the neurons involved and limit their activation.

Injection of the nerve in question with local anesthetic can provide relief for some patients (Chapter 5), although nerve ablation with drugs or by surgical means can be performed to alleviate symptoms.

Immunosuppression

Deliberate pharmacologic suppression of the immune system is used in the following three main clinical areas:

- To suppress inappropriate autoimmune responses (e.g., systemic lupus erythematosus or rheumatoid arthritis), where the host immune system is "attacking" host tissue.
- To suppress host immune rejection to donor organ grafts or transplants.
- To suppress donor immune responses against host antigens (prevention of graft-versus-host disease [GVHD] after bone marrow transplant).

The main pharmacologic agents used for immunosuppression are:

- Cyclosporine (cyclosporin A).
- Azathioprine.
- Glucocorticoids (Chapter 11).

Immunosuppressant drugs
Cyclosporine (cyclosporin A)

Mechanism of action: Cyclosporine is a cyclic peptide, derived from fungi, that has powerful immunosuppressive activity. It has a selective inhibitory effect on T cells by inhibiting the T-cell receptor (TCR)-mediated signal-transduction pathway. It is believed to exert its actions after entering the T cell and preventing the transcription of specific genes (Fig. 4.12).

After entry into the T cell, cyclosporine specifically binds to its cytoplasmic-binding protein, cyclophilin. This cyclosporine–cyclophilin complex then binds to a serine/threonine phosphatase called calcineurin, inhibiting its phosphatase activity. Calcineurin is normally activated when intracellular calcium ion levels rise following T-cell receptor binding to the appropriate major histocompatibility complex:antigen complex. When calcineurin is active, it dephosphorylates the cytoplasmic component of the nuclear factor of activated T cells (NF-ATc) into a form that migrates to the nucleus and induces transcription of genes,

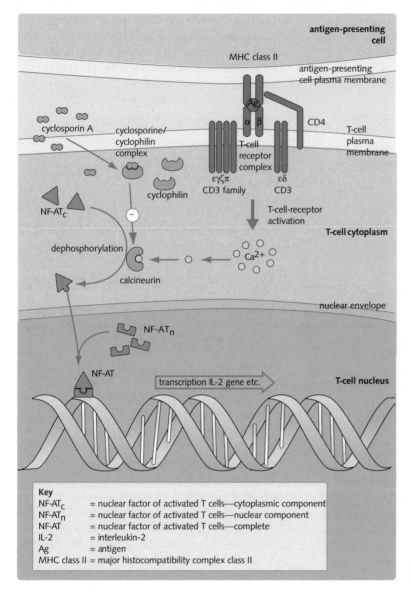

Fig. 4.12 Cyclosporine and T-cell suppression.

such as that for IL-2, that are involved in T-cell activation.

Inhibition of calcineurin by the cyclosporine–cyclophilin complex, therefore, prevents the nuclear translocation of NF-ATc and the transcription of certain genes essential for the activation of T cells. Hence, the production of IL-2 by T helper cells, the maturation of cytotoxic T cells, and the production of some other lymphokines, such as interferon-γ, are all inhibited.

The overall action of cyclosporine is to suppress reversibly both cell-mediated and antibody-specific adaptive immune responses.

Indications: Cyclosporine is used for the prevention of graft and transplant rejection, and for prevention of GVHD.

Route of administration: Oral, intravenous.

Adverse effects: Unlike most immunosuppressive agents, cyclosporine does not cause myelosuppression. It is markedly nephrotoxic to the proximal tubule of the kidney, and renal damage almost always occurs. This may be reversible or permanent. Hypertension occurs in 50% of people.

Less serious side effects include mild hepatotoxicity, anorexia, lethargy, gastrointestinal upsets, hirsutism, and gum hypertrophy.

Therapeutic notes: Cyclosporine is often used as part of a post-transplantation "triple therapy" regimen with oral corticosteroids and azathioprine.

Azathioprine

Mechanism of action: Azathioprine is a prodrug that is converted into the active component 6-mercaptopurine in the liver. Mercaptopurine is a fraudulent purine nucleotide that impairs DNA synthesis, and it has a cytotoxic action on dividing cells.

Indications: Azathioprine is used for the prevention of graft and transplant rejection and for autoimmune conditions when corticosteroid therapy alone is inadequate.

Route of administration: Oral, intravenous.

Adverse effects: Side effects of azathioprine include bone marrow suppression, which can lead to leukopenia, thrombocytopenia, and sometimes anemia. This is often the dose-limiting side effect.

Increased susceptibility to infections (often opportunistic pathogens) and to certain cancers (lymphomas) can occur. Common side effects include gastrointestinal disturbances, nausea, vomiting, and diarrhea. Loss of hair (alopecia) may be partial or complete, but this is usually reversible.

Drug interaction with allopurinol necessitates lowering the dose of azathioprine.

Therapeutic notes: Azathioprine is used as part of a post-transplantation "triple therapy" regimen with oral corticosteroids.

Immunosuppressant drugs are toxic agents with common, serious adverse effects that are frequently dose limiting. Knowledge of these adverse effects and their cause is, therefore, important.

Glucocorticoids

The use of glucocorticoids as immunosuppressant agents involves both their anti-inflammatory actions and their effects on the immune system (Chapter 11).

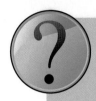

- What are the cardinal clinical features of inflammation?
- How do these arise physiologically?
- What are the principal chemical mediators of the acute inflammatory response?
- What are the steps in the conversion of arachidonic acid to its pro-inflammatory metabolites?
- How do nonsteroidal anti-inflammatory drugs act? (Name some examples of these drugs.)
- Why are cyclooxygenase 2 inhibitors believed to be superior to nonspecific inhibitors of cyclooxygenase?
- What are the common adverse effects and contraindications to nonsteroidal anti-inflammatory drugs?
- How do steroids act as anti-inflammatory agents?
- What are the classifications of the drugs used in the treatment of rheumatoid arthritis? What are their adverse effects?
- Why might the immunosuppressant drugs have a role to play in the management of rheumatoid arthritis?
- What is the underlying cause of gout? Which joints does it classically involve?
- What are the drugs used in the treatment of acute and chronic gout?
- What is pain, and what is the definition of an analgesic?
- How do opioid analgesic drugs act? What are their principal adverse effects?
- How can these adverse effects be minimized?
- What is an opioid antagonist, and what are indications for its use?
- What are the main treatment options for headache?
- What important clinical diagnoses should be excluded in the patient with headache? What are the likely differential diagnoses?
- What drugs are used to treat neuralgic pain? How might these act?
- What are the indications for immunosuppressant drugs? How do they act? (Give examples of such agents.)

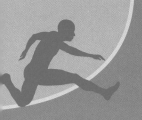

5. Peripheral Nervous System

Basic concepts

Nerve conduction

Conduction of impulses through nerves occurs as an all-or-none event called the action potential. The action potential is caused by voltage-dependent opening of sodium and potassium channels in the cell membrane.

The sodium equilibrium potential (Eq Na$^+$) is +60 mV, and the potassium equilibrium potential (Eq K$^+$) is −90 mV. Since a resting nerve has 50–75 more potassium channels open than sodium channels, the resting membrane potential is −70 mV.

Fig. 5.1 shows the concentrations of sodium and potassium inside and outside a resting nerve. The Na$^+$/K$^+$ pump (Na$^+$/K$^+$ ATPase) is an energy-dependent pump that functions to maintain the concentration gradient of these two ionic species across the membrane. Three sodium ions are pumped out of the cell for every two potassium ions pumped in, and thus the excitability of the cell is retained.

Figs. 5.2 and 5.3 summarize the events that occur during a nerve action potential. During a nerve action potential:

- The rate of sodium entry into the nerve axon becomes greater than the rate of potassium out of the axon, at which point the membrane becomes depolarized (the loss of a electrical gradient across the membrane).
- Depolarization sets off a sodium-positive feedback whereby more voltage-gated sodium channels open, and the membrane becomes more depolarized.

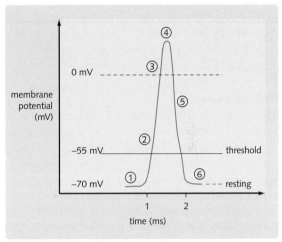

Fig. 5.2 Nerve action potential. For explanation of points 1–6, see Fig. 5.3.

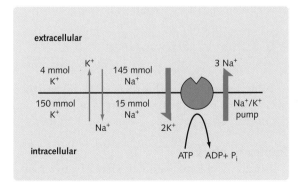

Fig. 5.1 Intracellular and extracellular sodium and potassium concentrations. The Na$^+$/K$^+$ ATPase pump maintains these concentration gradients across the cell membrane.

State of sodium and potassium channels and membrane potential at different stages of the nerve action potential		
Sodium channels	**Potassium channels**	**Membrane potential**
1 Closed resting	Closed resting	Resting (−70 mV)
2 Open	Closed resting	Depolarization (action potential upstroke)
3 More channels open	Closed resting	More depolarization
4 Channels close (inactive)	Special set of channels start oepning	Peak of action potential reached
5 All inactivated	More channels open	Re-polarization
6 Closed resting	Channels close	Resting membrane potential re-established

Fig. 5.3 State of sodium and potassium channels and membrane potential at different stages of the neuronal action potential.

- A threshold, which is usually 15 mV greater than the resting membrane potential, must be reached if an action potential is to be generated.
- The membrane repolarizes when the sodium channels become inactivated; a special set of potassium channels open, and potassium leaves the axon.
- The sodium channels eventually regain their resting excitable state, and the Na^+/K^+ ATPase restores the membrane potential back to -70 mV.

Fig. 5.4 shows the voltage-operated sodium channels in their inactivated, activated, and resting states. Two types of gate exist within the channel: the m-gates and the h-gates. These gates are open or closed according to the state of the channel.

Sodium channel

The voltage-operated sodium channel is present in all excitable tissues. It is a transmembrane protein made up of four domains, each with six transmembrane regions. It is sensitive to membrane potential and selectively passes sodium ions.

Local anesthetics block the sodium channel, and thus nerve conduction, by binding to the sixth transmembrane region of the fourth domain.

Size of the nerve fiber

Small nerve fibers are preferentially blocked because of their high surface-area-to-volume ratio. This results in a differential block whereby the small nociceptive (pain) and autonomic fibers are blocked but not the larger fibers responsible for the mediation of movement and touch.

Local anesthetics
History

Local anesthetics are drugs used to inhibit pain sensation. These drugs work by reversibly blocking nerve conduction.

South American Indians have been chewing the leaves of the coca plant, *Erythroxylon coca*, for thousands of years. When they chewed the plant, they found that their mouth and tongue went numb and that euphoria and excitement were induced. Cocaine was found to be the active ingredient, and it was first isolated from the coca plant in 1860.

Freud was the first to use cocaine clinically to treat patients, but this was unsuccessful. In 1884, however, Koller obtained some cocaine from Freud and was able to demonstrate its local anesthetic effects upon the cornea.

Procaine was first synthesized in 1905 as a synthetic substitute for cocaine.

Chemistry

All local anesthetics have the same basic structure:
- An aromatic group (lipophilic end) linked to a basic side chain (hydrophilic end) by an ester or amide bond (Fig. 5.5).
- The basic side chain (usually a secondary or tertiary amine) is important since only the uncharged molecule can enter the nerve axoplasm.

Potency and duration of action are correlated with high lipid solubility.

Pharmacokinetics

Elimination of local anesthetics is dependent on the nature of the chemical bond:
- Local anesthetics with ester bonds are inactivated by plasma cholinesterases.
- Local anesthetics with amide bonds are degraded by N-dealkylation in the liver.

Metabolites can often be pharmacologically active.

Mechanism of block
Importance of pH and ionization

Local anesthetics are weak bases ($pK_a = 8$–9). Only the uncharged form can penetrate lipid membranes; thus, quaternary ammonium compounds, which are fully protonated, must be injected directly into the nerve axon if they are to work.

The proportion of uncharged local anesthetic is governed by the pH, the pK_a, and the Henderson–Hasselbalch equation (Chapter 1):

$$B + H^+ = BH^+$$
$$pK_a = pH + \log\frac{[BH^+]}{[B]}$$

A local anesthetic with a pK_a of 8.0 will be 10% uncharged at pH 7.0, 50% uncharged at pH 8.0, and 5% uncharged at pH 6.0.

Routes of block

The majority of local anesthetics block by two routes (Fig. 5.6):
- By the hydrophobic route, the uncharged form enters the membrane and blocks the channel from a site in the protein membrane interface.

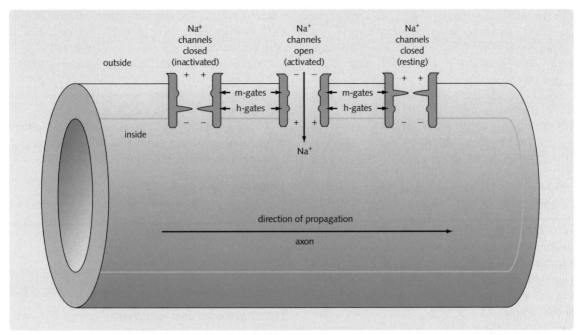

Fig. 5.4 Voltage-operated sodium channels in their inactivated, activated, and resting states. The m-gates and h-gates open or close according to the state of the channel. In the resting sodium channel, the m-gates are held closed by the strongly negative (−70 mV) electrical gradient across the membrane. Once an action potential begins to propagate, the loss of the membrane potential causes the m-gates to open, allowing sodium into the cell, further propagating the action potential. After a very short time, a further conformational change causes the h-gates to close, inactivating the sodium channel. The membrane then re-polarizes, and once at −70 mV, the m-gates again close, and the h-gates open so the sodium channel is back in its resting state.

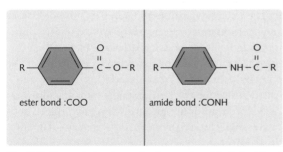

Fig. 5.5 General structure of ester- and amide-linked local anesthetics.

• By the hydrophilic route, the uncharged form crosses the membrane to the inside, where the charged form blocks the channel. This pathway depends on the channel being open, and, therefore, this type of block is use dependent. Use dependency is especially important in the antiarrhythmic action of local anesthetics.

Nerve block occurs when the number of noninactivated channels (those unaffected by the drug) is insufficient to bring about depolarization to threshold.

Routes of administration
Surface anesthesia
In surface anesthesia, the local anesthetic is applied directly to the mucous membranes (e.g., cornea, bronchial tree, esophagus, and genitourinary tract). The local anesthetic (e.g., lidocaine) must be able to penetrate the tissues easily. Tetracaine is used to anesthetize the skin prior to venipuncture, especially in children and anxious adults.

Problems occur when large areas (e.g., the bronchial tree) are anesthetized.

Infiltration anesthesia
Infiltration anesthesia involves direct injection of a local anesthetic into tissue. Often, a vasoconstrictor such as epinephrine is used with the local anesthetic to prevent the spread of the local anesthetic into the systemic circulation. Vasoconstrictors must never be used at extremities, as ischemia could result.

Intravenous regional anesthesia (IVRA) involves the injection of the local anesthetic distal to a cuff

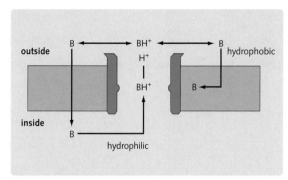

Fig. 5.6 Hydrophobic and hydrophilic routes of block for local anesthetics.

inflated above arterial pressure. It is important that the cuff not be released prematurely, as this could cause the release of a potentially toxic bolus into the circulation. This type of local anesthetic block is now seldom used.

Nerve block anesthesia
In nerve block anesthesia, local anesthetic is injected close to the appropriate nerve trunk (e.g., the brachial plexus). The injection must be accurate in location.

Spinal and epidural anesthesia
Spinal anesthesia involves the injection of a local anesthetic into the cerebrospinal fluid (CSF) in the subarachnoid space. A certain amount of spread can be controlled by increasing the specific gravity of the solution and tilting the patient.

In epidural anesthesia, the local anesthetic is injected into the space between the dura mater and the spinal cord.

In both spinal and epidural anesthesia, the local anesthetic acts by blocking mainly spinal roots, as opposed to the spinal cord itself. Problems arise from the block of preganglionic sympathetic fibers supplying the vasculature (causing vasodilatation) and the heart (causing bradycardia), both leading to hypotension. Rostral spread can lead to the blocking of intercostal and phrenic nerves, and can result in respiratory depression.

Unwanted effects
Unwanted effects of local anesthetics are mainly associated with the spread of the drug into the systemic circulation. These include:
- Effects on the central nervous system (CNS) such as restlessness, tremor, confusion, and agitation. At

high doses, CNS depression can occur. Procaine is worse than lidocaine or prilocaine for causing CNS depression and is seldom used. The exception is cocaine, which, owing to its monoamine-uptake blocking activity, produces euphoria.
- Respiratory depression.
- Possible effects on the cardiovascular system, including myocardial depression and vasodilation.
- Visual disturbances and twitching. Severe toxicity causes convulsions and coma.

Properties and uses
Fig. 5.7 shows the properties and uses of the main local anesthetics, and Fig. 5.8 lists other compounds that block sodium channels.

Somatic nervous system

Neuromuscular junction
Physiology of transduction
Skeletal (voluntary) muscle is innervated by motor neurons, the axons of which are able to propagate action potentials at high velocities.

The area of muscle that lies below the axon terminal is known as the motor end-plate, and the chemical synapse between the two is known as the neuromuscular junction (NMJ).

The axon terminal incorporates membrane-bound vesicles containing the neurotransmitter acetylcholine (ACh). Depolarization of the presynaptic terminal of the nerve by an action potential (generated by sodium influx) causes voltage-sensitive calcium channels to open, allowing calcium ions into the terminal. Normally, the level of calcium ions inside the nerves is very low—10,000 times lower than the external concentration. This calcium influx causes the release of ACh by exocytosis from vesicles. ACh diffuses across to the muscle membrane, where it binds to the nicotinic acetylcholine receptor (nicAChR) and/or is inactivated by acetylcholinesterase (Fig. 5.9). Several events then occur:
- During association, ACh binds to the nicAChR, which is an ion channel that allows cations into the muscle (mainly sodium but also potassium to a lesser extent).
- During the conformational change, the pore of the ion channel is open for 1 ms, during which approximately 20,000 sodium ions enter the cell. The resulting depolarization, called an end-plate

Properties and uses of the main local anesthetics

	Rate of onset	Duration	Tissue penetration	Chemistry	Common use
Cocaine	Rapid	Moderate	Rapid	Ester bond	ENT
Procaine	Moderate	Short	Slow	Ester bond	Little used, CNS effects
Tetracaine	Slow	Long	Moderate	Ester bond	Topical, pre-venepuncture
Oxybuprocine	Rapid	Short	Rapid	Ester bond	Surface, ophthalmology
Benzocaline	Very slow	Very long	Rapid	Ester bond, no basic side chain	Surface ENT
Lidocaine	Rapid	Moderate	Rapid	Amide bond	Widely used in all applications, EMLA
Prilocaine	Moderate	Moderate	Moderate	Amide bond	Many uses, IVRA, EMLA. Low toxicity
Bupivacaine	Slow	Long	Moderate	Amide bond	Epidural and spinal anaesthesia

Fig. 5.7 Properties and uses of the main local anesthetics (ENT, ear, nose and throat; IVRA, intravenous regional anesthetic).

Sodium channel blockers

Compound	Source	Type of block
Tetrodotoxin	Puffer fish	Outside only
Saxitoxin	Plankton	Outside only
μ-Conotoxins	Piscivorous marine snail	Affects inactivation
μ-Agatoxins	Funnel web spider	Affects inactivation
α-, β-, and γ-toxins	Scorpions	Complex
QX314 and QX222	Synthetic, permanently charged local anesthetics	Inside only (hydrophilic pathway)
Benzocaine	Synthetic, uncharged local anesthetic	From within the membrane (hydrophobic pathway)
Local anesthetics	Plant (cocaine), others synthetic	Inside and from within the membrane

Fig. 5.8 Naturally occurring and synthetic sodium channel blockers.

potential (EPP), depolarizes the adjacent muscle fiber.
• If the cellular response is large enough, an action potential is generated in the rest of the muscle fiber (sodium influx), resulting in the opening of voltage-operated calcium channels, but this time the calcium influx mediates contraction.
• ACh is rapidly inactivated by an enzyme called acetylcholinesterase (AChE), which hydrolyzes ACh into the inactive metabolites choline and acetic acid.
• In the synthesis of ACh, the choline generated is taken up by the nerve terminal, where another enzyme, choline acetyl transferase (ChAT), converts it back to ACh to be re-used.

Nicotinic acetylcholine receptor

The nicAChR is made up of five subunits (two α, one β, one γ, and one δ) that traverse the membrane and surround a central pore. The four different subunits show high sequence identity.

ACh must bind to both of the α-subunits in order to open a channel.

Each subunit has four membrane-spanning regions (helices); that is, each receptor has a total of 20. One of the transmembrane helices (M_2) from each subunit forms the lining of the channel pore.

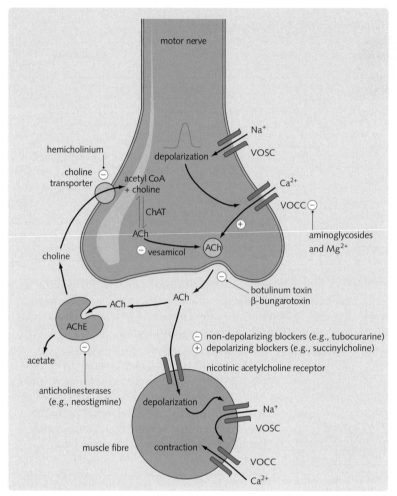

Fig. 5.9 Physiology of impulse transduction at the neuromuscular junction (NMJ) showing the site of action of drugs used in conjunction with the NMJ (VOSC, voltage-operated sodium channel; VOCC, voltage-operated calcium channel; AChE, acetylcholinesterase; ChAT, choline acetyl transferase; vesamicol, an experimental drug).

Pharmacologic targets

There are three major targets within the NMJ for clinically useful drugs (Fig. 5.10):

- The presynaptic release.
- The nicotinic acetylcholine (Nm) receptor.
- Acetylcholinesterase.

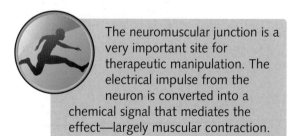

The neuromuscular junction is a very important site for therapeutic manipulation. The electrical impulse from the neuron is converted into a chemical signal that mediates the effect—largely muscular contraction.

Drugs affecting the neuromuscular junction

Presynaptic agents

Drugs inhibiting ACh synthesis: The rate-limiting step in the synthesis of ACh is the uptake of choline into the nerve terminal.

Hemicholinium is an analog of choline that blocks the choline transporter and causes a depletion of ACh stores. Because of the time taken for the stores to run down, the onset of this drug is slow. This, and the frequency-dependent nature of the block (depletion of stores is related to release of ACh), mean that it is not useful clinically. The block is reversed by the addition of choline.

Drugs inhibiting vesicular packaging of ACh: Vesamicol inhibits the active transport of ACh into storage vesicles and results in neuromuscular block.

Drugs inhibiting ACh release: Calcium entry into the nerve terminal is necessary for the release of ACh; thus, agents such as aminoglycoside antibiotics (e.g., streptomycin) that prevent this step will cause neuromuscular blockade. Muscle paralysis is occasionally a side effect of aminoglycoside

antibiotics, but it can be reversed by the administration of calcium salts.

Botulinum toxin is a neurotoxin produced by the anaerobic bacillus *Clostridium botulinum*. The toxin is very potent, and it is believed to inhibit ACh release by inactivating actin, which is necessary for exocytosis. In botulism, a serious type of food poisoning caused by this toxin, victims experience progressive parasympathetic and motor paralysis. Botulinum toxin type A is sometimes used clinically in the treatment of excessive muscle contraction disorders (dystonias) such as strabismus (squint), spasticity, and tremors.

Beta-bungarotoxin contained in snake venom acts in a similar manner to botulinum toxin.

Postsynaptic agents

Nondepolarizing blockers: These act as competitive antagonists by binding to the nicAChR but not activating it, producing motor paralysis. Details of the most commonly used non-depolarizing blockers are given in Fig. 5.11.

Approximately 80–90% of receptors must be blocked to prevent transmission, since the amount of ACh released by nerve terminal depolarization usually greatly exceeds that required to generate

Targets for clinically useful drugs at the neuromuscular junction		
Site	Action	Use
nicAChR	Block transmission	Neuromuscular blockers for surgery
AChE	Enhance transmission	Peripheral neuropathy (e.g., myasthenia gravis)
Release	Block transmission	Spasms (e.g., squints, tics, tremors)

Fig. 5.10 Targets for clinically useful drugs at the neuromuscular junction. Myasthenia gravis is an autoimmune disease in which there are decreased numbers of available receptors at the end-plate due to antibody binding. To allow normal neuromuscular function, drugs that increase the amount of acetylcholine in the cleft are given (AChE, acetylcholine esterase; nicAChR, nicotinic acetylcholine receptor).

Non-depolarizing blockers of postsynaptic receptors at the neuromuscular junction					
Drug	Approximate duration (mins)	Side effects			Elimination
		Ganglion block	Histamine release	Other	
Tubocurarine	60–120	Partial	Sometimes	Hypersensitivity (rare)	Mainly hepatic
Pancuronium	40–60	x	Minimal	Block of muscarinic receptors in the heart → tachycardia	Mainly renal
Gallamine	15	x	x	Block of muscarinic receptors in the heart → tachycardia	Mainly renal: avoid in patients with renal disease
Alcuronium	20	x	x	Dose dependency	Mainly hepatic
Vecuronium	20–30	x	x		Mainly hepatic
Atracurium	15–30	x	Sometimes		Degradation in plasma at body pH (Hofmann elimination)

Fig. 5.11 Nondepolarizing blockers of postsynaptic receptors at the neuromuscular junction.

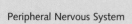
an action potential in the muscle. The drugs are all quaternary ammonium compounds and, therefore, do not cross the blood–brain barrier or the placenta. They are poorly absorbed orally, and they must be administered by intravenous injection. "Tetanic fade" (i.e., nonmaintained muscle tension during brief nerve stimulation) is seen with some of these drugs. This can be explained by the blocking of presynaptic autoreceptors which usually maintain the release of ACh during repeated stimulation.

The block can be reversed by anticholinesterases and depolarizing drugs. It is also enhanced in patients with myasthenia gravis. The main side effect from these drugs is hypotension caused by the blocking of ganglionic transmission. Histamine release from mast cells, resulting in bronchospasm, may be a problem in certain individuals (see Fig. 5.11).

Depolarizing (noncompetitive) blockers: Depolarizing blockers initially activate receptors, causing depolarization, but in doing so block further activation.

Depolarizing blockers act on the motor end-plate in the same manner as ACh (i.e., they are agonists and increase the cation permeability of the end-plate). However, unlike ACh, which is released in brief spurts and rapidly hydrolyzed, depolarizing blockers remain associated with the receptors long enough to cause a sustained depolarization and a resulting loss of electrical excitability (phase I).

Repeated or continuous administration of depolarizing blockers leads to the block becoming more characteristic of nondepolarizing drugs. This is known as phase II and is probably due to receptor desensitization, whereby the end-plate becomes less sensitive to ACh. The block starts to show tetanic fade, and it is partly reversed by anticholinesterase drugs.

Succinylcholine is the only depolarizing blocker used clinically because of its rapid onset time and short duration of action (approximately 6 minutes). Succinylcholine is a quaternary ammonium compound, and it must be given by intravenous injection. It is rapidly hydrolyzed by plasma cholinesterase, although certain people with a genetic variant of this enzyme may experience a neuromuscular block that may last for hours.

Depolarizing blockers have no effect in patients with myasthenia gravis, since these patients have a decreased number of receptors at the end-plate. In this instance, the blocking potency of depolarizing blockers is reduced.

The side effects of depolarizing blockers include:
- Initial spasms, which occur prior to paralysis, often resulting in postoperative muscle pain.
- Muscarinic receptor activation, resulting in bradycardia. Bradycardia can be prevented by the administration of atropine.
- Potassium release from muscle, resulting in elevated plasma potassium levels. This is usually a problem only in the case of trauma.

Anticholinesterases

Anticholinesterases inhibit AChE and thus increase the amount of ACh in the synaptic cleft and enhance cholinergic transmission.

Most of the anticholinesterases used are quaternary ammonium compounds and, therefore, do not penetrate the blood–brain barrier.

Short-acting anticholinesterases include edrophonium. This is selective for the NMJ and clinically relevant in the diagnosis of myasthenia gravis. Edrophonium's duration of action is only 2–10 minutes because it binds by electrostatic forces (no covalent bonds) to the active site of the enzyme. Edrophonium is, therefore, not used therapeutically.

Intermediate-acting anticholinesterases include neostigmine, pyridostigmine, and physostigmine.

Neostigmine is used intravenously to reverse the effects of nondepolarizing blockers. Its duration of action is 2–4 hours, and it is used orally in the treatment of myasthenia gravis. Although neostigmine shows some selectivity for the NMJ, atropine is sometimes coadministered to block the muscarinic effects of the drug.

Pyridostigmine has a duration of action of 3–6 hours, and it is also used orally in the treatment of myasthenia gravis. It has few parasympathetic actions.

Physostigmine shows selectivity for the postganglionic parasympathetic junction. It is a tertiary amine; its use, therefore, is associated with central effects such as initial excitation followed by depression and possibly respiratory depression and unconsciousness. The central effects can be antagonized by atropine. Physostigmine is used in the form of eye drops to constrict the pupil and contract the ciliary muscle in the treatment of glaucoma.

Most of the long-lasting or irreversible anticholinesterases are organophosphorus compounds. For example, sarin and tabun were developed as nerve gases, and parathion was developed as an insecticide, as well as for clinical use. These drugs have many adverse effects, such as bradycardia, hypotension, breathing problems, depolarizing neuromuscular block, central effects, and possible death from peripheral nerve demyelination. Echothiophate shows selectivity for the postganglionic parasympathetic junction, and it is used in the treatment of glaucoma.

While myasthenia gravis is a rare disease, its pathophysiology and clinical features are very interesting, and as such it is commonly asked about in exams.

Autonomic nervous system

Basic concepts

The autonomic nervous system is the means by which all tissues other than skeletal muscle are innervated (Fig. 5.12).

The axons of the autonomic nervous system leave their cell body, which is located in the CNS, as preganglionic fibers, synapse in the appropriate ganglion, and leave as postganglionic fibers. These postganglionic fibers reach the effector cells.

The neurotransmitter released by preganglionic fibers at autonomic ganglia, regardless of whether sympathetic or parasympathetic, is ACh.

The ACh receptors located on postganglionic fibers are of the nicotinic type.

In general, the sympathetic and parasympathetic systems mediate opposite effects (see Fig. 5.20).

Autonomic ganglia

Fig. 5.13 summarizes the differences between ganglionic nicAChR and those found on skeletal muscle at the NMJ.

Ganglion-stimulating drugs
Nicotinic agonists

There are few agonists that act selectively on the nicAChR without affecting muscarinic receptors. Carbachol is the best example of a drug that shows preference for the nicotinic receptor, but its action is not selective. Nicotine and lobeline both show

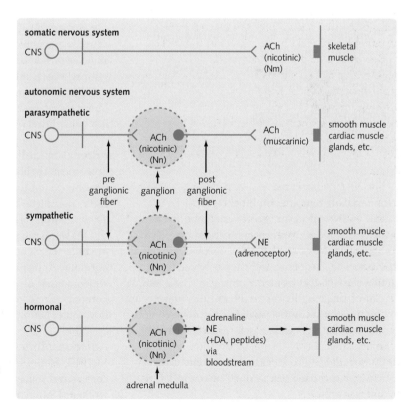

Fig. 5.12 Somatic and autonomic nervous systems: organization and neurotransmitters (ACh, acetylcholine; CNS, central nervous system; DA, dopamine; NE, norepinephrine).

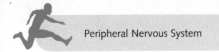

Distinguishing features of nicotinic acetylcholine receptors		
	Skeletal muscle	Neurons
Structure	2α 1β 1γ or ε 1δ	2α 3β
Specific agonists	Suxamethonium	DMPP
Specific antagonists	Gallamine Tubocurarine α-bungarotoxin	Hexamethonium Mecamylamine κ-bungarotoxin
Function	End-plate region depolarization at NMJ	Neuronal depolarizaton in ganglia and CNS

Fig. 5.13 Distinguishing features of the ganglionic nicotinic acetylcholine receptors and those found on skeletal muscle at the neuromuscular junction (DMPP, dimethylphenylpiperazinium).

preference for ganglionic nicotinic receptors, but at slightly higher concentrations than those needed to affect ganglionic transmission. Nicotine and lobeline are able to stimulate the NMJ.

These drugs have no clinical use, since their range of effects is vast, affecting both sympathetic and parasympathetic transmission:

- Sympathetic effects include tachycardia and vasoconstriction leading to hypertension.
- Parasympathetic effects include increased gastrointestinal motility and glandular secretions.

Ganglion-blocking drugs
Autonomic ganglia can be blocked presynaptically by inhibiting ACh synthesis, vesicular packaging, or release or postsynaptically by blocking the nicotinic (Nn) receptors.

Nondepolarizing ganglion blockers
A few of these drugs act solely as competitive antagonists, blocking receptors without depolarizing the ganglion. Most block the ion channel, as well as the associated receptor, and they produce their action through this former mechanism. For example:

- Some ganglion blockers, such as tubocurarine, are not antagonists at the ganglionic nicotinic receptor; they produce ganglion block through channel blockade.
- Tubocurarine also blocks transmission at the NMJ, but it does this through receptor antagonism.

- Hexamethonium was initially developed for use in treating hypertension, but it is no longer in clinical use.
- Trimethaphan and mecamylamine are the only clinically useful ganglion blockers. They have been used where controlled hypotension is needed, such as in anesthesia. They have a short duration of action and can be administered intravenously.

Ganglion-blocking drugs have a wide range of complex effects, although the sympathetic and parasympathetic systems tend to oppose one another. The effects of ganglion-blocking drugs include:

- Arteriolar vasodilatation leading to a marked reduction in blood pressure (block of sympathetic ganglia).
- Postural and postexercise hypotension (loss of cardiac reflexes).
- Slight reduction in cardiac output.
- Inhibition of gastrointestinal secretions and motility, leading to constipation, urinary retention, impotence, and failure of ejaculation.

Sympathetic nervous system
The fibers of the sympathetic nervous system leave the CNS from the thoracolumbar regions of the spinal cord (T1–L3). They synapse in ganglia located close to the spinal cord. These ganglia form a chain along each side of the spinal cord, which is known as sympathetic trunk.

The major transmitter released by postganglionic fibers at the junction with effector cells is norepinephrine (NE).

Adrenal medulla
Some postganglionic neurons in the sympathetic division do not have axons, but instead they release their transmitters directly into the bloodstream. These neurons are located in the adrenal medulla.

On stimulation by preganglionic fibers, the adrenal medulla acts as an endocrine gland, releasing its hormones/transmitters into the systemic circulation which consist of ~80% epinephrine, ~20% norepinephrine, as well as small amounts of dopamine, neuropeptides, and ATP.

Adrenoceptors
In 1913, Henry Dale observed that epinephrine constricted some blood vessels but relaxed others, while in 1948 Ahlquist defined two receptor

subtypes based on the rank order of potency of three agonists, namely isoproterenol, epinephrine, and norepinephrine. The two receptor subtypes were α and β. Potency at:

- α-receptors is norepinephrine ≥ epinephrine > isoproterenol.
- β-receptors is isoproterenol > epinephrine > norepinephrine.

Effects mediated by α-adrenoreceptors
Alpha$_1$-receptors
Alpha$_1$-receptors are located postsynaptically. Their activation causes smooth muscle contraction (except for the nonsphincter part of the gastrointestinal tract, where activation causes relaxation), glycogenolysis in the liver, and potassium release from the liver and salivary glands. Transduction is via G-proteins and an increase in the second messengers inositol (1,4,5), triphosphate (IP$_3$), and diacylglycerol (DAG).

Alpha$_2$-receptors
Alpha$_2$-receptors are located mainly presynaptically, but also postsynaptically on liver cells, platelets, and the smooth muscle of blood vessels. The activation of presynaptic α$_2$-receptors inhibits norepinephrine release and, therefore, provides a means of end-product negative feedback. Activation of postsynaptic α$_2$-receptors causes blood vessel constriction and platelet aggregation.
Transduction is via G-proteins and a decrease in the second messenger cyclic adenosine monophosphate (cAMP).

Effects mediated by β-adrenoceptors
Beta$_1$-receptors
Beta$_1$-receptors are mainly postsynaptic and located in the heart, platelets, and nonsphincter part of the gastrointestinal tract. They can, however, be found presynaptically. Activation causes an increase in the rate and force of contraction of the heart, relaxation of the non-sphincter part of the gastrointestinal tract, aggregation of platelets, an increase in the release of norepinephrine, lipolysis in fat, and amylase secretion from the salivary glands. Presynaptically, their activation causes an increase in norepinephrine release. Transduction is via G-proteins and an increase in the second messenger cAMP.

Beta$_2$-receptors
Beta$_2$-receptors are located postsynaptically. Their activation causes smooth muscle relaxation,

glycogenolysis in the liver, inhibition of histamine release from mast cells, and tremor in skeletal muscle. Transduction is via G-proteins and an increase in the second messenger cAMP.

Many of the adrenoceptor agonists and antagonists are not entirely specific for just the α- or the β-adrenoceptors, so side effects are common, and they should be remembered.

Drugs acting on the sympathetic system
Fig. 5.14 summarizes the drugs acting on the sympathetic system.

Presynaptic agents
Norepinephrine synthesis: The precursor to norepinephrine is L-tyrosine, which is taken up by adrenergic neurons.

Drugs decreasing norepinephrine synthesis: The rate-limiting step (RLS) is the conversion of tyrosine to dihydroxyphenylalanine (dopa), which is catalyzed by tyrosine hydroxylase and inhibited by a methyltyrosine. Norepinephrine provides a negative feedback upon this step. Carbidopa inhibits dopa decarboxylase and is used in Parkinson's disease to increase dopamine levels. Because this is not the RLS, drugs that inhibit dopa decarboxylase do not greatly affect norepinephrine synthesis. Administering α-methyldopa (used in hypertension) results in the formation of a false transmitter, α-methylnorepinephrine.

Drugs increasing norepinephrine synthesis: Levodopa (L-dopa) administration bypasses the RLS and is used in Parkinson's disease. Norepinephrine is stored in vesicles as a complex with ATP and a protein called chromogranin A.

Drugs inhibiting norepinephrine storage: Reserpine is a drug that was used in the treatment of hypertension and schizophrenia. It reduces stores of norepinephrine by preventing the accumulation of norepinephrine in vesicles. Its action is effectively irreversible since it has a very high affinity for the norepinephrine storage site. The displaced norepinephrine is immediately broken down by monoamine oxygenase (MAO) and is therefore unable to exert sympathetic effects.

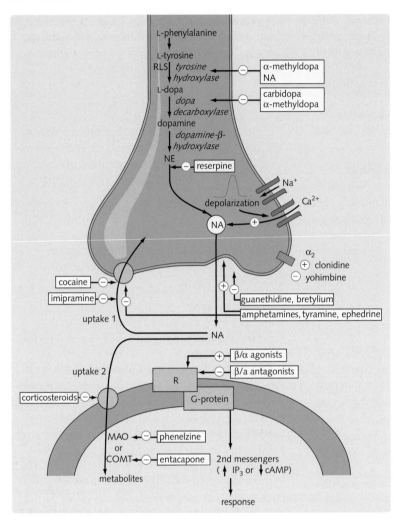

Fig. 5.14 Drugs affecting adrenergic transmission (cAMP, cyclic adenosine monophosphate; COMT, catechol-O-methyltransferase; IP$_3$, inositol triphosphate; MAO, monoamine oxidase; NE, norepinephrine; RLS, rate-limiting step).

Drugs inhibiting the breakdown of leaked norepinephrine stores: These include monoamine oxidase inhibitors (MAOIs) and catechol-O-methyltransferase (COMT) inhibitors. They prevent the breakdown of leaked catecholamines so that norepinephrine that leaves the vesicles is protected and eventually leaks out from the nerve ending.

Drugs inhibiting norepinephrine release: These include guanethidine and bretylium. These are adrenergic neuron-blocking drugs that prevent the exocytosis of norepinephrine from nerve terminals; they are used as hypotensive drugs. They are taken up by uptake 1 and concentrated in nerve terminals where they have a local anesthetic effect on impulse conduction. The tricyclic antidepressants, which inhibit uptake 1, prevent these drugs from exerting their effects. Clonidine is an α_2-receptor agonist and, therefore, inhibits norepinephrine release.

Drugs promoting norepinephrine release: These include amphetamines, tyramine, and ephedrine, which are sympathomimetic drugs that act indirectly. They are taken up by uptake 1 and displace norepinephrine from the vesicles. Because they also inhibit MAO, the displaced norepinephrine is not broken down, and it is able to exert sympathetic effects. These drugs act in part through a direct agonist effect on adrenoceptors. Yohimbine is an α_2-receptor antagonist and it, therefore, prevents norepinephrine from exerting a negative feedback effect on norepinephrine release.

Adrenoceptor agonists				
Drug	Receptor	Uses	Side effects	Phamacokinetics
Norepinephrine	α/β	No use clinically	Hypertension, tachycardia, ventricular arrhythmias	Poor oral absorption, metabolized by MAO and COMT, $t_{1/2}$ ~ 2 min
Epinephrine	α/β	Anaphylactic shock Cardiac resuscitation with local anaesthetics	Hypertension, tachycardia, ventricular arrhythmias	Poor oral absorption, metabolized by MAO and COMT, $t_{1/2}$ ~ 2 min given intravenously on intramuscularly
Oxymetazoline	α	Nasal decongestant	Rebound congestion	Given intranasally
Phenylephrine	α_1	Hypotension Nasal decongestant	Hypertension Reflex bradycardia	Metabolized by MAO $t_{1/2}$ < 1 min, given intramuscularly or intranasally
Clonidine	α_2	Hypertension Migraine	Drowsiness, hypotension	Good oral absorption, $t_{1/2}$ ~ 12 h
Isoproterenol	β	Asthma Cardiac resuscitation	Arrhythmias, tachycardia	Metabolized by COMT, given sublingually or as aerosol $t_{1/2}$ ~ 2 h
Dobutamine	β_1	Heart failure	Tachycardia	
Salmeterol	β_2	Asthma Premature labour	Arrhythmias, tachycardia, vasodilatation	Given by aerosol $t_{1/2}$ ~ 4 h

Fig. 5.15 Adrenoceptor agonists and their clinical uses (COMT, catechol-O-methyltransferase; MAO, monoamine oxidase).

Postsynaptic agents

Adrenoceptor agonists: These are termed "sympathomimetics." They activate postsynaptic receptors, eliciting a response (Fig. 5.15).

Adrenoceptor antagonists: These are termed "sympatholytics." They block postsynaptic receptors (Fig. 5.16).

Inactivation

Uptake 1: This is located on neuronal terminals, and it is the main mechanism for norepinephrine inactivation. Uptake 1 has a high affinity for the uptake of norepinephrine (K = 0.3 mmol/L in the rat), but the maximum rate of uptake is low (V_{max} = 1.2 nmol/g per minute in the rat). It has a specificity rank of norepinephrine > epinephrine > isoproterenol. It is blocked by cocaine, amphetamines, and tricyclic antidepressants (e.g., imipramine), which therefore potentiate the actions of norepinephrine.

Uptake 2: This is located outside neurons (e.g., in smooth muscle, cardiac muscle, and endothelium),

and it is the main mechanism for the removal of circulating epinephrine from the bloodstream. It has a low affinity for the uptake of norepinephrine (K = 250 mmol/L in the rat) but a high maximum rate of uptake (V_{max} = 100 nmol/g per minute in the rat). Uptake 2 has a specificity rank of epinephrine > norepinephrine > isoproterenol, and it is blocked by corticosteroids.

Metabolism of catecholamines by monoamine oxidase: MAO is found on the surface of mitochondria, principally within adrenergic nerve terminals but also in other cells, such as those of the liver and intestines. MAO metabolizes catecholamines into their corresponding aldehydes. It comprises two major forms: MAO_A and MAO_B. Norepinephrine is mainly broken down by MAO_A in nerve terminals. Inhibitors of MAO increase the releasable store of norepinephrine, but they do not greatly potentiate sympathetic transmission, since catecholamines are mainly inactivated by reuptake. MAOIs include the antidepressant drugs phenelzine and tranylcypromine.

Adrenoceptor antagonists				
Drug	Receptor	Uses	Side effects	Pharmacokinetics
Labetalol	α/β	Hypertension	Postural hypotension	Oral absorption $t_{1/2} \sim 4$ h
Phentolamine	α	No clinical use	Hypotension Tachycardia Nasal congestion	Metabolized by the liver, given intravenously $t_{1/2} \sim 2$ h
Prazosin	α_1	Hypertension	Hypotension Tachycardia Nasal congestion Drowsiness	Oral absorption, metabolized by the liver $t_{1/2} \sim 4$ h
Yohimbine	α_2	No clinical use	Hypertension Excitement	Oral absorption, metabolized by the liver $t_{1/2} \sim 4$ h
Propranolol	β	Hypertension Angina Arrhythmias	Bronchoconstriction Heart failure	Oral absorption, first-pass metabolism, 90% plasma-protein-bound $t_{1/2} \sim 4$ h
Butoxamine	β_2	No clinical use		

Fig. 5.16 Adrenoceptor antagonists and their clinical uses (COMT, catechol-O-methyltransferase; MAO, monoamine oxidase).

Metabolism of catecholamines by catechol-O-methyltransferase: Catechol-O-methyltransferase (COMT) is found in all tissues and breaks down most catecholamines and the byproducts of the actions of MAO. COMT metabolizes catecholamines to give a methoxy derivative. Entacapone is a drug used clinically for parkinsonism, and it is a COMT inhibitor.

Parasympathetic nervous system

The fibers of the parasympathetic nervous system leave the CNS from the sacral region (S3 and S4) of the spinal cord and via cranial nerves III, VII, IX, and X. The fibers synapse in ganglia, which, unlike the sympathetic system, are located within the innervated organs themselves.

The major transmitter released by postganglionic fibers at the junction with effector cells is ACh.

Parasympathetic receptors

The ACh released by postganglionic nerve fibers acts on muscarinic (M) receptors, of which between three and five subtypes exist.

"Neuroparietal" M₁ receptors

M_1 "neuroparietal" receptors are principally found in the CNS, peripheral neurons, and gastric

parietal cells. Their effects tend to be excitatory, depolarizing membranes through a decrease in potassium conductance. Activation causes central excitation and gastric acid secretion, while transduction is via G-proteins and an increase in the second messengers IP_3 and DAG through stimulation of phospholipase C.

"Neurocardiac" M₂ receptors

M_2 "neurocardiac" receptors are found in the heart and on peripheral neurons. Their effects are inhibitory, increasing potassium conductance and inhibiting calcium channels. In the heart, their activation causes a decrease in the rate (via potassium) and force (via calcium) of contraction. Transduction is via G-proteins and a decrease in the second messenger cAMP through inhibition of adenylyl cyclase.

"Smooth muscle–glandular" M₃ receptors

M_3 "smooth muscle–glandular" receptors are found in smooth muscle and glands. Their effects tend to be excitatory, increasing sodium conductance. Activation causes glandular secretions such as saliva and sweat, and smooth muscle contraction. Transduction is via G-proteins and an increase in the second messengers IP_3 and DAG. M_3 receptors are also located on vascular endothelium,

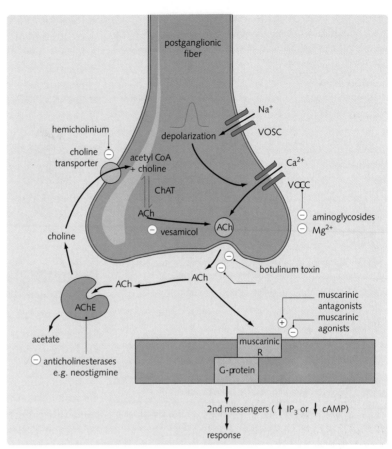

Fig. 5.17 Drugs acting on the parasympathetic nerve transmission (VOSC, voltage-operated sodium channel; VOCC, voltage-operated calcium channel; AChE, acetylcholinesterase; ChAT, choline acetyl transferase).

activation of which causes vasodilatation, through the release of endothelium-derived relaxing factor (EDRF).

"Eye" M_4 receptors

M_4 "eye" receptors are believed to be exclusive to the eye. Their activation causes constriction of the pupil and accommodation for near vision. Transduction is via G-proteins and a decrease in the second messenger cAMP through inhibition of adenylyl cyclase.

Drugs acting on the parasympathetic system

Fig. 5.17 summarizes the drugs that act on the parasympathetic system.

Presynaptic agents

For information regarding presynaptic agents, see pp. 78–79.

Anticholinesterases

For information regarding anticholinesterases, see pp. 80–81.

Postsynaptic agents

Muscarinic-receptor agonists: These are termed "parasympathomimetic." They activate postsynaptic receptors (Fig. 5.18).

Muscarinic-receptor antagonists: These are termed "parasympatholytic" and block postsynaptic receptors (Fig. 5.19).

Nonselective antagonists can be used in anesthesia to prevent bronchial secretions and vagal slowing of heart rate.

Different tissues respond differently to muscarinic antagonists (Fig. 5.20). Salivary, sweat, and bronchial glands are the most sensitive and can be blocked by very low doses of atropine. In contrast, the parietal

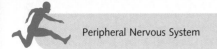

Drugs acting on the parasympathetic nervous system			
Drug	Muscarinic receptors	Nicotinic receptors	Uses
Carbachol	++	+++	Gut and bladder stimulation postoperatively
Methacholine	++++	–	
Bethanechol	+++	–	Gut and bladder stimulation postoperatively
Muscarine	+++	–	
Pilocarpine	++	–	To decrease intraocular pressure in glaucoma

Fig. 5.18 Muscarinic agonists and their clinical uses.

Muscarinic antagonists		
Drug	Muscarinic receptor	Specific uses
Atropine	Nonselective	Reduces gastrointestinal motility Cardiac arrest
Hyoscine	Nonselective	Motion sickness
Ipratropium	Nonselective	Bronchodilator
Cyclopentolate	M_4	Dilation of pupil
Tropicamide	M_4	Dilation of pupil
Pirenzepine	M_1	Reduces gastric acid secretion
Trihexyphenidyl	M_1	Parkinson's disease

Fig. 5.19 Muscarinic antagonists and their clinical uses.

cells are the most resistant, and the block of gastric acid secretion requires high doses of atropine.

The side effects of muscarinic antagonists include:
- Dry mouth and skin and increased body temperature (inhibition of salivary and sweat glands).
- Blurred vision and pupil no longer responsive to light (dilation of pupil).

- Paralysis of accommodation: cycloplegia (relaxation of ciliary muscle).
- Urinary retention.
- Central excitation: irritability and hyperactivity.
- Sedation (hyoscine).

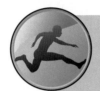

Sympathetic transmission is enhanced under conditions of stress, known as the "fight-or-flight response."

Nitrergic nervous system

Nitric oxide is now well recognized as a neurotransmitter in the CNS, and more recently it has been attributed to have numerous roles to play in the peripheral nervous system too.

Nitric oxide is generated by the action of the enzyme nitric oxide synthase (NOS), of which constitutive and inducible isoforms exist. L-Arginine is the amino acid precursor of nitric oxide synthesis.

Nitric oxide activates the guanylyl cyclase enzyme, which is responsible for generating cyclic guanosine monophosphate (cGMP). The synthesis of cGMP in turn activates a protein kinase, which phosphorylates ion channels in the plasma membrane and causes hyperpolarization of the smooth muscle cell. Intracellular calcium ions are consequently sequestered into the endoplasmic reticulum, and further calcium influx into the cell is inhibited by the closure of calcium channels. The overall effect of a fall in intracellular calcium is a relaxation of the smooth muscle.

The smooth-muscle effects of nitric oxide in the peripheral nervous system are now recognized to be important in the gastrointestinal system and in sexual arousal in both sexes, particularly in males.

Therapeutic manipulation of the nitrergic nervous system is confined to the male reproductive system at present, and the agents currently used in the management of erectile dysfunction (e.g., sildenafil or Viagra®) are discussed in Chapter 9.

Effects of sympathetic and parasympathetic nerve stimulation					
Target tissue	Sympathetic		Paraympathetic		Overall effect
Nerve terminals	α_2	Decresed release	M_2	Decreased release	Decreased transmission
Smooth muscle					
Blood vessels	$\alpha_{1/2}$ b_2	Contraction Relaxation	M_3	Relaxation (via EDRF)	Vasoconstriction Vasodilatation
Bronchi	β_2 α_1	Relaxation Contraction	M_3 M_3	Contraction Secretion	Bronchodilatation Bronchoconstriction Bronchosecretion
Gastrointestinal tract: nonsphincter sphincter secretions	β_1/α_1 α_1	Relaxation Contraction	M_3 M_3 M_3	Contraction Relaxation Secretion	Increased/decreased motility and tone GI secretions
Parietal cells			M_1	Contraction	Gastric and secretion
Pancreas			M_3	Contraction	Increased secretions
Uterus	α_1 β_2	Contraction Relaxation	M_3 M_3		
Bladder: detrusor sphincter	β_2 α_1	Relaxation Contraction	M_3 M_3	Contraction Relaxation	Micturition Urine retention
Seminal tract Vas deferens Penis venous sphincter	α_1 β_2 α_1	Contraction Relaxation Contraction	M_3	Vasodilatation	Ejaculation Ejaculation Erection
Radial muscle (iris) Ciliary muscle Lacrimal gland	α_1 β_2	Contraction Relaxation	M_4 M_4 M_4	Relaxation Contraction Contraction	Pupil relaxation/constriction Accommodation Tear secretion
Heart	β_1	Increased rate and force	M_2	Decreased rate and force	
Liver	α_1/β_2	Glycogenolysis			
Fat	β_1	Lipolysis			
Salivary glands	α_1/β_1	Secretion of thick saliva	M_3	Abundant secretion of watery saliva	
Platelets	α_2	Platelet aggregation			
Mast cells	β_2	Inhibition of histamine release			

Fig. 5.20 Summary table of the opposing effects of sympathetic and parasympathetic nerve stimulation on body tissues.

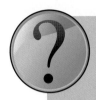

- How does the size of a nerve fiber affect its potential to be blocked?
- What are the mechanism of action of local anesthetics, the importance of pH, and the two routes by which block occurs?
- How can presynaptic agents be used to block transmission at the neuromuscular junction? (Give examples and describe their clinical use.)
- By which routes can local anesthetics be administered? (Give a clinical use for each example given.)
- What are the distinguishing characteristics between nondepolarizing and polarizing postsynaptic blocking drugs? (Give examples and describe their clinical use.)
- What are the clinical features of the adverse reactions to local anesthetics? Why are local anesthetic drugs not used in end arteries?
- What are the effects of anticholinesterases and how they are used clinically? (Give examples.)
- What are the events that occur during transmission across the neuromuscular junction?
- How do nicotinic and muscarinic acetylcholine receptors differ in the location and mechanism of action?
- What are the function and divisions of the autonomic nervous system?
- What are the actions and counteractions of the sympathetic and parasympathetic nervous systems on the major organs of the body?
- What are the mediators involved in presynaptic and postsynaptic transmission and the receptors involved in the sympathetic nervous system?
- What are the mediators involved in presynaptic and postsynaptic transmission and the receptors involved in the parasympathetic nervous system?
- What is the role of the adrenal gland in promoting a systemic response other than its synthesis and release of steroids? What innervates this?
- What are the main classes of adrenoceptors, their subdivisions, and the tissues in which they predominate?
- What are the classes of adrenoceptor, and their naturally occurring agonist(s) and physiologic roles in humans?
- What are the common adrenoceptor agonist and antagonist drugs, their route of administration, adverse effects, and clinical uses?
- By what mechanisms is acetylcholine cleared from the synaptic cleft and from the synaptic terminal? (Name the drugs which inhibit these pathways.)
- What are the mechanisms of action of the different classes of muscarinic receptors and their likely physiologic roles?
- What are the side effects most commonly reported by patients taking anticholinergic drugs?

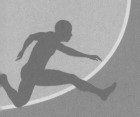

6. Central Nervous System

Parkinsonism

Parkinson's disease and parkinsonism
Definitions
Parkinson's disease is a progressive neurologic disorder of the basal ganglia that occurs most commonly in the elderly.

Parkinsonism is most commonly caused by Parkinson's disease, although numerous other causes do exist. Parkinsonism is characterized by a resting tremor, slow initiation of movements (bradykinesia), and muscle rigidity known collectively as the ''parkinsonian triad.'' A patient with parkinsonism will present with characteristic signs:
• A shuffling gait.
• A blank ''mask-like'' facial expression.
• Speech impairment.
• An inability to perform skilled tasks.

Pathogenesis
Analysis of brains of parkinsonian patients post mortem shows a substantially reduced concentration of dopamine (less than 10% of normal) in the basal ganglia. The basal ganglia exert an extrapyramidal neural influence that normally acts to maintain smooth voluntary movement.

The main pathology in Parkinson's disease is a progressive degeneration of the dopaminergic neurons of the substantia nigra, which project in the nigrostriatal pathway to the corpus striatum (Fig. 6.1). The inhibitory dopaminergic activity of the nigrostriatal pathway is, therefore, considerably reduced (by 20–40%) in people with Parkinson's disease.

The reduction in the inhibitory dopaminergic activity of the nigrostriatal pathway results in unopposed cholinergic neuron hyperactivity from the corpus striatum, which contributes to the pathological features of parkinsonism. Frank symptoms of parkinsonism appear only when more than 80% of the dopaminergic neurons of the substantia nigra have degenerated.

Parkinson's disease is progressive, with continued loss of dopaminergic neurons in the substantia nigra correlating well with worsening of clinical symptoms. Untreated Parkinson's eventually results in dementia and death.

Etiology
The cause of Parkinson's disease is unknown in most cases (idiopathic), although both endogenous and environmental neurotoxins are known to be responsible in causing parkinsonism (Fig. 6.2).

The possibility of a neurotoxic cause has been strengthened by the finding that 1-methyl–4-phenyl–1,2,3,6-tetrahydropyridine (MPTP), a chemical

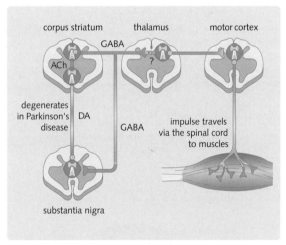

Fig. 6.1 Basal ganglia systems involved in Parkinson's disease (ACh, acetylcholine; DA, dopamine; GABA, γ-aminobutyric acid). (Redrawn from Page et al., 2002.)

Etiology of parkinsonism
• Mostly unknown (idiopathic Parkinson's disease) • Toxin induced: MPTP; carbon monoxide, manganese • Drug induced: neuroleptics (dopamine antagonists) • Rare causes: cerebral ischemia; viral encephalitis and others?

Fig. 6.2 Etiologic mechanisms in the development of parkinsonism (MPTP, methyl–4-phenyl–1,2,3,6-tetrahydropyridine).

contaminant of heroin, causes irreversible damage to the nigrostriatal dopaminergic pathway. This damage can lead to the development of symptoms similar to those of idiopathic Parkinson's disease; it has been seen in Californian drug users and induced in experimental primates.

Drugs that block dopamine receptors can also induce parkinsonism. Neuroleptic drugs used in the treatment of schizophrenia can produce parkinsonian symptoms as an adverse effect.

Rare causes of parkinsonism are cerebral ischemia (progressive atherosclerosis or stroke), viral encephalitis, or other pathological damage.

Treatment of parkinsonism

The treatment of parkinsonism is based on correcting the imbalance between the dopaminergic and cholinergic systems at the basal ganglia (Fig. 6.3). Two major groups of drugs are used: drugs that increase dopaminergic activity between the substantia nigra and the corpus striatum, and anticholinergic drugs that inhibit striatal cholinergic activity.

Drugs that increase dopaminergic activity
Dopamine precursors

An example of a dopamine precursor is levodopa (L-dopa).

Mechanism of action: L-dopa is the immediate precursor of dopamine and is able to penetrate the blood–brain barrier to replenish the dopamine content of the corpus striatum. L-dopa is decarboxylated to dopamine in the brain by dopa

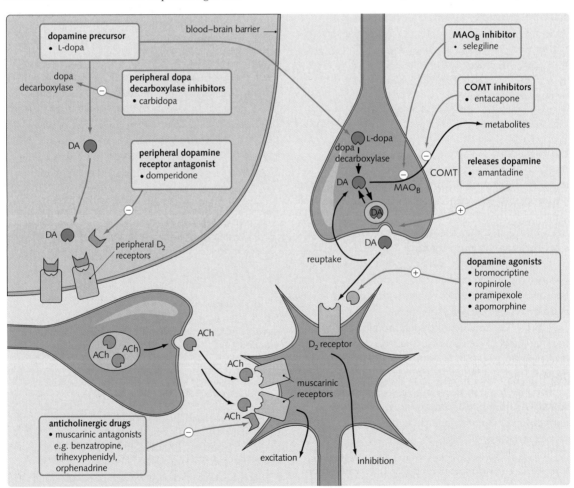

Fig. 6.3 Drugs used to treat parkinsonism and their site of action (ACh, acetylcholine; L-dopa, levodopa; MAO_B, monoamine oxidase B; COMT, catechol-O-methyl transferase; DA, dopamine).

decarboxylase, and it has beneficial effects produced through the actions of dopamine on D_2 receptors (see Fig. 6.3). Dopamine itself is not used, owing to its inability to cross the blood–brain barrier.

Route of administration: L-dopa is administered orally. It reaches peak plasma concentrations after 1–2 hours, and only 1% reaches the brain, owing to peripheral metabolism.

Indications: L-dopa is used in the treatment of parkinsonism (excluding drug-induced extrapyramidal symptoms).

Contraindications: Closed-angle glaucoma.

Adverse effects: The extensive peripheral metabolism of L-dopa means that large doses have to be given to produce therapeutic effects in the brain. Large doses are more likely to produce adverse effects. These include:

- Nausea and vomiting.
- Psychiatric side effects (schizophrenia-like symptoms).
- Cardiovascular effects (hypotension).
- Dyskinesias.

Nausea and vomiting are caused by stimulation of dopamine receptors in the chemoreceptor trigger zone in the area postrema, which lies outside the blood–brain barrier.

Psychiatric side effects are common limiting factors in L-dopa treatment; these include vivid dreams, confusion, and psychotic symptoms more commonly seen in schizophrenia. These effects are probably a result of increased dopaminergic activity in the mesolimbic area of the brain, possibly similar to that found pathologically in schizophrenia (dopaminergic overactivity is implicated in schizophrenia).

Hypotension is common but usually asymptomatic. Cardiac arrhythmias are due to increased catecholamine stimulation following the excessive peripheral metabolism of L-dopa. Dyskinesias can often develop and tend to involve the face and limbs. They usually reflect over-treatment and respond to simple dose reduction.

Three strategies have been developed to optimize L-dopa treatment, to maximize the central effects of L-dopa within the brain, and to minimize its unwanted peripheral effects. These strategies involve coadministration of:

- Carbidopa, an inhibitor of dopa decarboxylase in the periphery, which cannot penetrate the blood–brain barrier. Hence, extracerebral conversion of L-dopa to dopamine is inhibited.
- Domperidone, a dopamine antagonist, which does not penetrate the blood–brain barrier and can, therefore, block the stimulation of dopamine receptors in the periphery.
- Selegiline and entacapone, MAO_B and COMT inhibitors, respectively, which inhibit dopamine degradation in the central nervous system (CNS).

Therapeutic effects: Initially, treatment with L-dopa is effective in 80% of patients with possible restoration of near-normal motor function, but although L-dopa restores dopamine levels in the short term, therapy has no effect on the underlying degenerative disease process.

As progressive neuronal degeneration continues, the capacity of the corpus striatum to covert L-dopa to dopamine diminishes. This affects the majority of patients within 5 years and manifests itself as "end of dose deterioration" (a shortening of duration of each dose of L-dopa) and the "on–off effect" (rapid fluctuations in clinical state, varying from increased mobility and a general improvement to increased rigidity and hypokinesia). The latter effect occurs suddenly and for short periods from a few minutes to a few hours, tending to worsen with length of treatment.

Dopamine agonists

Examples of dopamine agonists include bromocriptine, ropinirole, pergolide, pramipexole, and apomorphine.

Mechanism of action: Bromocriptine, ropinirole, pergolide, pramipexole, and apomorphine are dopamine agonists selective for the D_2 receptor (see Fig. 6.3). Apomorphine also has agonist action at D_1 receptors.

Route of administration: Oral. Apomorphine is given by the subcutaneous route.

Indications: Dopamine agonists are used in combination with L-dopa in an attempt to reduce the late adverse effects of L-dopa therapy ("end of dose deterioration" and "on–off effect") or when L-dopa alone does not adequately control the symptoms.

Adverse effects: The adverse effects of dopamine agonists are essentially similar to those of L-dopa (i.e., nausea, postural hypotension, psychiatric

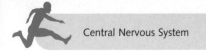

symptoms), but they tend to be more common and more severe. Apomorphine produces profound nausea and vomiting.

Therapeutic notes: Currently, bromocriptine is the most clinically used of the dopamine agonists in the treatment of Parkinson's disease.

Drugs stimulating release of dopamine
Amantadine is an example of a drug that stimulates the release of dopamine (see Fig. 6.3).

Mechanism of action: Facilitation of neuronal dopamine release and inhibition of its reuptake into nerves and additional muscarinic blocking actions.

Route of administration: Oral.

Indications: Amantadine has a synergistic effect when used in conjunction with L-dopa therapy in Parkinson's disease.

Adverse effects: Anorexia, nausea, and hallucinations.

Therapeutic notes: Amantadine has modest antiparkinsonian effects, but it is only of short-term benefit, since most of its effectiveness is lost within 6 months of initiating treatment.

Monoamine oxidase B inhibitors
Selegiline is an example of a MAO_B inhibitor.

Mechanism of action: Selegiline selectively inhibits the MAO_B enzyme in the brain that is normally responsible for the degradation of dopamine (see Fig. 6.3). By reducing the catabolism of dopamine, the actions of L-dopa are potentiated, thus allowing the dose to be reduced by up to one third. There is evidence to suggest that selegiline may slow the progression of the underlying neuronal degeneration in Parkinson's disease.

Route of administration: Oral.

Indications: MAO_B inhibitors can be used on their own in mild cases of parkinsonism or in conjunction with L-dopa to reduce "end of dose deterioration" in severe parkinsonism.

Adverse effects: The adverse effects of MAO_B inhibitors are those that might be expected by potentiation of L-dopa.

Catechol-O-methyl transferase inhibitors
Entacapone has recently been introduced as a catechol-O-methyl transferase (COMT) inhibitor.

Mechanism of action: Dopamine is broken down by a second pathway, in addition to that of MAO_B. The enzyme COMT is responsible for the degradation of dopamine to inactive methylated metabolites. COMT inhibitors specifically inhibit this enzyme.

Route of administration: Oral.

Indications: As an adjunct to L-dopa preparations when "end of dose deterioration" is problematic.

Contraindications: Pheochromocytoma.

Adverse effects: Nausea, vomiting, abdominal pain, and diarrhea.

Therapeutic notes: An earlier COMT inhibitor was withdrawn due to hepatotoxicity, and so liver monitoring with serum enzymes is recommended.

Drugs that inhibit striatal cholinergic activity
Anticholinergic agents
Benztropine, trihexyphenidyl, procyclidine, and orphenadrine are examples of anticholinergic (antimuscarinic) agents.

Mechanism of action: Benztropine, trihexyphenidyl, procyclidine, and orphenadrine are antagonists at the muscarinic receptors that mediate striatal cholinergic excitation (see Fig. 6.3). Their major action in the treatment of Parkinson's disease is to reduce the excessive striatal cholinergic activity that characterizes the disease.

Route of administration: Oral.

Adverse effects: Typical peripheral anticholinergic effects, such as a dry mouth and blurred vision, are less common. More often, patients experience a variety of CNS effects, ranging from mild memory loss to acute confusional states.

Therapeutic notes: Termination of anticholinergic treatment should be gradual, as parkinsonism can worsen when these drugs are withdrawn. Anticholinergic drugs are most effective in controlling tremor rather than other symptoms of Parkinson's disease.

Transplantation
The transplantation of cells from the substantia nigra of human fetuses into the putamen of patients with Parkinson's disease has shown some success in controlling parkinsonian symptoms. Transplantation in the treatment of Parkinson's disease is still experimental, and its role is highly controversial.

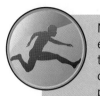

Note that with the possible exception of selegiline, none of the drugs used in Parkinson's disease affect the inevitable progressive degeneration of nigrostriatal dopaminergic neurons. The disease process is unaffected, just compensated for by drug therapy.

Dementia

Alzheimer's disease is a specific process that results in dementia and is unrelated to the dementias associated with stroke, brain trauma, and alcohol. Alzheimer's disease is very common in the elderly, and its prevalence increases markedly with age.

Alzheimer's disease is progressive, and it is associated with shrinkage of the brain substance, loss of neuronal tissue, and deposition of so-called amyloid plaques. The clinical features include deterioration in cognitive function, disorientation, and generalized confusion.

Neuropharmacologic studies have shown that despite widespread shrinkage of the brain, loss of neurons in the forebrain is most marked, and a relative selective loss of cholinergic neurons most likely accounts for the features of this dementia.

The obvious therapeutic target is, therefore, restoration of cholinergic function.

Certain cholinesterase inhibitors appear to improve cognitive functioning in as many as 50% of patients and delay subsequent deterioration in mental capacity.

Cholinesterase inhibitors

Donepezil, galantamine, and rivastigmine are cholinesterase inhibitors, licensed for use in Alzheimer's disease.

Mechanism of action: The cholinesterase inhibitors prevent the breakdown of acetylcholine within the synaptic cleft, and they enhance endogenous cholinergic activity within the CNS and peripheral tissues.

Route of administration: Oral.

Indications: Mild to moderate dementia in Alzheimer's disease.

Contraindications: Pregnancy, breastfeeding, hepatic and renal impairment.

Adverse effects: Nausea, vomiting, diarrhea, anorexia, and agitation.

NMDA receptor channel blocker

Memantine is a low-affinity blocker recently approved for Alzheimer's disease.

Anxiety and sleep disorders

Anxiety and anxiolytics

Anxiety is a state characterized by psychological symptoms such as a diffuse, unpleasant, and vague feeling of apprehension, often accompanied by physical symptoms of autonomic arousal such as palpitations, light-headedness, perspiration, "butterflies," and, in some people, restlessness.

While occasional anxiety is perfectly normal, it is a common and disabling symptom in a variety of mental illnesses including phobias, panic disorders, and obsessive compulsive disorders. Drugs used to treat such anxiety disorders are called anxiolytics.

Sleep disorders and hypnotics

Insomnia is a common and nonspecific disorder that may be reported by 40–50% of people at any given time.

Causes of insomnia include medical illness, alcohol or drugs, periodic limb movement disorder, sleep apnea, and psychiatric illness. Without an obvious underlying cause, it is known as primary or psychophysiologic.

Hypnotics are drugs used to treat psychophysiologic (primary) insomnia. The distinction between the treatment of anxiety and that of sleep disorders is not clear cut, particularly if anxiety is the main impediment to sleep.

Gamma-aminobutyric acid (GABA) receptor

The γ-aminobutyric (GABA) receptors of the $GABA_A$ type are involved in the actions of some classes of hypnotic/anxiolytic drugs, notably:

- The benzodiazepines (BDZs), which are currently the most commonly used clinically.
- Newer nonbenzodiazepine hypnotics (e.g., zolpidem).
- The now-obsolete barbiturates.

The $GABA_A$ receptor belongs to the superfamily of ligand-gated ion channels. It consists of several

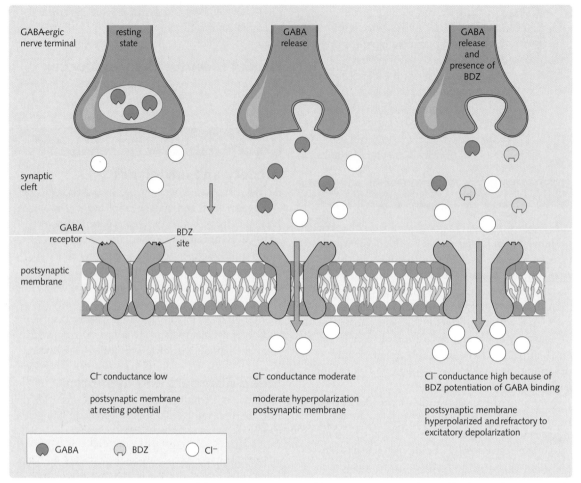

Fig. 6.4 Diagrammatic representation of the GABA$_A$ receptor and how its activity is enhanced by benzodiazepines and similarly by barbiturates (BDZ, benzodiazepine; GABA, γ-aminobutyric acid; Cl$^-$, chloride ion). (Redrawn from Page et al., 2002.)

subunits—α, β, γ, and δ—which form the GABA/Cl$^-$ channel complex, as well as containing benzodiazepine and barbiturate modulatory receptor sites. The GABA site appears to be located on the α- and β-subunits while the benzodiazepine modulatory site is distinct and located on the γ-subunit.

GABA released from nerve terminals binds to postsynaptic GABA$_A$ receptors, the activation of which increases the Cl– conductance of the neuron.

Occupation of the benzodiazepine sites by benzodiazepine receptor agonists enhances the actions of GABA on the Cl$^-$ conductance of the neuronal membrane. The barbiturates similarly enhance the action of GABA, but by occupying a distinct modulatory site (Fig. 6.4).

Anxiolytic and hypnotic drugs

The pharmacotherapy of anxiety and sleep disorders involves several different classes of drug, as shown in Fig. 6.5, and nonpharmacologic management relying upon cognitive and behavior psychotherapy.

Benzodiazepines

Benzodiazepines are drugs with anxiolytic, hypnotic, muscle relaxant, and anticonvulsant actions that are used in the treatment of both anxiety states and insomnia.

Different benzodiazepines are marked as hypnotics and anxiolytics. It is mainly the duration of action that determines the choice of drug (see below).

Anxiolytics and hypnotics	
Anxiolytics	**Hypnotics**
Benzodiazepines (act on GABA$_A$ receptors) e.g., diazepam, lorazepam	Benzodiazepines (act on GABA$_A$ receptors) e.g., triazolam, temazepam, lormetazepam, nitrazepam
Acting on serotonergic receptors (act on 5-HT$_{1A}$ or 5-HT$_3$ receptors) e.g., buspirone	Non-benzodiazepine hypnotics (act on GABA$_A$ receptors) e.g., zopiclone and zolpidem
Other drugs e.g., propranolol antidepressants	Other drugs e.g., choral hydrate chlormethiazole barbiturates (obsolete) sedative antidepressants sedative antihistamines

Fig. 6.5 Drugs used to treat anxiety and sleep disorders (GABA, γ-aminobutyric acid; 5-HT, 5-hydroxytryptamine).

Approximate elimination half-lives of benzodiazepines	
Benzodiazepine	**Approximate half-life (hours)**
Midazolam	2 – 4
Temazepam	8 – 12
Alprazolam	12
Lorazepam	12
Clonazepam	23
Diazepam	32 (one metabolite is active for up to 200 hours)

Fig. 6.6 Approximate elimination half-lives of the benzodiazepines.

Mechanism of action: Benzodiazepines potentiate the action of GABA, the primary inhibitory neurotransmitter in the CNS. They do this by binding to a site on GABA$_A$ receptors, increasing their affinity for GABA. This results in an increased opening frequency of these ligand-gated Cl$^-$ channels, thus potentiating the effect of GABA release in terms of inhibitory effects on the postsynaptic cell (see Fig. 6.4).

Indications: Benzodiazepines are used clinically in the short-term relief of severe anxiety and severe insomnia, preoperative sedation, status epilepticus, and acute alcohol withdrawal.

Route of administration: Oral is the usual route. Intravenous, intramuscular, and rectal preparations are available.

Contraindications: Benzodiazepines should not be given to people with bronchopulmonary disease, and they have additive or synergistic effects with other central depressants such as alcohol, barbiturates, and antihistamines.

Adverse effects: Benzodiazepines have several adverse effects:

- Drowsiness, ataxia, and reduced psychomotor performance are common; therefore, care is necessary when driving or operating machinery.
- Dependence becomes apparent after 4–6 weeks, and is both physical and psychological. The withdrawal syndrome (in 30% of patients)

comprises rebound anxiety and insomnia, tremulousness, and twitching.

Although in overdose benzodiazepines alone are relatively safe when compared with other sedatives (e.g., barbiturates), if benzodiazepines are taken in combination with alcohol, the CNS-depressant effects are potentiated, and fatal respiratory depression can result. Treatment is with the benzodiazepine antagonist flumazenil.

Therapeutic notes: Benzodiazepines are active orally, and they differ mainly in respect of their duration of action (Fig. 6.6). Short-acting agents (e.g., lorazepam and temazepam) are metabolized to inactive compounds, and these are used mainly as sleeping pills because of the relative lack of "hangover" effects in the morning. Some long-acting agents (e.g., diazepam) are converted to long-lasting active metabolites with half-lives longer than the administered parent drug. With others (e.g., nitrazepam), it is the parent drug itself that is metabolized slowly. Such drugs are more suitable for an anxiolytic effect maintained all day long, or when early morning waking is the problem.

Nonbenzodiazepine hypnotics

Zolpidem and zaleplon are new-generation hypnotics that have a short duration of action with little or no hangover effect.

Although these drugs are not benzodiazepines, they act in a comparable manner to benzodiazepines on the GABA$_A$ receptor, although (it is thought) at a different site.

Anxiolytic drugs acting at serotonergic receptors

The serotonergic theory of anxiety suggests that serotonergic transmission is involved in anxiety as, in general, stimulation of this system causes anxiety, while a reduction in serotonergic neuronal activity reduces anxiety.

The serotonergic theory prompted the development of anxiolytic drugs that act to moderate serotonergic neurotransmission while not causing sedation and incoordination.

5-hydroxytryptamine 1A agonists

Buspirone is a serotonergic (5-hydroxytryptamine 1A; 5-HT1$_A$) agonist.

Mechanism of action: In the raphe nucleus, the dendrites of serotonergic neurons possess inhibitory presynaptic autoreceptors of the 5-HT$_{1A}$ subtype that, when stimulated, decrease the firing of 5-HT neurons. This class of anxiolytic agents called the azapirones is thought to reduce 5-HT transmission by acting as partial agonists at these 5-HT$_{1A}$ receptors. Buspirone is the first of this new class of anxiolytics. Sumatriptan is similar.

Route of administration: Oral.

Indications: Buspirone is indicated for the short-term relief of generalized anxiety disorder.

Contraindications: 5-HT$_{1A}$ agonists should not be used in people with epilepsy.

Adverse effects: The adverse effects of 5-HT$_{1A}$ agonists include nervousness, dizziness, headache, and light-headedness.

In contrast to benzodiazepines, buspirone does not cause significant sedation or cognitive impairment, and it carries only a minimal risk of dependence and withdrawal. It does not potentiate the effects of alcohol.

Therapeutic notes: The anxiolytic effects of buspirone gradually evolve over 1–3 weeks.

5-hydroxytryptamine 3 antagonists

Ondansetron is a 5-HT$_3$ receptor antagonist that is well established for use as an antiemetic drug. Ondansetron also has anxiolytic properties by virtue of its antagonism at the excitatory postsynaptic 5-HT$_3$ receptor.

Beta-adrenoreceptor blockers

Beta-adrenoreceptor blockers or β-blockers (e.g., propranolol) can be very effective in alleviating the somatic manifestations of anxiety caused by marked sympathetic arousal, such as palpitations, tremor, sweating, and diarrhea.

Mechanism of action: Beta blockers act by antagonism at β-adrenoreceptors so that excessive catecholamine release does not produce the sympathetic responses of tachycardia, sweating, etc. Beta blockers are also used in cardiovascular disease.

Route of administration: Oral.

Indications: Beta blockers are indicated in patients with predominantly somatic symptoms; this, in turn, may prevent the onset of worry and fear. Patients with predominantly psychological symptoms may obtain no benefit. Beta blockers can be useful in social phobias and to reduce performance anxiety in musicians, for whom fine motor control may be critical.

Contraindications: Beta blockers should not be used in people with asthma or heart failure.

Adverse effects: Beta blockers can cause bradycardia, heart failure, bronchospasm, and peripheral vasoconstriction.

Barbiturates

Barbiturates are nonselective CNS depressants that produce effects ranging from sedation and reduction of anxiety to unconsciousness and death from respiratory and cardiovascular failure. Barbiturates increase GABA-mediated inhibition by acting on the same receptor as benzodiazepines, though at a different site.

At low doses, barbiturates prolong the duration of individual Cl$^-$ channel openings triggered by a given GABA stimulus (benzodiazepines increase the frequency of Cl$^-$ channel openings). At high doses, they are far more depressant than benzodiazepines because they start to increase Cl$^-$ conductance directly, thus decreasing the sensitivity of the postsynaptic membrane to excitatory transmitters.

While very popular until the 1960s as sedative/hypnotic agents, they are now obsolete since they readily lead to psychological and physical dependence, and a relatively small overdose can be fatal. Conversely, benzodiazepines, which have largely replaced barbiturates as sedative/hypnotics, have been taken in huge overdoses without serious long-term effects.

Barbiturates are still important in anesthesia and to a lesser extent in the treatment of epilepsy.

Miscellaneous agents

There are a number of miscellaneous hypnotic agents that have been used historically and which are still prescribed under certain circumstances.

Chloral hydrate and derivatives

Chloral hydrate is metabolized to trichloroethanol, which is an effective hypnotic. It is cheap, but it causes gastric irritation, and there is no convincing evidence that it has any advantage over the newer benzodiazepines.

Chloral hydrate and its derivatives were previously popular hypnotics for children. Current thinking does not justify the use of hypnotics in children, and these drugs now have very limited uses.

Antidepressants

If the underlying cause of insomnia is associated with depression, or particularly in depressed patients exhibiting anxiety and agitation, then tricyclic antidepressants (TCAs) with sedative actions (e.g., amitriptyline) may be useful, as they act as a hypnotic when given at bedtime. Alternatively, selective serotonin reuptake inhibitors (SSRIs) may correct the mood disorder and lessen the symptoms of anxiety or insomnia.

Sedative antihistamines

The older antihistamine drugs (e.g., diphenhydramine) have antimuscarinic actions and pass the blood–brain barrier, commonly causing drowsiness and psychomotor impairment.

Proprietary brands of diphenhydramine are on sale to the public to relieve temporary sleep disturbances, as these drugs are relatively safe.

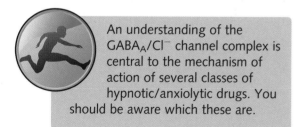

An understanding of the GABA$_A$/Cl$^-$ channel complex is central to the mechanism of action of several classes of hypnotic/anxiolytic drugs. You should be aware which these are.

Affective disorders

Affective disorders involve a disturbance of mood (cognitive/emotional symptoms) associated with changes in behavior, energy, appetite, and sleep (biologic symptoms).

Affective disorders can be thought of as pathologic extremes of the normal continuum of human moods, from extreme excitement and elation (mania) to severe depressive states.

There are two types of affective disorder, unipolar affective disorders and bipolar affective disorders.

Unipolar affective disorders

Unipolar affective disorder is characterized by misery, malaise, despair, guilt, apathy, indecisiveness, low energy and fatigue, changes in sleeping pattern, loss of appetite, and suicidal thoughts.

Attempts have been made to classify types of depression as either "reactive" or "endogenous" in origin.

Reactive depression is attributable to a clear psychological cause (e.g., bereavement). It involves less severe symptoms and less likelihood of biologic disturbance. It affects 3–10% of the population, with the incidence increasing with age, and it is more common in females.

Endogenous depression is associated with no clear cause, more severe symptoms (e.g., suicidal thought), and a greater likelihood of biologic disturbance (e.g., insomnia, anorexia). It affects 1% of the population, usually starting in early adulthood, and affects both sexes equally.

The distinction between reactive and endogenous depression is of importance since there is some evidence that depressions with endogenous features tend to respond better to drug therapy.

Bipolar affective disorders

Bipolar affective disorder (BPAD) presents with mood and behavior oscillating between depression and mania, and it is, therefore, also known as manic–depressive disorder.

Bipolar affective disorder develops earlier in life than unipolar depressive disorders, and it tends to be inherited. It affects 1% of the population, and it can have associated elements of psychotic phenomena.

Monoamine theory of depression

The etiology of major depressive disorders is not clear. Genetic, environmental, and neurochemical influences have all been examined as possible etiological factors.

The most widely accepted neurochemical explanation of endogenous depression involves the monoamines (norepinephrine, NE; serotonin, 5-HT;

dopamine, DA). The original hypothesis of depression, "the monoamine theory," stated that depression resulted from a functional deficit of these transmitter amines, while conversely mania was caused by an excess.

The monoamine theory explains why:
- Drugs that deplete monoamines are depressant (e.g., reserpine and methyldopa).
- A wide range of drugs that increase the functional availability of monoamine neurotransmitters improve mood in depressed patients (e.g., tricyclics [TCA] and monoamine oxidase inhibitors [MAOIs]).
- The concentration of monoamines and their metabolites is reduced in the cerebrospinal fluid (CSF) of depressed patients.
- In some post-mortem studies, the most consistent finding is an elevation in cortical 5-HT$_2$ binding.

The monoamine theory cannot explain why:
- A number of compounds that increase the functional availability of monoamines (e.g., amphetamines, cocaine, and L-dopa) have no effect on the mood of depressed patients.
- Some older, atypical antidepressants (e.g., iprindole) worked without manipulating monoaminergic systems.
- There is a "therapeutic delay" of 2 weeks between the full neurochemical effects of antidepressants and the start of their therapeutic effect.

It is unlikely, therefore, that monoamine mechanisms alone are responsible for the symptoms of depression. Other systems that may be involved in depression include:
- The GABA system.
- The neuropeptide systems, particularly vasopressin and the endogenous opiates.
- Secondary-messenger systems, which also appear to have a crucial role in some treatments.

Treatment of unipolar depressive disorders

The major classes of drug that are used to treat depression, and their mechanisms of action, are summarized in Fig. 6.7.

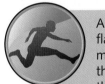 Although almost certainly flawed and incomplete, the monoamine theory is probably the best way to rationalize your thinking about affective disorders and to understand the mechanism of action of the drugs used in their treatment.

Major classes of antidepressant drug and mechanism of action		
Class of antidepressant drug	**Examples**	**Mode of action**
Tricyclic antidepressants (TCAs)	Amitriptyline Imipramine Lofepramine	Nonspecific blockers of monoamine uptake
Selective serotonin reuptake inhibitors (SSRIs)	Fluoxetine Paroxetine Sertraline	Selective blockers of 5-HT reuptake
Serotonin norepinephrine reuptake inhibitors (SNRIs)	Venlafaxine	Selective blockers of 5-HT and norepinephrine uptake
Monoamine oxidase inhibitors (MAOIs)	Phenelzine Tranylcypromine	Noncompetitive, nonselective irreversible blockers of MAO$_A$ and MAO$_B$
Reversible inhibitors of MAO$_A$ (RIMAs)	Moclobemide	Reversibly inhibit MAO$_A$ selectively
Atypical	Reboxetine Mirtazapine	Act by various mechanisms that are poorly understood

Fig. 6.7 Major classes of antidepressant drugs and their mechanism of action (5-HT, 5-hydroxytryptamine; MAO, monoamine oxidase).

Tricyclic antidepressants and related drugs

Examples of TCAs and related drugs include amitriptyline, imipramine, and lofepramine.

Mechanism of action: TCAs act by blocking 5-HT and noradrenaline uptake into the presynaptic terminal from the synaptic cleft (Fig. 6.8). They have a certain affinity for H_1 and muscarinic receptors, and for α_1- and α_2-receptors.

Contraindications: TCAs and related drugs should not be used in:

- Recent myocardial infarction or arrhythmias (especially heart block), since TCAs increase the risk of conduction abnormalities.
- Manic phase.
- Severe liver disease.
- Epilepsy, where TCAs lower the seizure threshold.
- Patients taking other anticholinergic drugs, alcohol, or epinephrine, as TCAs potentiate the effects of these. Lidocaine is contraindicated in combination with TCAs, owing to a potentially fatal drug interaction.

Adverse effects: While TCAs are an effective therapy for depression, the adverse effects can reduce patient compliance and acceptability. Side effects include:

- Muscarinic blocking effects such as a dry mouth, blurred vision, and constipation.
- Alpha-adrenergic blocking effects causing postural hypotension.
- Norepinephrine uptake block in the heart, increasing the risk of arrhythmias.
- Histamine-blocking effects leading to sedation.
- Weight gain.

TCAs are relatively dangerous in overdose. Patients present with confusion, mania, and potentially fatal arrhythmias due to the cardiotoxic nature of the drug.

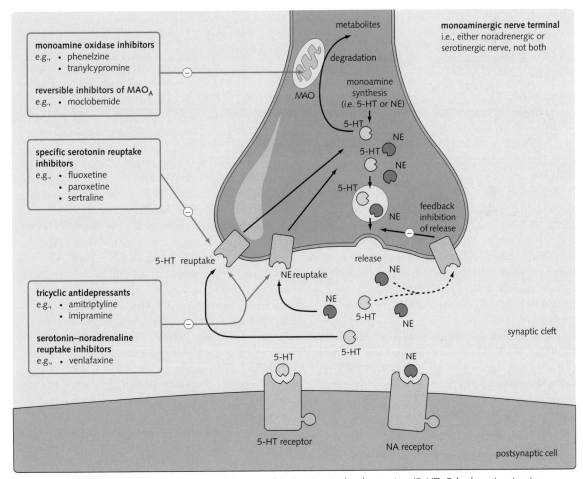

Fig. 6.8 Site of action of the major classes of drug used to treat unipolar depression (5-HT, 5-hydroxytryptamine [serotonin]; MAO, monoamine oxidase; NE, norepinephrine).

Therapeutic notes: No individual TCA has superior antidepressant activity, and the choice of drug is usually determined by the most acceptable or desired side effects. For example, drugs with sedative actions, such as amitriptyline, are the TCAs of choice for patients in agitated or anxious states. The most recent TCA is lofepramine, which causes fewer antimuscarinic side effects and is less dangerous if taken in overdose.

Therapeutic effects take 2–3 weeks to develop. TCA-related antidepressants should be withdrawn slowly.

Selective serotonin reuptake inhibitors

Selective serotonin (5-HT) reuptake inhibitors (SSRIs) are the most recently introduced class of antidepressant agent. Fluoxetine (Prozac®) is an SSRI. Other examples include citalopram, fluvoxamine, paroxetine, and sertraline.

Mechanism of action: SSRIs act with a high specificity for potent inhibition of serotonin reuptake into nerve terminals from the synaptic cleft, while having only minimal effects on noradrenaline uptake (see Fig. 6.8). They block serotonin transporters, which belong to a class of Na^+/Cl^--coupled transporters.

Contraindications: Contraindications with SSRIs are few. They should not be used with MAOIs, as the combination can cause a potentially fatal serotonergic syndrome of hyperthermia and cardiovascular collapse.

Adverse effects: The side-effect profile of SSRIs is much better than that of TCAs and MAOIs, as there are no amine interactions, anticholinergic actions, adrenergic blockade, or toxic effects in overdose. Adverse effects, however, caused by their effect on serotonergic nerves throughout the body, include nausea, diarrhea, insomnia, anxiety, and agitation. Sexual dysfunction is sometimes a problem.

Therapeutic notes: SSRIs have a similar efficacy to that of TCAs. Their clinical advantages and lack of side effects have led to their popularity. These include no anticholinergic effects, no toxicity in overdose, and no cardiotoxic effects. SSRIs are now the most widely prescribed antidepressants.

Serotonin–norepinephrine reuptake inhibitors

The only drug currently in the serotonin–norepinephrine reuptake inhibitor (SNRIs) new class of antidepressants is venlafaxine.

Mechanism of action: SNRIs cause potentiation of neurotransmitter activity in the CNS, probably by inhibiting reuptake of both serotonin and norepinephrine (see Fig. 6.8).

Contraindications: The drug interactions of SNRIs are much like those of SSRIs; however, extra care must be taken with hypertensive patients, as venlafaxine raises blood pressure.

Adverse effects: The adverse effects of SNRIs are similar to those of SSRIs, but they occur with lower frequency.

Therapeutic notes: The pharmacologic effects of venlafaxine are similar to those of the TCAs, but adverse effects are reduced because it has little affinity for cholinergic and histaminergic receptors or α-adrenoreceptors.

Monoamine oxidase inhibitors

Examples of irreversible monoamine oxidase inhibitors (MAOIs) include phenelzine, tranylcypromine, and isocarboxazid; and examples of reversible inhibitors of MAO_A (RIMAs) include moclobemide.

Mechanism of action: MAOIs block the action of MAO_A and MAO_B, which are neuron enzymes that metabolize (degrade) the monoamines (norepinephrine, 5-HT, and dopamine) (see Fig. 6.8). MAO has two main isoforms, MAO_A and MAO_B, which differ in terms of substrate preference; inhibition of the MAO_A form correlates best with antidepressant efficacy. Both non-selective irreversible blockers of MAO_A and MAO_B, and drugs that reversibly inhibit MAO_A are available.

Adverse effects: Dietary interactions may occur, such as the "cheese reaction." MAO in the gut wall and liver normally breaks down ingested tyramine. When the enzyme is inhibited, tyramine reaches the circulation and causes the release of norepinephrine from sympathetic nerve terminals; this can lead to a severe and potentially fatal rise in blood pressure. Patients on MAOIs must, therefore, avoid foods rich in tyramine, which include cheese, game, and alcoholic drinks. Preparations containing sympathomimetic amines (e.g., cough mixtures and nasal decongestants) should also be avoided. MAOIs are not specific, and they reduce the metabolism of barbiturates, opioids, and alcohol. Side effects include CNS stimulation causing excitement and tremor, sympathetic blockade causing postural hypotension, and muscarinic blockade causing a dry mouth and blurred vision. Phenelzine can be hepatotoxic.

Therapeutic notes: Response to treatment with MAOIs may be delayed for 3 weeks or more. Phobic and depressed patients with atypical, hypochondriacal, or hysterical features are said to respond best to MAOIs. Because of the dietary and drug restrictions outlined above, MAOIs are largely reserved for depression refractory to other antidepressants and treatment.

Atypical antidepressants

Examples of atypical antidepressants include reboxetine and mirtazapine.

Mechanism of action: Reboxetine is a selective inhibitor of norepinephrine reuptake, increasing the concentration of this mediator in the synaptic cleft. Mirtazapine has α_2-adrenoreceptor-blocking activity, which, by acting on inhibitory α_2-autoreceptors on central noradrenergic nerve endings, may increase the amount of norepinephrine in the synaptic cleft.

Contraindications: The contraindications for atypical antidepressants are similar to those for TCAs.

Adverse effects: Atypical antidepressants generally cause less autonomic side effects and are less dangerous in overdose, owing to their lower cardiotoxicity compared with TCAs. Mirtazapine may cause agranulocytosis.

Therapeutic notes: Mirtazapine is sedative and is, therefore, used in depression when a degree of sedation is desirable. Neither reboxetine nor mirtazapine is currently a first-line drug for the treatment of depression.

Treatment of bipolar affective disorders

Bipolar affective disorder (BPAD) is treated with a combination of mood stabilizers and antidepressants, and sometimes antipsychotics. Mood stabilizers include lithium and carbamazepine.

Lithium

Lithium is administered as lithium carbonate, and it is the most widely used mood stabilizer, with antimanic and antidepressant activity.

Mechanism of action: The mechanism of action of lithium is unclear, but it probably involves modulation of secondary-messenger pathways of cAMP and inositol triphosphate (IP_3). It is known that lithium inhibits the pathway for recapturing inositol for the resynthesis of polyphosphoinositides. It may exert its effect by reducing the concentrations of lipids important in secondary signal transduction in the brain.

Indications: Lithium salts are mainly used in the prophylaxis and treatment of BPAD, but also in the prophylaxis and treatment of acute mania and in the prophylaxis of resistant recurrent depression.

Contraindications: Some drugs may interact, causing a rise in plasma lithium concentration and so should be avoided. Such drugs include antipsychotics, non-steroidal anti-inflammatory drugs (NSAIDs), diuretics, and cardioactive drugs. Lithium is excreted via the kidney, and caution should be employed in patients with renal impairment.

Adverse effects: Lithium has a long plasma half-life and a narrow therapeutic window; therefore, side effects are common, and plasma concentration monitoring is essential. Early side effects include thirst, nausea, diarrhea, tremor, and polyuria; late side effects include weight gain, edema, acne, nephrogenic diabetes insipidus, and hypothyroidism. Toxicity/overdose (serum level >2–3 mmol/L) effects include vomiting, diarrhea, tremor, ataxia, confusion, and coma.

Therapeutic notes: The decision to give prophylactic lithium requires specialist advice, and careful monitoring after initiation of treatment is essential.

Carbamazepine

Carbamazepine is as effective as lithium in the prophylaxis of BPAD and acute mania, particularly in rapidly alternating BPAD.

Mechanism of action: Carbamazepine is a GABA agonist, and this may be the basis of its antimanic properties. The relevance of its effect in stabilizing neuronal sodium and on calcium channels is unclear.

Adverse effects: Drowsiness, diplopia, nausea, ataxia, rashes, and headache; blood disorders such as agranulocytosis and leukopenia; and drug interactions with lithium, antipsychotics, TCAs, and MAOIs. Many other drugs can be affected by the effect of carbamazepine on inducing hepatic enzymes. Diplopia, ataxia, clonus, tremor, and sedation are associated with acute carbamazepine toxicity.

Therapeutic notes: At the start of treatment with carbamazepine, plasma concentrations should be monitored to establish a maintenance dose.

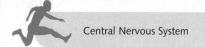
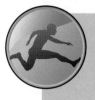
Mania hardly ever exists in isolation from depression, which is why it is referred to as bipolar affective disorder, as it has two faces.

Psychotic disorders

Basic concepts
Psychotic disorders are characterized by a mental state that is out of touch with reality, involving a variety of abnormalities of perception, thought, and ideas.

Psychotic illnesses include:
• Schizophrenia.
• Schizoaffective disorder.
• Delusional disorders.
• Some depressive and manic illnesses.

Schizophrenia is the most important of these psychotic illnesses because of its prevalence, young age of onset, and chronic and disabling nature.

Neuroleptics, or antipsychotics, are drugs used in the treatment of psychotic disorders.

Schizophrenia
Epidemiology
Schizophrenia characteristically develops in people aged 15–45 years; it has a relatively stable cross-cultural incidence affecting 1% of the population; 64% of cases are male.

Symptoms and signs
Schizophrenia is a psychotic illness characterized by multiple symptoms affecting thought, perceptions, emotion, and volition.

Symptoms fall into two groups (positive and negative) that may have different underlying causes.
Positive symptoms include:
• Delusions, which are false personal beliefs held with absolute conviction.
• Hallucinations, which are false perceptions in the absence of a real external stimulus; most commonly, these are auditory (hearing voices) and occur in 60–70% of schizophrenics, but they can be visual, tactile, or olfactory.
• Thought alienation and disordered thought, which is the belief that one's thoughts are under the control of an outside agency (e.g., aliens, CIA).

This type of belief is common, and thought processes are often incomprehensible.

Negative symptoms include:
• Poverty of speech, which is a restriction in the amount of spontaneous speech.
• Flattening of affect, which is a loss of normal experience and expression of emotion.
• Social withdrawal.
• Anhedonia, which is an inability to experience pleasure.
• Apathy, involving reduced drive, energy, and interest.
• Attention deficit, manifested by inattentiveness at work or on interview.

The distinction between the positive and negative symptoms found in schizophrenia is of importance, as neuroleptic drugs tend to have most effect on positive symptoms, while negative symptoms are fairly refractory to treatment and carry a worse prognosis.

Theories of schizophrenia
The cause of schizophrenia remains mysterious. Any theory of the cause of schizophrenia must take into account the strong, though not invariable, hereditary tendency (50% concurrence in monozygotic twins), as well as the environmental factors known to predispose toward its development.

Many hypotheses have been suggested to explain the manifestations of schizophrenia at the level of neurotransmitters in the brain. The potential role of excessive dopaminergic activity, in particular, has attracted considerable attention. Evidence for this theory includes the following:
• Most antipsychotic drugs block dopamine receptors, the clinical dose being proportional to the ability to block D_2 receptors.
• Single positive electron tomography ligand scans show that there are increased D_2 receptors in the nucleus accumbens of schizophrenic patients.
• Psychotic symptoms can be induced by drugs that increase dopaminergic activity, such as some of the anti-parkinsonian agents.

However, there is much evidence that the dopaminergic theory fails to explain. Current research indicates a likely role for other neurotransmitters in schizophrenia, including 5-HT, GABA, and glutamate. Although the dopamine theory cannot explain many of the features and

Dopamine receptors		
Type	2nd messengers + cellular effects	Location in CNS and postulated function
D_1	cAMP increase	• Mainly postsynaptic inhibition • Functions unclear
D_2	cAMP decrease K^+ conductance up Ca^{2+} conductance down	• Mainly presynaptic inhibition of dopamine synthesis/release in nigrostriatal, mesolimbic, and tuberoinfundibular systems • Affinity of neuroleptics for D_2 receptors correlates with antipsychotic potency.
D_3	Unknown	• Localized mainly in limbic and cortical structures concerned with cognitive functions and emotional behaviour • Not clear whether antipsychotic effects of neuroleptics are mediated by the D_3 type
D_4	Unknown	• Similar to D_3 type; clozapine has particular affinity for D_4 receptors

Fig. 6.9 Classes of dopamine receptor (CNS, central nervous system).

Neuroleptic drugs		
Class	Chemical classification	Examples
Typical anti-psychotics	Phenothiazines: • propylamine side chains • piperidine side chains • piperazine side chains	Chlorpromazine Thioridazine Fluphenazine
	Butyrophenones	Haloperidol
	Thioxanthines	Flupentixol
Atypical anti-psychotics	Dibenzodiazepines	Clozapine, olanzapine
	Dopamine/5-HT blockers; • diphenylbutylpiperidines • substituted benzamides • benzixasoles	Pimozide Sulpiride Risperidone

Fig. 6.10 Classes of neuroleptic drugs (5-HT, 5-hydroxytryptamine).

findings in schizophrenia, most current pharmacological treatment (typical neuroleptics) is aimed at dopaminergic transmission (Fig. 6.9).

Neuroleptic drugs

The treatment of schizophrenia and all other psychotic illnesses involves the use of antipsychotic medication, the neuroleptic drugs. Neuroleptic drugs produce a general improvement in all the acute

positive symptoms of schizophrenia, but it is less clear how effective they are in the treatment of chronic schizophrenia and negative symptoms.

Mechanism of action: Antipsychotic drugs have a variety of structures and fall into various classes (Fig. 6.10). There is a strong correlation between clinical potency and affinity for D_2 receptors among the typical neuroleptics.

Neuroleptics take days or weeks to work, suggesting that secondary effects (e.g., increase in number of D_2 receptors in limbic structure) may be more important than a direct effect of D_2 receptor block. It was once thought, therefore, that neuroleptics exerted their antipsychotic effect by interfering with dopamine transmission at D_2 receptors in the mesocortical and mesolimbic systems. The development of newer atypical neuroleptics that are not very active at the D_2 receptor but which are still clinically effective has challenged this hypothesis.

Most neuroleptics also block other monoamine receptors, and this is often the cause of some of the side effects of these drugs.

The distinction between typical and atypical groups is not clearly defined, but it rests partly on the incidence of extrapyramidal motor side effects and partly on receptor specificity. Atypical neuroleptics are less prone to producing motor disorders than other drugs, and they tend to have different pharmacologic profiles with respect to dopamine and other receptor specificity.

Route of administration: All the neuroleptic drugs can be given orally, though some of the typical drugs can be given by the intramuscular route, which prolongs their release and aids drug compliance.

Typical neuroleptics
Phenothiazines

This class of compounds is subdivided into three groups by the type of side chain attached to the mother structure (phenothiazine ring) (see Fig. 6.10). Side-effect patterns vary with the different side chains:

- Propylamine side chains (e.g., in chlorpromazine) produce strong sedation, a moderate muscarinic block, and moderate motor disturbance. Indicated for violent patients, owing to their sedative effect.
- Piperidine side chains (e.g., in thioridazine) produce moderate sedation, strong muscarinic block, and low motor disturbance. Favored for use in the elderly.
- Piperazine side chains (e.g., in fluphenazine) produce low sedation, low muscarinic block, and strong motor disturbance. Contraindicated for use in the elderly, owing to the motor effects.

Butyrophenones and thioxanthenes

The butyrophenone and thioxanthene groups of compounds have the same profile of low sedation, low muscarinic block, and high incidence of motor disturbance.

An example of a butyrophenone compound is haloperidol; thiothixene is an example of the thioxanthenes.

Atypical neuroleptics
Dibenzodiazepines

Dibenzodiazepines such as clozapine and olanzapine have a low affinity for the D_2 receptor and a higher affinity for D_1 and D_4 receptors.

Indications: Atypical neuroleptics are indicated only in chronic cases refractory to other drugs or with severe motor disturbance. This is due to a 1% risk of potentially fatal neutropenia in those patients on these agents.

Adverse effects: Clozapine has a low incidence of adverse motor effects because of its low affinity for the D_2 receptor. Side effects of dibenzodiazepines

Adverse effects of neuroleptics
• Acute neurological effects: acute dystonia, akathisia, parkinsonism
• Chronic neurological effects: tardive dyskinesia, tardive dystonia
• Neuroendocrine effects: amenorrhea, galactorrhea, infertility
• Idiosyncratic: neuroleptic malignant syndrome
• Anticholinergic: dry mouth, blurred vision, constipation, urinary retention, ejaculatory failure
• Antihistaminergic: sedation
• Antiadrenergic: hypotension, arrhythmia
• Miscellaneous: photosensitivity, heat sensitivity, cholestatic jaundice, retinal pigmentation

Fig. 6.11 Adverse effects of the neuroleptics (Adapted from Page *et al.*, 2002).

include hypersalivation, sedation, weight gain, tachycardia, and hypotension.

Therapeutic notes: Olanzapine is similar to clozapine but carries less risk of agranulocytosis.

Dopamine/5-HT blockers

Examples of dopamine/5-HT blockers include the diphenylbutylpiperidines and the benzixasoles. Examples of the former include pimozide; examples of the latter include risperidone.

Pimozide shows high selectivity for D_2 receptors compared with D_1 or other neurotransmitter receptors. Pimozide appears to be similar to conventional neuroleptic agents, but it has a longer duration of action, allowing once daily medication.

Benzixasoles such as risperidone show a high affinity for 5-HT receptors and a lower affinity for D_2 receptors. With this class of drugs, extrapyramidal motor side effects occur with less frequency than with classic neuroleptics.

Adverse effects of neuroleptics

Neuroleptic drugs cause a variety of adverse effects (Fig. 6.11).

The majority of the unwanted effects of neuroleptics can be inferred from their pharmacologic actions, such as the disruption of dopaminergic pathways (the major action of most neuroleptics) and the blockade of monoamine and other receptors, including muscarinic receptors, α-adrenoreceptors, and histamine receptors.

In addition, individual drugs may cause immunological reactions or have their own characteristic side-effect profile.

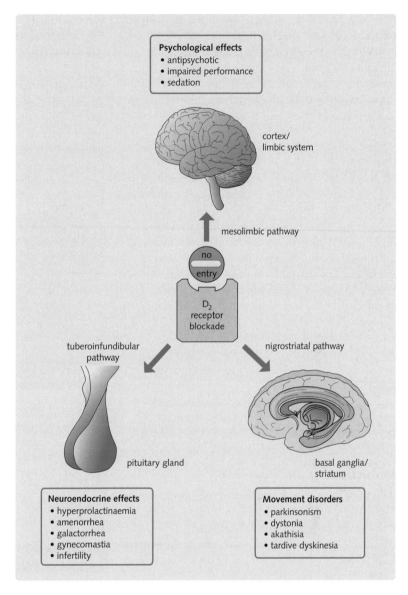

Fig. 6.12 Effect of D$_2$ dopamine receptor blockade on the dopaminergic pathways in the brain.

Adverse effects on the dopaminergic pathways

There are three main dopaminergic pathways in the brain (Fig. 6.12):

- Mesolimbic and/or mesocortical dopamine pathways running from groups of cells in the midbrain to the nucleus accumbens and amygdala. This pathway affects thoughts and motivation.
- Nigrostriatal dopamine pathways running from the midbrain to the caudate nuclei. This pathway is important in smooth motor control.
- Tuberoinfundibular neurons running from the hypothalamus to the pituitary gland, the secretions of which they regulate.

Antagonism of dopamine receptors leads to interference with the normal functioning of these pathways, bringing about unwanted side effects as well as the desired antipsychotic effect. This antagonism is the cause of the most serious side effects associated with neuroleptic use, which include:

- Psychological effects due to D$_2$ receptor blockade of the mesolimbic/mesocortical pathway.
- Movement disorders due to D$_2$ receptor blockade of the nigrostriatal pathways.
- Neuroendocrine disorders due to D$_2$ receptor blockade of the tuberoinfundibular pathway.

It is by dopaminergic antagonism of the mesolimbic mesocortical pathway that it is thought that typical neuroleptics exert their antipsychotic effects. However, as a side effect of mesolimbic and mesocortical dopaminergic inhibition, sedation and impaired performance are common.

Blocking of dopamine receptors in the basal ganglia (corpus striatum) frequently results in distressing and disabling movement disorders. Two main types of movement disorder occur. Acute reversible parkinsonian-like symptoms (tremor, rigidity, and akinesia) are treated by dose reduction, anticholinergic drugs, or switching to an atypical neuroleptic. Slowly developing tardive dyskinesia, often irreversible, and manifesting as involuntary movements of the face, trunk, and limbs, appears months or years after the start of neuroleptic treatment. It may be a result of proliferation or sensitization of dopamine receptors. Incidence is unpredictable, and it affects approximately 20% of long-term users of neuroleptics. Treatment is generally unsuccessful. The newer atypical neuroleptics may be less likely to induce tardive dyskinesia.

By reducing the negative feedback on the anterior pituitary, over-secretion of prolactin can result (hyperprolactinemia). This can lead to gynecomastia, galactorrhea, menstrual irregularities, impotence, and weight gain in some patients (see Fig. 6.12).

Adverse effects from nonselective receptor blockade
The adverse effects of neuroleptics from nonselective receptor blockade include:
- Anticholinergic effects due to muscarinic-receptor blockade, such as dry mouth, urinary retention, constipation, blurred vision, etc.
- Adverse effects due to α-adrenoreceptor blockade. Many neuroleptics have the capacity to block α-adrenoreceptors and cause postural hypotension.
- Adverse effects due to histamine-receptor blockade. Antagonism of central histamine H_1 receptors may contribute to sedation.

Adverse effects due to individual drugs or immune reactions
The neuroleptic drug clozapine can cause neutropenia due to toxic bone marrow suppression, while pimozide can cause sudden death secondary to cardiac arrhythmia.

Immune reactions to neuroleptic drugs can include dermatitis, rashes, photosensitivity, and urticaria. Such reactions are more common with the phenothiazines, which can also cause deposits in the cornea and lens.

Neuroleptic malignant syndrome
Neuroleptic malignant syndrome is the most lethal adverse effect of neuroleptic use. It is an idiosyncratic reaction of unknown pathophysiology. Symptoms include fever, extrapyramidal motor disturbance, muscle rigidity, and coma. Urgent treatment is indicated.

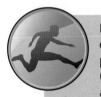

Neuroleptics have many side effects, some related to their principal mechanism of action (dopamine receptor antagonism) and some unrelated to this. Learn these well, as they are a popular examination topic.

Nausea and vertigo

Nausea and vertigo are common clinical problems, and they may represent a whole array of pathologies. The use of antiemetic drugs can be very effective at alleviating these symptoms, though caution must be taken to ensure that the underlying mechanism for the symptoms is investigated.

Antiemetic drugs are discussed in the gastrointestinal chapter (Chapter 10).

Epilepsy

Definitions
Epilepsy is a chronic disease in which seizures result from the abnormal discharge of cerebral neurons.

A seizure is a particular behavior produced by an abnormal high-frequency discharge of a group of neurons, starting focally and spreading to a varying extent to affect other parts of the brain. According to the focus and spread of discharges, seizures may be classified as:
- Partial (focal), which originate at a specific focus and do not spread to involve other cortical areas.
- Generalized, which usually have a focus (often in the temporal lobe) and then spread to other areas.

Classification of common epileptic syndromes	
Partial (local, focal) seizures	**Generalized seizures**
• Psychomotor (temporal lobe) epilepsy	• Tonic–clonic seizure or grand-mal epilepsy
• Partial motor epilepsy	• Absence seizure or petit-mal epilepsy

Fig. 6.13 Classification of common epileptic syndromes.

Different epileptic syndromes can be classified on the basis of seizure type and pattern, with other clinical features (such as age of onset), anatomic location of focus, and etiology taken into account.

Common types of epileptic syndromes
Epileptic syndromes result from either generalized seizures or focal seizures (Fig. 6.13).

Generalized seizure involves loss of consciousness, and it may be convulsive or nonconvulsive:
- Tonic–clonic, or grand-mal, epilepsy is a convulsive generalized seizure characterized by periods of tonic muscle rigidity followed later by massive jerking of the body (clonus).
- Absence, or petit-mal, seizures are generalized seizures characterized by changes in consciousness lasting less than 10 seconds. They occur most commonly in children, where they can be confused with day dreaming.

The effect on the body of focal seizures depends on the location of the abnormal signal focus. For example, involvement of the motor cortex will produce convulsions, whereas involvement of the brainstem can produce unconsciousness.

Psychomotor or temporal lobe epilepsy results from a partial seizure with cortical activity localized to the temporal lobe. Such seizures are characterized by features including impaired consciousness or confusion, amnesia, emotional instability, atypical behavior, and outbursts.

Partial motor seizures have their focus in cortical motor regions, and they present with convulsive or tonic activity corresponding to the neurons involved (e.g., the left arm).

Another type of epileptic syndrome is status epilepticus. This is a state in which fits follow each other without consciousness being regained. Status epilepticus constitutes a medical emergency because of possible exhaustion of vital centers.

Causes of epilepsy
The etiology of epilepsy is unknown in 60–70% of cases, but heredity is an important factor.

Damage to the brain—for example, by tumors, head injury, infections, or cerebrovascular accident—may subsequently cause epilepsy.

The neurochemical basis of the abnormal discharges in epilepsy is not known, but it may involve altered GABA metabolism.

Treatment of epilepsy
Drugs used to treat epilepsy are termed antiepileptics; the term anticonvulsant is also used.

The aim of pharmacologic treatment of epilepsy is to minimize seizure activity/frequency, without producing adverse drug effects.

Mechanisms of action of antiepileptics
Antiepileptic drugs act generically to inhibit the rapid, repetitive neuronal firing that characterizes seizures. There are three established mechanisms of action by which the antiepileptic drugs achieve this (Fig. 6.14).

Inhibition of ionic channels involved in neuronal excitability
Drugs such as phenytoin, carbamazepine, and valproate inhibit the "fast" sodium current. These drugs bind preferentially to inactivated (closed) sodium channels, preventing them from opening. The high-frequency repetitive depolarization of neurons during a seizure increases the proportion of sodium channels in the inactivated state susceptible to blockade. Eventually, sufficient sodium channels become blocked so that the "fast" neuronal sodium current is insufficient to cause a depolarization. Note that neuronal transmission at normal frequencies is relatively unaffected because a much smaller proportion of the sodium channels are in the inactivated state.

Ethosuximide inhibits "T-type" low-threshold, fast-inactivating calcium. Absence seizures involve oscillatory neuronal activity between the thalamus and the cerebral cortex. The oscillation involves "T-type" calcium channels, which produce low-threshold spikes, thus allowing groups of cells to fire in bursts. It appears that the anti-absence drug ethosuximide reduces this fast-inactivating calcium current, dampening the thalamocortical oscillations that are critical in the generation of such absence seizures.

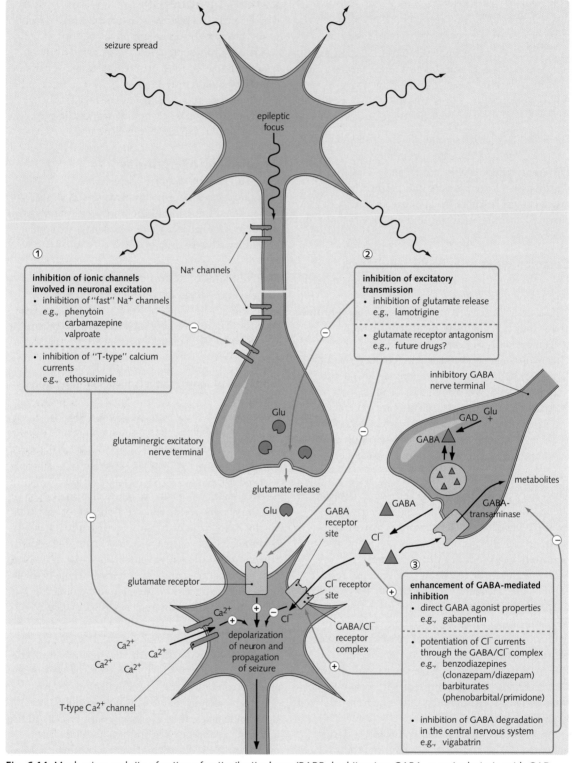

Fig. 6.14 Mechanism and site of action of antiepileptic drugs (BARB, barbiturates; GABA, γ-aminobutyric acid; GAD, glutamic acid decarboxylase; Glu, glutamate).

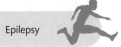

Inhibition of excitatory transmission

Drugs that block excitatory amino acid receptors (N-methyl-D-aspartate [NMDA] antagonists) have been shown to be antiepileptic in animal models. Such drugs may prove useful in the clinical treatment of epilepsy in the future. Lamotrigine, one of the newer antiepileptic agents, inhibits the release of glutamate as one of its actions, and this may contribute to its antiepileptic activity.

Enhancement of GABA-mediated inhibition

This can take any of the following forms:

- Enhancement by direct GABA agonist properties (e.g., by gabapentin, another of the newer antiepileptics, an agent which has been designed to mimic GABA in the CNS).
- Potentiation of chloride currents through the $GABA_A/Cl^-$ channel complex (e.g., by benzodiazepines and barbiturates). The increased postsynaptic inhibitory chloride current at $GABA_A$ receptors hyperpolarizes neurons and makes them refractory to excitation (see Fig. 6.4).
- Inhibition of GABA degradation in the CNS (e.g., by vigabatrin, which is an irreversible inhibitor of GABA transaminase [$GABA_T$], the enzyme normally responsible for metabolism of GABA in the neuron.) Inhibition of $GABA_T$, therefore, leads to an increase in synaptic levels of GABA and so enhances GABA-mediated inhibition.

Remember that epilepsy is simply aberrant electrical activity spreading throughout an area of or the whole of the brain. Antiepileptic medications limit the propagation of this spread and inhibit symptoms developing.

Antiepileptic drugs (anticonvulsants)

Antiepileptic drugs can be classified according to their mechanism of action, but in clinical practice it is useful to think of the drugs according to their use (Fig. 6.15; see also Fig. 6.14).

Phenytoin

Mechanism of action: This involves use-dependent block of voltage-gated sodium channels. Phenytoin reduces the spread of a seizure. Electroencephalographic (EEG) recordings show that phenytoin does not stop the "spiking" at a focus (i.e., it does not prevent the ignition of an epileptic discharge), but it does stop it spreading and causing overt clinical symptoms.

Route of administration: Oral, intravenous.

Indications: Phenytoin is indicated in all forms of epilepsy except absence seizures. Phenytoin has also shown efficacy in the treatment of neuralgic pain.

Contraindications: Phenytoin has many contraindications, mainly because it induces the hepatic cytochrome P450 oxidase system, increasing the metabolism of oral contraceptives, anticoagulants, dexamethasone, and meperidine.

Adverse effects: The adverse effects of phenytoin may be dosage- or non-dosage-related. The dosage-related effects of phenytoin affect the cerebellovestibular system, leading to ataxia, blurred vision, and hyperactivity. Acute toxicity causes sedation and confusion. The non-dosage-related effects include collagen effects such as gum hypertrophy and coarsening of facial features; allergic reaction (e.g., rash, hepatitis, and lymphadenopathy); hematologic effects (e.g., megaloblastic anemia); endocrine effects, such as hirsutism; and teratogenic effects, including congenital malformations).

Therapeutic notes: The use of phenytoin is complicated by its zero-order pharmacokinetics, characteristic toxicities, and necessity for long-term administration. Phenytoin has a narrow therapeutic index, and the relationship between dose and plasma concentration is nonlinear. This is due to the fact that phenytoin is metabolized by a hepatic enzyme system that is saturated at therapeutic levels. Small dosage increases may, therefore, produce large rises in plasma concentrations with acute side effects. Monitoring of plasma concentration greatly assists dosage adjustment. Because of its adverse effects and

Drugs used for epilepsy classified by clinical use		
Seizure type	Primary drugs	Secondary drugs
Partial and/or generalized tonic–clonic seizures	• Sodium valproate • Carbamazepine	• Phenytoin • Vigabatrin • Gabapentin • Lamotrigine • Phenobarbital
Absence seizures	• Ethosuximide • Sodium valproate	• Phenobarbital • Lamotrigine
Status epilepticus	• Lorazepam	• Diazepam • Clonazepam

Fig. 6.15 Drugs used for epilepsy, classified by clinical use.

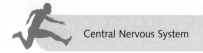

narrow therapeutic window, phenytoin is no longer a first-line treatment for any of the seizure syndromes.

Sodium valproate

Mechanism of action: Sodium valproate has two mechanisms of action: like phenytoin, it causes use-dependent block of voltage-gated sodium channels; it also increases the GABA content of the brain when given over a prolonged period.

Route of administration: Oral, intravenous.

Indications: Sodium valproate is useful in all forms of epilepsy.

Contraindications: Sodium valproate should not be given to people with acute liver disease or a history of hepatic dysfunction.

Adverse effects: Sodium valproate has many fewer side effects than other antiepileptics; the main problems are gastrointestinal upset and, more importantly, liver failure. Hepatic toxicity appears to be more common when sodium valproate is used in combination with other antiepileptics.

Therapeutic notes: Sodium valproate is well absorbed orally and has a half-life of 10–15 hours. Sodium valproate is now the first-line drug for most types of seizure syndromes.

Carbamazepine

Mechanism of action: Like phenytoin, carbamazepine causes use-dependent block of voltage-gated sodium channels.

Route of administration: Oral, rectal.

Indications: Carbamazepine can be used in all forms of epilepsy except absence seizures. It may also be useful for neuralgic pain.

Contraindications: Like phenytoin, carbamazepine is a strong cytochrome P450 enzyme inducer and so causes similar drug interactions.

Adverse effects: The adverse effects of carbamazepine are really limited to the nervous system—ataxia, nystagmus, dysarthria, vertigo, and sedation.

Therapeutic notes: Carbamazepine is well absorbed orally with a long half-life (25–60 hours) when first given. Enzyme induction subsequently reduces this half-life.

Ethosuximide

Mechanism of action: Ethosuximide exerts its effects by inhibition of low-threshold calcium currents ("T-currents").

Route of administration: Oral.

Indications: Ethosuximide is the drug of choice in simple absence seizures and is particularly well tolerated in children.

Contraindications: Ethosuximide may make tonic–clonic attacks worse.

Adverse effects: The adverse effects of ethosuximide include gastrointestinal upset, drowsiness, mood swings, and skin rashes. Rarely, it causes serious bone marrow depression.

Vigabatrin

Mechanism of action: Vigabatrin exerts its effects by irreversible inhibition of GABA transaminase.

Route of administration: Oral.

Indications: Vigabatrin is indicated in epilepsy not satisfactorily controlled by other drugs.

Contraindications: Vigabatrin should not be used in people with a history of psychosis because of the side effect of hallucinations.

Adverse effects: Drowsiness, dizziness, depression, and visual hallucinations.

Therapeutic notes: Vigabatrin is a new drug, used as an adjunct to other therapies.

Lamotrigine

Mechanism of action: Lamotrigine appears to act via an effect on sodium channels and by inhibiting the release of excitatory amino acids.

Route of administration: Oral.

Indications: Monotherapy and adjunctive treatment of partial seizures and generalized tonic–clonic seizures. It may also be useful for neuralgic pain.

Contraindications: Hepatic impairment.

Adverse effects: Rashes, fever, malaise, drowsiness, and, rarely, hepatic dysfunction.

Therapeutic notes: Lamotrigine is one of the newer classes of antiepileptic agents, and its use in practice is gradually increasing.

Gabapentin

Mechanism of action: Gabapentin is a lipophilic drug that was designed to act like GABA in the CNS (agonist), although it does not appear to have GABA-mimetic actions. Its mechanism of action remains elusive.

Route of administration: Oral.

Indications: As an adjunct to therapy in partial epilepsy with or without secondary generalization. It is also useful in some cases of neuropathic pain.

Contraindications: Caution to avoid sudden withdrawal, in the elderly and in those with renal impairment.

Adverse effects: Somnolence, dizziness, ataxia, fatigue, and, rarely, cerebellar signs.

Therapeutic notes: Like lamotrigine, gabapentin is a relatively new drug, and it is not as widely used as other, more traditional agents.

Barbiturates

Examples of barbiturates include phenobarbital and primidone.

Mechanism of action: Barbiturates cause potentiation of chloride currents through the GABA$_A$/Cl$^-$ channel complex.

Route of administration: Oral, intravenous.

Indications: Barbiturates are used in all forms of epilepsy, including status epilepticus.

Contraindications: Barbiturates should not be used in children, the elderly, and people with respiratory depression.

Adverse effects: The main side effect of barbiturates is sedation, which limits their use clinically, along with the danger of potentially fatal CNS depression in overdose. Phenobarbital is a good inducer of cytochrome P450, and so it can be involved in drug interactions.

Therapeutic notes: Only the long-acting barbiturates are antiepileptic. Phenobarbital has a plasma half-life of 10 hours. The strong sedative nature of these drugs now limits their use in the management of epilepsy.

Benzodiazepines

Examples of benzodiazepines include clonazepam and diazepam.

Mechanism of action: Benzodiazepines cause potentiation of chloride currents through the GABA$_A$/Cl$^-$ channel complex (see Fig. 6.4).

Route of administration: Oral, intravenously.

Indications: Clonazepam is useful for tonic–clonic and partial seizures. Lorazepam and diazepam are effective in the management of status epilepticus.

Contraindications: Benzodiazepines should not be used in people with respiratory depression.

Adverse effects: The most common adverse effect of the benzodiazepines is sedation. Intravenous lorazepam and diazepam can depress respiration.

Therapeutic notes: The repeated seizures of status epilepticus can damage the brain and be potentially life threatening, so they should be controlled by administration of intravenous diazepam. Lorazepam has a longer half-life than diazepam.

Other anticonvulsants

Other agents used as antiepileptics include levetiracetam, tiagabine, topiramate, acetazolamide, and felbamate.

Status epilepticus

Intravenous benzodiazepines (lorazepam or diazepam) are first-line drugs in status epilepticus. If these fail to bring an end to seizure activity, intravenous sodium valproate or phenytoin or carbamazepine via a nasogastric tube should be attempted, ideally in an intensive care setting. Other options include intravenous thiopental.

General anesthetics

Concepts of general anesthesia

General anesthesia is the absence of sensation associated with a reversible loss of consciousness.

General anesthetics are used as an adjunct to surgical procedures in order to render the patient unaware of, and unresponsive to, painful stimuli. Modern anesthesia is characterized by the so-called balanced technique, in which drugs and anesthetic agents are used specifically to produce:
- Analgesia.
- Sleep/sedation.
- Muscle relaxation and abolition of reflexes.

No one drug or anesthetic agent can produce all these effects, and so a combination of agents is used in the three clinical stages of surgical general anesthesia. The three stages are:
- Premedication.
- Induction.
- Maintenance.

Some may argue that a fourth stage exists, in which drugs are used to reverse the action of agents given in the previous three stages.

Premedication

Premedication is often given on the ward before the patient is taken to the operating room (Fig. 6.16), and it has four component aims:
- Relief from anxiety.
- Reduction of parasympathetic bradycardia and secretions.

- Analgesia.
- Prevention of postoperative emesis.

Relief from anxiety
Oral benzodiazepines (e.g., diazepam and lorazepam) are most effective and perform three useful functions:
- To relieve apprehension and anxiety before anesthesia.
- To lessen the amount of general anesthetic required to achieve and to maintain unconsciousness.
- Possibly, to sedate postoperatively.

Reduction of parasympathetic bradycardia and secretions
Muscarinic antagonists (e.g., atropine and hyoscine; see Chapter 5) are used to prevent salivation and bronchial secretions, and, more importantly, to protect the heart from arrhythmias, particularly bradycardia caused by some inhalation agents and neuromuscular blockers.

Analgesia
Opioid analgesics (e.g., fentanyl; see Chapter 4) are often given prior to an operation. Although the patient is unconscious during surgery, adequate analgesia is important to stop physiologic stress reactions to pain. Nonsteroidal anti-inflammatory drugs are useful alternatives and adjuncts to opiates, although they are likely to be inadequate for severe postoperative pain used alone.

Postoperative antiemesis
Drugs that provide postoperative antiemesis include metoclopramide and prochlorperazine. Nausea and vomiting are common after general anesthesia, often because of the administration of opioid drugs peri- and postoperatively. Antiemetic drugs can be given with the premedication to inhibit this.

Induction
Intravenous agents are used to produce a rapid induction of unconsciousness. Intravenous agents are preferred by patients, since injection lacks the menacing quality of having a mask placed over the face (see Fig. 6.16).

Prevention of acid aspiration in emergency and obstetric operations is crucial, and it relies on the administration of either an H_2-receptor antagonist or a proton pump inhibitor prior to induction (Chapter 10).

Maintenance
Inhalation anesthetic agents are used to maintain a state of general anesthesia after induction in most patients, although intravenous agents can be used via a continuous pump (see Fig. 6.16).

Anesthetic agents
Anesthetic agents depress all excitable tissues including central neurons, cardiac muscle, and smooth and striated muscle. Different parts of the CNS have different sensitivities to anesthetics, and the reticular activating system, which is responsible for consciousness, is among the most sensitive. Hence, it is possible to use anesthetics at a concentration that produces unconsciousness without unduly depressing the cardiovascular or respiratory centers of the brain, or the myocardium. However, for the majority of anesthetics the margin of safety is small.

General anesthetics		
Premedication	**Induction/ intravenous agents**	**Maintenance/ inhalation agents**
· Relief from anxiety (e.g., diazepam, lorazepam) · Reduction of parasympathetic bradycardia and secretions (e.g., atropine, hyoscine) · Analgesia (e.g., NSAIDs, fentanyl) · Postoperative antiemesis (e.g., metoclopramide, prochlorperazine)	· Barbiturates (e.g., thiopental) · Non-barbiturates (e.g., propofol, ketamine)	Nitrous oxide Halothane Enflurane Isoflurane

Fig. 6.16 General anesthetic agents.

Intravenous anesthetics

Intravenous anesthetics (e.g., thiopental, propofol, and ketamine) are all CNS depressants. They produce anesthesia by relatively selective depression of the reticular activating system of the brain. They may be used alone for short surgical procedures, but they are used mainly for the induction of anesthesia; therefore, rapidity of onset is the desirable feature.

Intravenous anesthetics are all highly lipid-soluble agents and cross the blood–brain barrier rapidly; their rapid onset (<30 seconds) results from this rapid transfer into the brain and high cerebral blood flow. Duration of action is short (minutes) and terminated by redistribution of the drug from the CNS into less-well-perfused tissues (Fig. 6.17); drug metabolism is irrelevant to recovery.

Thiopental

Mechanism of action: Thiopental is a highly lipophilic member of the barbiturate group of CNS depressants that act to potentiate the inhibitory effect of GABA on the $GABA_A/Cl^-$ receptor channel complex.

Route of administration: Intravenous.

Indications: Rapid induction of general anesthesia.

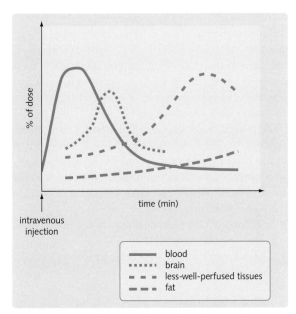

Fig. 6.17 Graph illustrating how redistribution of intravenous anesthetic agents causes a short central duration of action (Adapted from *Pharmacology* by H Rang, M Dale, J Ritter. Churchill Livingstone, 1995).

Contraindications: Thiopental should not be given to a patient with a previous allergy to it. Porphyria.

Adverse effects: Respiratory depression, myocardial depression (bradycardia), vasodilatation, and anaphylaxis. There is a risk of severe vasospasm if it is accidentally injected into an artery.

Therapeutic notes: Thiopental is a widely used induction agent, but it has no analgesic properties. It provides smooth and rapid (<30 seconds) induction, but, owing to its narrow therapeutic margin, overdosage with consequent cardiorespiratory depression can occur. Thiopental is given as the sodium salt, which is unstable in solution, and so it must be made up immediately before use.

Propofol

Mechanism of action: Propofol is similar to thiopental in its mechanism of action.

Route of administration: Intravenous.

Indications: Rapid induction of general anesthesia.

Contraindications: Propofol should not be given to patients with a previous allergy to it.

Adverse effects: Convulsions, anaphylaxis, and delayed recovery from anesthesia have occasionally been reported as side effects.

Therapeutic notes: Propofol is associated with rapid recovery without nausea or hangover, and it is very widely used. Propofol is the drug of choice if an intravenous agent is to be used to maintain anesthesia by a continuous infusion.

Etomidate

Mechanisms of action: The mechanism of action of etomidate is similar to that of thiopental.

Route of administration: Intravenous.

Indications: Rapid induction of general anesthesia.

Contraindications: Etomidate should not be given to patients with a previous allergy to it.

Adverse effects: Extraneous muscle movement and pain on injection and possible adrenocortical suppression.

Therapeutic notes: Etomidate is an induction agent that gained favor over thiopental because of its larger therapeutic margin and faster metabolism leading to fewer hangover effects. Etomidate is more prone to causing extraneous muscle movement and pain on injection compared with other agents.

115

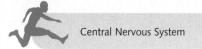

Ketamine

Mechanism of action: Ketamine produces full surgical anesthesia, but the form of the anesthesia is known as dissociative anesthesia, as the patient may remain conscious though amnesic and insensitive to pain. This effect is probably related to an action on NMDA-type glutamate receptors.

Ketamine is a derivative of the street drug phencyclidine (PCP/"angel dust").

Route of administration: Intravenous, intramuscular.

Indications: Ketamine is used in the induction and maintenance of anesthesia, especially in children.

Contraindications: Ketamine should not be given to people with hypertension or psychosis.

Adverse effects: These include cardiovascular stimulation, tachycardia, and raised arterial blood pressure, as well as transient psychotic sequelae such as vivid dreams and hallucinations.

Therapeutic notes: Ketamine is not often used as an induction agent, owing to the high incidence of dysphoria and hallucinations during recovery in adults. These effects are much less marked in children; and ketamine, in conjunction with a benzodiazepine, is often used for minor procedures in pediatrics.

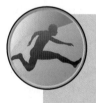 Like the benzodiazepines and the barbiturates, thiopental and propofol act via the $GABA_A/Cl^-$ receptor in causing CNS depression.

Inhalation anesthetics

Examples of inhalation anesthetics include halothane, enflurane, isoflurane, sevoflurane, and desflurane. Nitrous oxide also has anesthetic properties.

Inhalation anesthetics may be gases or volatile liquids. They are commonly used for the maintenance of anesthesia after induction with an intravenous agent.

Mechanism of action: It is not known exactly how inhalation anesthetic agents produce their effects. Unlike most drugs, inhalation anesthetics do not all belong to one recognizable chemical class. The shape and electronic configuration of the molecule are evidently unimportant. A distinct anesthetic "receptor" is, therefore, unlikely; it would seem that the pharmacologic action of inhalation anesthetics is dependent on the physicochemical properties of the molecule.

Three theories of anesthesia have received the most attention—the lipid, hydrate, and protein theories.

The lipid theory arose because a close correlation was noticed between anesthetic potency and lipid solubility. It has been suggested that anesthetics dissolve in membrane lipid and affect its physical state by two possible mechanisms. These are:

• Volume expansion, which is supported by pressure reversal of anesthesia, but qualitative inconsistencies exist.

• Membrane fluidization, although the high concentrations required and weak effect of temperature make this difficult to accept.

The hydrate theory arose because anesthetic molecules stabilize water molecules in their vicinity. It has been suggested that this alteration of the membrane accounts for the effects of anesthetics.

While there is some correlation between potency and the ability to form hydrates, anomalous compounds such as sulfur hexafluoride do not form hydrates, but they do have anesthetic properties.

The protein theory arose because there is increasing evidence that anesthetics may act by binding to discrete hydrophobic domains of membrane proteins. This would explain the "cut-off" phenomenon and the stereoselectivity of anesthetics. The protein theory is currently popular, but the nature of the target protein(s) in the CNS has not been identified. Possible targets include voltage-operated channels, receptor-operated channels, or secondary-messenger systems.

Pharmacokinetic aspects: The depth of anesthesia produced by inhalation anesthetics is directly related to the partial pressure (tension) of the agent in the arterial blood, as this determines the concentration of agent in the CNS. The concentration of anesthetic in the blood is in turn determined by:

• The concentration of anesthetic in the inspired gas (alveolar concentration).

• The solubility of the anesthetic in blood (blood/gas partition coefficient).

• Cardiac output.

• Alveolar ventilation.

Rapid induction and recovery are important properties of an anesthetic agent, allowing flexible control over the arterial tension (and hence brain tension) and, therefore, the depth of anesthesia. The speed at which induction of anesthesia occurs is determined by two properties of the anesthetic: its solubility in blood (blood/gas partition coefficient) and its solubility in fat (lipid solubility). Therefore:

- Agents of low blood solubility (e.g., nitrous oxide, enflurane) produce rapid induction and recovery because relatively small amounts are required to saturate the blood, and so the arterial tension (and hence brain tension) rises and falls quickly.
- Agents of high blood solubility (e.g., halothane) have much slower induction and recovery times because much more anesthetic solution is required before the arterial anesthetic tension approaches that of the inspired gas.

Agents with high lipid solubility (e.g., ether) accumulate gradually in the body fat during prolonged anesthesia and so may produce a prolonged hangover if used for a long operation.

Nitrous oxide
Mechanism of action: See above.

Route of administration: Inhalation.

Indications: Nitrous oxide is used in the maintenance of anesthesia (in combination with other agents) and for analgesia (50% mixture in oxygen).

Contraindications: Pneumothorax: nitrous oxide diffuses into air containing closed spaces resulting in an increased pressure; in the case of pneumothorax, this may compromise breathing.

Adverse effects: Nitrous oxide was thought to be relatively free of side effects—it has little effect on cardiovascular and respiratory systems—but the risk of bone marrow suppression is now a known factor.

Therapeutic notes: Nitrous oxide cannot produce surgical anesthesia when administered alone because of a lack of potency. It is commonly used as a nonflammable carrier gas for volatile agents, allowing their concentration to be reduced. As a 50% mixture in oxygen, nitrous oxide is a good analgesic. It is used in childbirth and by dentists and paramedics.

Halothane
Mechanism of action: See above.

Route of administration: Inhalation.

Indications: Halothane is used in the maintenance of anesthesia.

Contraindications: Halothane should not be given to people with a previous reaction to halothane or exposure to halothane in the previous 3 months.

Adverse effects: Like most volatile anesthetics, halothane causes cardiorespiratory depression. Respiratory depression results in elevated pCO_2 and perhaps ventricular arrhythmias. Halothane also depresses cardiac muscle fibers and may cause bradycardia. The result of this is a concentration-dependent hypotension.

The most significant toxic effect of halothane is severe hepatic necrosis, which occurs in 1 in 35,000 cases. Lesser degrees of liver damage may occur more frequently. The damage is caused by metabolites of the 20% of administered halothane that is biotransformed in the liver (80% of an administered dose is excreted by the lungs).

Therapeutic notes: Halothane is a halogenated hydrocarbon, and it is probably the most widely used inhalation agent.

Enflurane
Mechanism of action: See above.

Route of administration: Inhalation.

Indications: Enflurane is used in the maintenance of anesthesia.

Contraindications: Enflurane should not be given to people with epilepsy.

Adverse effects: Enflurane causes cardiorespiratory depression similar to that with halothane, although the incidence of arrhythmias is much lower than with halothane.

Enflurane undergoes only 2% metabolism in the liver, so it is much less likely than halothane to cause hepatotoxicity. The disadvantage of enflurane is that it may cause electroencephalogram (EEG) changes and muscle twitching, and special caution is needed in epileptic subjects.

Therapeutic notes: Enflurane is a volatile anesthetic similar to, but less potent than, halothane, about twice the concentration being necessary for maintenance. Induction and recovery times are faster than for halothane.

Isoflurane
Mechanism of action: See above.

Route of administration: Inhalation.

Indications: It is used in the maintenance of anesthesia.

Contraindications: Susceptibility to malignant hyperthermia.

Adverse effects: Isoflurane has actions similar to those of halothane, but it has fewer effects upon the cardiorespiratory system. Hypotension is caused by a dose-related decrease in systemic vascular resistance

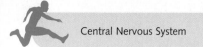

rather than a marked fall in cardiac output. Less hepatic metabolism (0.2%) occurs than with enflurane, so hepatotoxicity is even rarer.

Therapeutic notes: Isoflurane is an isomer of enflurane. It has a potency intermediate between that of halothane and enflurane.

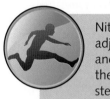 Nitrous oxide is used as an adjunct to other inhaled anesthetic agents, as it reduces the dose required to maintain a steady state of anesthesia, thus limiting side effects and allowing more rapid recovery.

Use of neuromuscular blockers in anesthesia

For some operations (e.g., intra-abdominal) complete relaxation of skeletal muscle is essential. Some general anesthetic agents have significant neuromuscular blocking actions, but drugs that specifically block the neuromuscular junction are frequently employed (e.g., succinylcholine, rocuronium, vecuronium, and atracurium; see Chapter 5).

Drug misuse

Concepts of drug misuse

Historically, there has been a long relationship between humans and the nontherapeutic use of drugs that act on the mind and body. Virtually all cultures have used drugs for nontherapeutic purposes. For instance, the Incas used psychoactive fungi, and the ancient Egyptians (and many other cultures since) used alcohol.

It is important to realize that the misuse of drugs is a socially defined concept that has as much to do with the legal, religious, moral, and cultural framework of a society as the pharmacologic properties of the drug itself. Drugs now banned (e.g., opium) were once popular and legal in the nineteenth century, while attitudes to alcohol vary both historically and geographically from total prohibition to deep entrenchment in the culture.

Humans show great ingenuity in creating, harvesting, obtaining, and taking drugs for nontherapeutic reasons, and they go to great lengths to do so. The sheer prevalence and associated comorbidity make drug misuse an important medical subject.

Definitions
Drug misuse

Drug misuse is defined as the use of drugs that cause actual physical or mental harm to an individual or to society or that are illegal. Therefore, drug misuse includes alcohol, nicotine, and the damaging overprescription of tranquilizers as well as the more obvious illicit drugs such as ecstasy or amphetamines.

The term "drug abuse" is synonymous with "drug misuse."

Drug dependence

Drug dependence is defined as the compulsion to take a drug repeatedly, with distress being caused if this is prevented.

Drugs of dependence all have rewarding effects (this is why they are taken), but they also have unpleasant (aversive) effects, often as the drug leaves the brain.

Dependence involves psychological factors as well as physical aspects. These are not exclusive, and there is a mixture of both in most people who are dependent upon drugs.

Psychological dependence occurs when the rewarding effects (positive reinforcement) predominate to cause a compulsion to continue taking the drug.

Physical dependence occurs when the distress on stopping the drug (negative reinforcement) is the main reason for continuing to take it (i.e., avoidance of the "withdrawal syndrome").

Drug tolerance

Drug tolerance is the necessity to increase the dose of an administered drug progressively in order to maintain the effect that was produced by the (smaller) original doses. Drug tolerance is a phenomenon that develops with chronic administration of a drug.

Many different mechanisms can give rise to drug tolerance, though they are rather poorly understood. These include:
• Downregulation of receptors.
• Changes in receptors.
• Exhaustion of biologic mediators or transmitters.
• Increased metabolic degradation (enzyme induction).
• Physiologic adaptation.

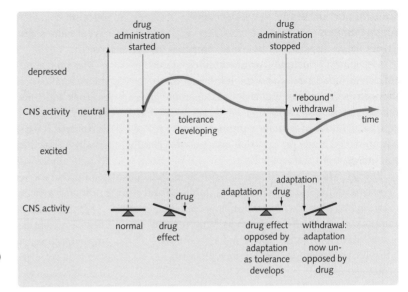

Fig. 6.18 Tolerance to and withdrawal from central nervous system (CNS) depressant drugs (e.g., alcohol). The graph for tolerance of and withdrawal from CNS stimulant drugs (e.g., cocaine) would be a mirror image in the x-axis of what is shown.

Summary table of drugs with a high misuse potential	
Drug class	**Examples**
Central stimulants	Cocaine Amphetamines MDMA (ecstasy) Nicotine
Central depressants	Alcohol Benzodiazepines Barbiturates
Opioid analgesics	Morphine Heroin (diacetylmorphine) Methadone Oxycodone
Cannabinoids	Cannabis Tetrahydrocannabinoids (THCs)
Hallucinogens	LSD Mescaline Psilocybin
Dissociative anesthetics	Ketamine Phencyclidine

Fig. 6.19 Drugs with high potential for misuse (LSD, lysergic acid diethylamide; MDMA, methylenedioxymethamphetamine).

Withdrawal
Withdrawal is the term used to describe the syndrome of effects caused by stopping administration of a drug. It results from the change of (neuro)physiologic equilibrium induced by the presence of the drug (Fig. 6.18).

Legal aspects of drugs of abuse
Scheduled drugs
The use of drugs with potential for abuse is restricted by the FDA under the Control Substance Act of 1970. These drugs are termed "controlled drugs" and are classified as "scheduled drugs" as follows:

Schedule I: High abuse potential, no accepted medical use in the U.S. (e.g., heroin, PCP, marijuana, MDMA ["ecstasy"], LSD, and others).

Schedule II: High abuse potential, accepted medical uses (e.g., strong opioid agonists such as morphine, cocaine, amphetamines, methylphenidate, short-acting barbiturates, and others). These drugs must have a written prescription with the physician's DEA number and cannot be prescribed or refilled over the telephone.

Schedule III: Moderate abuse potential, accepted medical uses (moderate opioid antagonists such as codeine, anabolic steroids, some barbiturates, and others).

Schedule IV: Low abuse potential, accepted medical uses (e.g., weak opioid agonists, benzodiazepines, zolpidem, and others).

Schedule V: Drugs without abuse potential, not classified as "controlled" drugs.

Drugs of misuse
Drugs with a high potential for misuse fall into many distinct pharmacologic categories. They may or may not be used therapeutically, and they may be illegal or legal (Fig. 6.19).

119

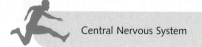

Central stimulants
Amphetamines
Street names: Speed, Whizz, Billy, Uppers.

Mechanism of action: Amphetamines cause the release of monoamines and the inhibition of monoamine reuptake, especially of dopamine and noradrenaline in neurons.

Route of administration: Amphetamines are administered orally or "snorted" as a powder nasally; sometimes used intravenously.

Effects: The effects of amphetamines include the following: increased motor activity; euphoria and excitement; anorexia and insomnia; peripheral sympathomimetic effects, such as hypertension and inhibition of gut motility; and stereotyped behavior and psychosis, which develop with prolonged usage.

Clinical uses: The (very few) clinical uses of amphetamines are for narcolepsy and for hyperkinesis in children. They are no longer recommended as appetite suppressants, owing to their adverse effects.

Tolerance, dependence, and withdrawal: Tolerance to the peripheral sympathomimetic stimulant effects of amphetamines develops rapidly, but it develops much more slowly to other effects such as locomotor stimulation. Amphetamines cause strong psychological dependence but no real physical dependence. After stopping chronic use, the individual will usually enter a deep, long sleep ("REM rebound") and awaken feeling tired, depressed, and hungry. This state may reflect the depletion of the normal monoamine stores.

Adverse effects: Acute amphetamine toxicity causes cardiac arrhythmias, hypertension, and stroke. Chronic toxicity causes paranoid psychosis, vasoconstriction, tissue anoxia at sites of injection or snorting, and damage to the fetal brain *in utero*.

> Try to use the correct chemical name when describing drugs of misuse, rather than a street name or personal favorite—i.e., amphetamines rather than Whizz or Speed. It tends to go down better with examiners!

Cocaine
Street names: Coke, Charlie, Snow, Crack (free base).

Mechanism of action: Cocaine strongly inhibits the reuptake of catecholamines at noradrenergic neurons and thus strongly enhances sympathetic activity.

Route of administration: Cocaine hydrochloride is usually snorted nasally. "Crack" is the free base, which is more volatile and which does not decompose on heating. It can, therefore, be smoked, producing a brief intense "rush."

Effects: The behavioral effects produced by cocaine are similar to those produced by amphetamines, such as euphoria. The euphoric effects may be greater, and there is less of a tendency for stereotypical behavior and paranoid delusions.

The effects of cocaine hydrochloride (lasting about an hour) are not as long lasting as those of amphetamine, while those obtained from crack are brief (minutes).

Clinical uses: Cocaine is occasionally used as a topical anesthetic by ear, nose, and throat specialists.

Tolerance, dependence, and withdrawal: Cocaine causes strong psychological dependence but no real physical dependence. Withdrawal causes a marked deterioration in motor performance, which is restorable on provision of the drug.

Adverse effects: Acute cocaine toxicity causes toxic psychosis, cardiac arrhythmias, hypertension, and stroke. Chronic toxicity causes paranoid psychosis, vasoconstriction, tissue anoxia at sites of injection or snorting, and damage to the fetal brain.

Methylenedioxymethamphetamine
Street names: Ecstasy, E, Disco Biscuits, Pills.

Mechanism of action: Methylenedioxymethamphetamine (MDMA) is an amphetamine derivative that has a mechanism of action similar to that of amphetamines (release of monoamines, inhibition of monoamine reuptake). MDMA especially has actions on serotonergic neurons, potentiating 5-HT.

Route of administration: MDMA is usually taken as a pill containing other psychoactive drugs, such as amphetamine or ketamine.

Effects: MDMA has mixed stimulant and hallucinogenic properties, especially in its pure form. Euphoria, arousal, and perceptual disturbances are common. Uniquely, MDMA has the effect of creating a feeling of euphoric empathy, so that social barriers are reduced.

Clinical uses: MDMA has no clinical use. Trials have been licensed for its evaluation as a treatment for people with social avoidant personality disorders.

Tolerance, dependence, and withdrawal: It is not currently known to what extent tolerance and dependence occur with MDMA. The withdrawal syndrome is similar to that with amphetamines.

Adverse effects: The most serious consequences of acute MDMA toxicity appear to be hyperthermia, exhaustion, and dehydration caused indirectly by the repetitive locomotor behavior induced (dancing!), which can be fatal. Chronic MDMA toxicity causes neurodegeneration of serotonergic nerves in the brains of experimental primates. The correlation to humans is not known.

Nicotine

Nicotine is found in cigarettes, cigars, pipes, and chewing tobacco. Various therapeutic products are available which contain nicotine as part of nicotine replacement therapy for those wishing to withdraw from their nicotine addiction. These are discussed at the end of the chapter.

Mechanism of action: Nicotine exerts its effects by causing nicotinic acetylcholine receptor (nicAChR) excitation, leading to neurotransmitter release and nicAChR desensitization.

Route of administration: Nicotine is usually inhaled, although it can be chewed.

Effects: Nicotine has both stimulant and relaxant properties. Physiologically, nicotine increases alertness, decreases irritability, and relaxes skeletal muscle tone.

Peripheral effects due to ganglionic stimulation include tachycardia, increased blood pressure, and decreased gastrointestinal motility.

Clinical uses: Nicotine has no clinical use.

Tolerance, dependence, and withdrawal: Tolerance to nicotine occurs rapidly, first to peripheral effects but later to central effects.

Nicotine is highly addictive, causing both physical and psychological dependence.

Withdrawal from tobacco often leads to a syndrome of craving, irritability, anxiety, and increased appetite for approximately 2–3 weeks.

Adverse effects: Acute nicotine toxicity causes nausea and vomiting. Chronic toxicity caused by smoking leads to more morbidity than all other drugs combined, predisposing to all of the following diseases, often greatly so:
- Cardiovascular diseases, including atherosclerosis, hypertension, and coronary heart disease.
- Cancer of the lung, bladder, and mouth.
- Respiratory diseases such as bronchitis, emphysema, and asthma.
- Fetal growth retardation.

Central depressants
Ethanol

Mechanism of action: Ethanol, or alcohol, acts in a similar way to volatile anesthetic agents, as a general CNS depressant. The cellular mechanisms involved may include inhibition of calcium entry, hence reduction in transmitter release, as well as potentiation of inhibitory GABA transmission.

Route of administration: Ethanol is administered orally.

Effects: The familiar effects of ethanol intoxication range from increased self-confidence and motor incoordination to unconsciousness and coma. Peripheral effects include a self-limiting diuresis and vasodilatation.

Clinical uses: Ethanol is used as an antidote to methanol poisoning.

Tolerance, dependence, and withdrawal: Tolerance and physical and psychological dependence all occur with ethanol, such that thousands of people a year are admitted to psychiatric hospitals for alcohol dependence and psychosis, and up to 20% of males on a medical ward have alcohol-related disabilities.

The alcohol withdrawal syndrome is a rebound of the nervous system after adaptation to the depression caused by alcohol. This syndrome occurs in two stages:
- Early stage ("hangover"), which is common and starts 6–8 hours after cessation of drinking. It involves tremulousness, nausea, retching, and sweating.
- Late stage (delirium tremens), which is much less common and starts 48–72 hours after cessation of drinking. It involves delirium, tremor, hallucinations, and confusion.

Management of these late withdrawal symptoms involves sedation with benzodiazepines; clonidine may be useful.

Adverse effects: Acute ethanol toxicity causes ataxia, nystagmus, coma, respiratory depression, and death. Chronic ethanol toxicity causes neurodegeneration (potentiated by vitamin deficiency), dementia, liver damage, pancreatitis, and so forth, as well as accompanying psychiatric illness—depression/psychosis is common.

Benzodiazepines

Mechanism of action: Benzodiazepines exert their effects by potentiation of inhibitory GABA transmission.

Route of administration: Benzodiazepines are usually administered orally.

Effects: The effects of benzodiazepines include sedation, agitation, and ataxia.

Clinical uses: Benzodiazepines are heavily prescribed as anxiolytics and hypnotics.

Tolerance, dependence, and withdrawal: Benzodiazepines have a potential for misuse—tolerance and dependence are common.

A physical withdrawal syndrome can occur in patients given benzodiazepines, even for short periods. Symptoms include rebound anxiety and insomnia with depression, nausea, and perceptual changes that may last from weeks to months.

Adverse effects: The adverse effects of acute benzodiazepine toxicity include hypotension and confusion. Cognitive impairment occurs in chronic benzodiazepine toxicity.

Opioid analgesics

Heroin (diacetylmorphine) and other opioids

Street names: Smack, Dragon, Brown.

Mechanism of action: Opioids (e.g., heroin and morphine) show agonist action at opioid receptors.

Note that the sense of euphoria and well-being produced by strong opioids undoubtedly contributes to their analgesic activity by helping to reduce the anxiety and stress associated with pain. This effect also accounts for the illicit use of these drugs by addicts.

Route of administration: Opioids are generally taken intravenously by misusers, as this produces the most intense sense of euphoria ("rush").

Effects: Opioids produce feelings of euphoria and well-being. Other effects are mentioned on page 64.

Clinical uses: Opioids are used in analgesia for moderate to severe pain.

Tolerance, dependence, and withdrawal: Tolerance to opioid analgesics develops quickly in addicts and results in larger and larger doses of the drug being needed to achieve the same effect.

Dependence involves both psychological factors and physical factors. Psychological dependence is based on the positive reinforcement provided by euphoria.

There is a definite physical withdrawal syndrome in addicts following cessation of drug treatment with opioids. This syndrome comprises a complex mixture of irritable and sometimes aggressive behavior, combined with extremely unpleasant autonomic symptoms such as fever, sweating, yawning, pupillary dilatation, and piloerection that gives the state its colloquial name of "cold turkey." Patients are extremely distressed and restless and strongly crave the drug. Symptoms are maximal at 2 days and largely disappear in 7–10 days.

Treatment of withdrawal: Methadone is a long-acting opioid, active orally, that is used to wean addicts from their addiction. The withdrawal symptoms from this longer-acting compound are more prolonged, but less intense than, for example, those of heroin. Treatment usually involves substitution of methadone followed by a slow reduction in dose over time.

Clonidine, an α_2-adrenoreceptor agonist, inhibits firing of locus ceruleus neurons, and it is effective in suppressing some components of the opioid withdrawal syndrome, especially the nausea, vomiting, and diarrhea.

Adverse effects: Acute opioid toxicity causes the following:

- Confusion, drowsiness, and sedation. Initial excitement is followed by sedation and finally coma on overdose.
- Shallow and slow respiration, due to reduction of sensitivity of the respiratory centre to CO_2.
- Vomiting, due to stimulation of the chemoreceptor trigger zone.
- Autonomic effects such as tremor and pupillary constriction.
- Bronchospasm, flushing, and arteriolar dilatation due to histamine release.

Acute toxicity may be countered by use of an opioid antagonist such as naloxone or naltrexone.

The adverse effects of direct chronic toxicity are minor.

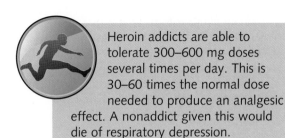

Heroin addicts are able to tolerate 300–600 mg doses several times per day. This is 30–60 times the normal dose needed to produce an analgesic effect. A nonaddict given this would die of respiratory depression.

Cannabinoids
Cannabis
Street names: Puff, Weed, Pot, Dope, Gear, Grass, Resin, Ganja, Blow.

There are two forms of cannabis: marijuana is the dried leaves and flowers of the cannabis plant, and hashish is the extracted resin of the cannabis plant.

Mechanism of action: How cannabis exerts its effects is not clearly defined, but it includes both depressant, stimulant, and psychomimetic effects.

The active constituent of cannabis is delta–9-tetrahydrocannabinol (THC), although metabolites that also have activity may be important.

Route of administration: Cannabis is usually smoked, although it may be eaten.

Effects: Cannabis has several effects:
- Subjectively, users feel relaxed and mildly euphoric.
- Perception is altered, with apparent sharpening of sensory experience.
- Appetite is enhanced.
- Peripheral actions include vasodilation and bronchodilatation and a reduction in intraocular pressure.

Clinical uses: Cannabis is being evaluated for palliative or symptomatic relief use in certain conditions (e.g., for the antiemetic effect of THC and a possible role in treatment of multiple sclerosis and glaucoma).

Tolerance, dependence, and withdrawal: Tolerance to cannabis occurs to a minor degree. It is not dangerously addictive, with only moderate physical and psychological withdrawal effects noted, such as mild anxiety/dysphoria and sleep disturbances.

Adverse effects: Acute cannabis toxicity causes confusion and hallucinations. Chronic toxicity may cause flashbacks, memory loss, and "demotivational syndrome."

Psychotomimetic drugs or hallucinogens
Street names: Acid, Trips, Magic Mushrooms.

Examples of psychotomimetic drugs include LSD, mescaline, and psilocybin.

Mechanism of action: How LSD, mescaline, and psilocybin produce changes in perception is not well understood but seems to involve serotonin. LSD appears to affect serotonergic systems by acting on 5-HT$_2$ inhibitory autoreceptors on serotonergic neurons to reduce their firing. Whether LSD is an agonist, an antagonist, or both is not clear.

Route of administration: Psychotomimetic drugs are administered orally as a liquid, pills, or paper stamps.

Effects: Psychotomimetic drugs cause a dramatically altered state of perception—vivid and unusual sensory experiences combined with euphoric sensations. Hallucinations, delusions, and panic can occur; this is known as a "bad trip," and it can be terrifying.

Clinical uses: Psychotomimetic drugs have no clinical uses.

Tolerance, dependence, and withdrawal: Tolerance to, dependence on, and withdrawal from psychotomimetic drugs are not significant.

Adverse effects: Acute toxicity from psychotomimetic drugs causes frightening delusions or hallucinations that can lead to accidents or violence. In chronic toxicity, "flashbacks" (a recurrence of hallucination) may occur long after the "trip." Other psychotic symptoms may also occur.

Smoking cessation
The most successful smoking cures combine psychological and pharmacologic treatments.

Pharmacologic options largely rely on nicotine replacement, once the patient has stopped smoking, with gradual reduction in nicotine. The latest drug to be used to help cigarette smokers is bupropion (Zyban®), which is derived from an antidepressant.

Nicotine products
Mechanism of action: Measured doses of nicotine are used to replace nicotine derived from cigarettes once

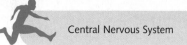

the patient has stopped smoking, meeting the physical nicotine needs. The dose of nicotine is gradually reduced over 10–12 weeks.

Route of administration: Oral (chewing gum, sublingual tablets), transdermal (patches), nasal (spray), inhalation.

Indications: Adjunct to smoking cessation.

Contraindications: Severe cardiovascular disease, recent cerebrovascular accident, pregnancy, and breastfeeding.

Adverse effects: Nausea, dizziness, headache and cold and influenza-like symptoms, palpitations.

Bupropion (Zyban®)

Mechanism of action: Bupropion is a selective inhibitor of the neuronal uptake of norepinephrine and dopamine. This is believed to reduce nicotine craving and withdrawal symptoms.

Route of administration: Oral.

Indications: Adjunct to smoking cessation.

Contraindications: History of epilepsy and eating disorders, pregnancy, and breastfeeding.

Adverse effects: Dry mouth, gastrointestinal disturbances, insomnia, tremor, and impaired concentration.

While smoking may be more socially acceptable than taking heroin, the difficulties faced by those wishing to stop their habit can be enormous, which is why psychological intervention has a role to play alongside pharmacologic methods.

124

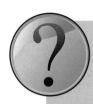

- What are the signs and symptoms of parkinsonism and the etiologic factors in its pathogenesis?
- What are the more common classes of drugs used to treat Parkinson's disease, their route of administration, mechanism of action, and adverse effects?
- What mechanisms are available to optimize L-dopa treatment, without enhancing its adverse effects?
- What are the psychological and somatic symptoms of anxiety? (Name the classes of drugs used in its management.)
- By what mechanism do anxiolytics exert their effect? What are their routes of administration and adverse effects?
- What classes of drugs are used to treat insomnia? Under what circumstances should hypnotic drugs be prescribed?
- What are the affective disorders? What are their proposed biochemical abnormalities?
- What are the main classes of drugs used in the management of mood disorders, their mechanisms of action, and adverse effects?
- What are the advantages of the selective serotonin reuptake inhibitors over the tricyclic antidepressants?
- What is the concept of psychotic disorders? What are examples of two positive and two negative symptoms?
- What is the underlying pathophysiology of psychotic disease and the rationale for drug treatment?
- What are the more common typical and atypical drugs used in psychotic disease? What are their mechanisms of action and adverse effects?
- What is epilepsy? What are the biochemical/structural causes for its clinical features?
- What are the more common antiepileptic drugs, their routes of administration, and major adverse effects? (Summarize their general mechanism of action.)
- What are the principles and drugs used in the management of status epilepticus?
- What is the incidence of teratogenesis associated with anticonvulsant use in pregnancy?
- What are the components needed for adequate general anesthesia prior to surgery?
- What is one drug used in each stage of anesthesia, from premedication, induction, and maintenance? What are their routes of administration, general mechanisms of action, and adverse effects?
- What is the role of nitrous oxide as an anesthetic gas?
- Which drugs are commonly misused? What forms of classification exist for drugs of misuse?
- What treatment options are available to people who wish to stop smoking, but who suffer from nicotine withdrawal? How do these agents act, and what are their main adverse effects?

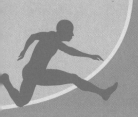

7. Cardiovascular System

Heart

Cardiac anatomy and physiology
The heart as a pump
The heart functions as a pump that, together with the vascular system, supplies the tissues with blood containing oxygen and nutrients as well as removing waste products.

The flow of blood around the body is as follows (Fig. 7.1):
- Deoxygenated blood from body tissues reaches the right atrium through the systemic veins (the superior and inferior vena cava).
- Blood flows into the right ventricle, which then pumps the deoxygenated blood via the pulmonary circulation to the lungs, where the blood becomes oxygenated before reaching the left atrium.
- Blood flows from the left atrium into the left ventricle, where it is pumped into the systemic circulation, via the aorta, to supply the tissues of the body.

Cardiac rate and rhythm
The sinoatrial node (SAN), located in the roof of the right atrium near the entrance of the superior vena cava, and the atrioventricular node (AVN), located at the base of the right atrium, possess a spontaneous intrinsic rhythm.

Since the SAN discharges at a frequency higher than other regions of the heart (80 impulses/minute), it is the pacemaker for the heart and as such determines the heart rate.

The action potential generated by the SAN spreads throughout both atria, reaching the AVN, from which it enters the interventricular septum by means of the bundle of His. The bundle of His splits into left and right branches, making contact with the Purkinje fibers, which conduct the impulse throughout the ventricles, causing the ventricles to contract (Fig. 7.2).

Cardiac action potential
The shape of the action potential is characteristic of the location of its origin (i.e., whether from nodal tissue, the atria, or the ventricles) (see Fig. 7.2).

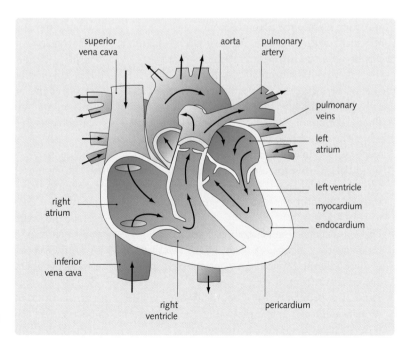

Fig. 7.1 Blood flow through the heart chambers (redrawn from Page et al., 2002).

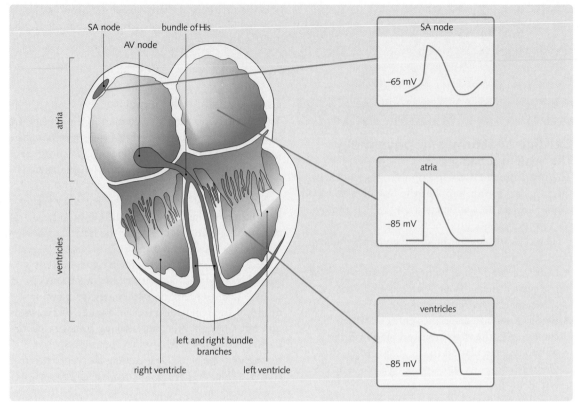

Fig. 7.2 Regional variation in action potential configuration throughout the heart (AV, atrioventricular; SA, sinoatrial). (Redrawn from Page et al., 2002.)

Nonnodal cells

The resting membrane potential across the ventricular cell membrane is approximately −85 mV; this is because the resting membrane is more permeable to potassium than to other ions. Four phases occurring at the ventricular cell membrane are:

- Phase 0 or depolarization. Depolarization occurs when the membrane potential reaches a critical value of −60 mV. The upstroke of the action potential is due to the transient opening of voltage-gated sodium channels, allowing sodium ions into the cell. In addition, potassium conductance falls to very low levels.
- Phase 1 or partial repolarization. Partial repolarization occurs as a result of the inactivation of the sodium current and a transient outward potassium current.
- Phase 2 or plateau phase. The membrane remains depolarized at a plateau of approximately 0 mV. This is due to the activation of a

voltage-dependent slow inward calcium current, conducting positive charge into the cell, and a delayed rectifier potassium current, conducting positive charge out of the cell.
- Phase 3 or repolarization. Repolarization is a result of the inactivation of the calcium current and an increase in potassium conductance (Fig. 7.3).

Nodal cells

The resting membrane potential of nodal cells is approximately −60 mV.

In nodal cells, there is no fast sodium current. Instead, the action potential is initiated by an inward calcium current, and because calcium spikes conduct slowly, there is a delay of approximately 0.1 seconds between atrial and ventricular contraction.

Nodal cells have a phase known as phase 4 or the pacemaker potential. This phase involves a gradual depolarization that occurs during diastole and is known as the f current (I_f, funny). The f current is

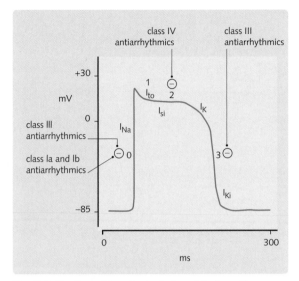

Fig. 7.3 Configuration of a typical ventricular action potential showing the ionic currents, the phases, and where class I, III, and IV antiarrhythmic drugs act (1, 2, and 3, phases of the action potential; I_{Na}, fast inward Na^+ current; I_{si}, slow inward Ca^{2+} current; I_{to}, transient outward K^+ current; I_K, delayed rectifier K^+ current; I_{Ki}, inward rectifier K^+ current). (Redrawn from Page et al., 2002.)

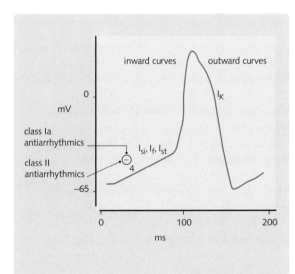

Fig. 7.4 Configuration of a typical sinoatrial node action potential showing the ionic currents, the phases, and where class Ia and II antiarrhythmic drugs act (4, phase of the action potential; I_{si}, an inward current carried by Ca^{2+} ions; I_f, a "funny" current carried by Na^+ and Ca^{2+} ions; I_{st}, the sustained inward Na^+ current; I_K, the delayed rectifier current which is an outward K^+ current). (Redrawn from Page et al., 2002.)

activated by hyperpolarization at -45 mV and consists of sodium and calcium ions entering the cell (Fig. 7.4).

Autonomic control of the heart

Both the parasympathetic and sympathetic nervous systems influence the heart, though parasympathetic activity predominates, which explains why the heart rate is lower than the inherent firing frequency of the SAN.

The sympathetic nervous system mediates its effects through the cardiac nerve and activation of β_1-adrenoceptors. These are linked to adenylyl cyclase, and their activation causes increased levels of cyclic adenosine monophosphate (cAMP) and a subsequent increase in intracellular calcium levels.

The parasympathetic nervous system mediates its effects through the vagus nerve and activation of M_2-receptors. These are also linked to adenylyl cyclase, but their activation causes decreased levels of cAMP and a subsequent decrease in intracellular calcium levels.

The effects of the sympathetic and parasympathetic nervous systems on the heart are summarized in Fig. 7.5.

Cardiac contractility

Myocardial contraction is the result of calcium entry through L-type channels, giving rise to an increase in cytosolic calcium (Fig. 7.6).

The calcium is derived from two sources: the sarcoplasmic reticulum within the cell and the extracellular medium.

Extracellular calcium enters the cell, triggering larger amounts of calcium to be released from the

Effects of the sympathetic and parasympathetic systems on the heart		
	Sympathetic	Parasympathetic
Heart rate	Increased	Decreased
Force of contraction	Increased	Decreased
Automaticity	Increased	Reduced
AV node conduction	Facilitated	Inhibited
Cardiac efficiency	Reduced	Increased

Fig. 7.5 Effects of the sympathetic and parasympathetic system on the heart (AV, atrioventricular).

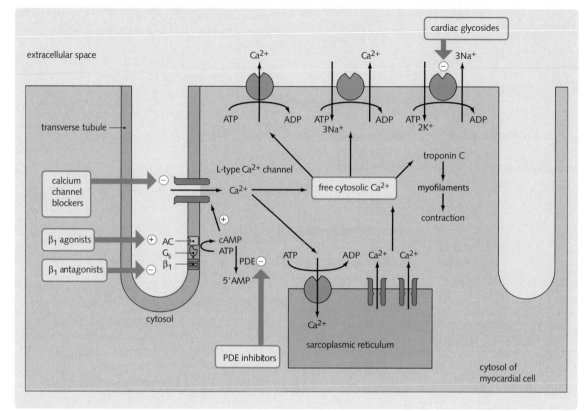

Fig. 7.6 Effects of drugs on cardiac contractility (AC, adenylyl cyclase; β1, β1-adrenoceptor; G_s, stimulatory G-protein; PDE, phosphodiesterase).

sarcoplasmic reticulum, a process known as calcium-induced calcium release.

During contraction, the intracellular levels of calcium rise to levels 10,000 times greater than those at rest. Calcium binds to troponin C, thus modifying the position of actin and myosin filaments, and allowing the cell to contract.

Contraction ceases only once calcium has been removed from the cytoplasm. This occurs through two mechanisms:

- Calcium is pumped out of the cell via the electrogenic Na^+/Ca^{2+} exchanger, which pumps one calcium ion out for every three sodium ions in.
- Calcium is resequestered into sarcoplasmic reticulum stores by a Ca^{2+} ATPase pump.

Cardiac dysfunction
Congestive heart failure
Congestive heart failure (CHF) is the combined failure of both the left and right sides of the heart.

The incidence of heart failure is between 1–5 per 1000 per year, and this doubles for each decade of life after the age of 45; over 100,000 hospital admissions annually are directly related to heart failure.

CHF occurs when the cardiac output does not meet the needs of the tissues. This is thought to result from defective excitation–contraction coupling, with progressive systolic and diastolic ventricular dysfunction.

Some of the causes, symptoms, and signs of acute and chronic heart failure are listed in Fig. 7.7.

The characteristics of left and right ventricular failure are listed in Fig. 7.8.

The body attempts to compensate for the effects of CHF by two processes—extrinsic and intrinsic.

Extrinsic neurohumoral reflexes: Extrinsic neurohumoral reflexes aim to maintain cardiac output and blood pressure such that hypotension → activation of baroreceptors (receptors responding to changes in pressure) → increased sympathetic

Causes and symptoms/signs of acute and chronic heart failure			
Causes		Symptoms/signs	
Acute HF	Chronic HF	Acute HF	Chronic HF
Myocardial infarction Acute valvular lesion	Systemic hypertension Myocardial infarction Valvular lesions Cardiomyopathies	Tachycardia Hypotension Dyspnea Pulmonary edema Systemic edema	Exertional dyspnea Systemic edema Cardiomegaly Fatigue Orthopnea

Fig. 7.7 Causes and symptoms/signs of acute and heart failure (HF).

Characteristics of right and left ventricular failure	
Right ventricular failure	Left ventricular failure
Reduced cardiac output Hypotension	Reduced cardiac output Hypotension
Peripheral edema Raised jugular venous pressure Hepatomegaly Ascites	Pulmonary edema Dyspnea Fatigue

Fig. 7.8 Characteristics of right and left ventricular failure.

activity → increased heart rate and vasoconstriction → increased cardiac contractility and vascular tone → increased arterial pressure.

However, the greater resistance (arterial pressure) against which the heart must pump reduces both the ejection fraction and the perfusion of the tissues.

The reduced perfusion of the kidneys activates the renin–angiotensin system, leading to renin secretion and subsequent elevation of plasma angiotensin II and aldosterone levels (see Fig. 7.14).

Angiotensin II causes peripheral vasoconstriction, and aldosterone increases sodium retention, leading to increased water retention, edema, and an increased preload.

Intrinsic cardiac compensation: The increased cardiac preload leads to incomplete emptying of the ventricles and an increase in end-diastolic pressure.

The heart eventually fails, owing to the massive increase in myocardial energy requirements.

Arrhythmias

Sudden death as a result of arrhythmias is the most common cause of death in developed countries, and it usually results from underlying cardiovascular pathology such as atherosclerosis.

Myocardial ischaemia is one of the most important causes of arrhythmias, and it occurs when a coronary artery becomes occluded, thus preventing sufficient blood from reaching the myocardium. Accumulation of endogenous biological mediators, including potassium, cAMP, thromboxane A_2, and free radicals, are believed to initiate arrhythmias.

Reperfusion after coronary occlusion is necessary for tissue recovery and prevention of myocardial necrosis, but spontaneous resumption of coronary flow is often itself a cause of arrhythmias.

Arrhythmias have been defined according to their appearance on the electrocardiogram (ECG) by the Lambeth Conventions. These include:

- Ventricular: premature beats, tachycardia, fibrillation, and *torsade de pointes*.
- Atrial: premature beats, tachycardia, flutter, and fibrillation.

The two main mechanisms by which cardiac rhythm becomes dysfunctional are abnormal impulse generation (automatic or triggered) and abnormal impulse conduction.

Abnormal impulse generation

Automatic: Automatic abnormal impulse generation is likely to cause sinus and atrial tachycardia, and ventricular premature beats. It can be:

- Enhanced: pathologic conditions, such as ischemia, may affect nodal and conducting tissue so that their inherent pacemaker frequency is greater than that of the SAN. Ischemia causes partial depolarization of tissues (owing to a decrease in the activity of the electrogenic sodium pump) and catecholamine release, thus enhancing the automaticity of the slow pacemakers (AVN, Purkinje fibers, bundle of His), and often giving rise to an ectopic focus triggering the development of a premature beat.
- Abnormal: a premature beat may also develop in atrial or ventricular tissue, which is not normally automatic.

131

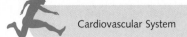
Triggered: Forms of triggered abnormal impulse generation are:

- Early after-depolarizations (EADs), which are likely to cause *torsade de pointes* and reperfusion-induced arrhythmias. EADs are triggered during repolarization (i.e., phase 2 or 3) of a previously normal impulse. They may result from a decrease in the delayed rectifier K^+ current, and they are associated with abnormally long action potentials. They are, therefore, more likely to occur during bradycardia and class III antiarrhythmic drug treatment.
- Delayed after-depolarizations (DADs) are triggered once the action potential has ended (i.e., during phase 4) of a previously normal impulse. DADs usually result from cellular calcium overload, associated with ischaemia, reperfusion, and cardiac glycoside intoxication.

Abnormal impulse conduction

Heart block: Heart block is likely to cause ventricular premature beats, and it results from damage to nodal tissue (most commonly the AVN) caused by conditions such as infarction. AV block may be first, second, or third degree, manifesting itself from slowed conduction to complete block of conduction, where the atria and ventricles beat independently.

Re-entry: Re-entry is likely to cause ventricular and atrial tachycardia and fibrillation, atrial flutter, and Wolff–Parkinson–White syndrome. Re-entry is of two types: circus movement and reflection.

In circus movement, an impulse re-excites an area of the myocardium, recently excited, after the refractory period has ended. This usually occurs in a ring of tissue in which a unidirectional block is present, preventing anterograde conduction of the impulse, but allowing retrograde conduction of the same impulse. This results in its continuous circulation, termed circus movement. The time taken for the impulse to propagate around the ring must exceed the refractory period; therefore, administration of drugs that prolong the refractory period will interrupt the circuit and terminate re-entry.

Reflection occurs in nonbranching bundles within which electrical dissociation has taken place. Owing to this electrical dissociation, an impulse can return over the same bundle.

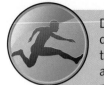

Don't panic. Arrhythmias are difficult to understand fully. Aim to know the more common arrhythmias, their causes and presentations, and their immediate and subsequent long-term management. If you master that, then try to add the cellular events and mechanism of drug action.

Angina pectoris

Angina is associated with acute myocardial ischaemia, and it results from underlying cardiovascular pathology. When coronary flow does not meet the metabolic needs of the heart, a radiating chest pain results; this is angina pectoris.

Stable or classical angina is due to fixed stenosis of the coronary arteries, and it is brought on by exercise and stress.

Unstable angina or crescendo angina can occur suddenly at rest, and it becomes progressively worse, with an increase in the number and severity of attacks. The following conditions can all cause unstable angina:

- Coronary atherosclerosis.
- Coronary artery spasm.
- Transient platelet aggregation and coronary thrombosis.
- Endothelial injury causing the accumulation of vasoconstrictor substances.
- Coronary vasoconstriction following adrenergic stimulation.

Variant angina or Prinzmetal's angina occurs at rest, at the same time each day, and it is usually due to coronary artery spasm. It is characterized by an elevated ST segment on the ECG during chest pain, and it may be accompanied by ventricular arrhythmias.

Treatment of cardiac dysfunction
Drugs used in heart failure
Cardiac glycosides

Examples of cardiac glycosides include digoxin and digitoxin.

Cardiac glycosides possess an aglycone steroid nucleus, conveying the pharmacologic activity of these compounds; an unsaturated lactone ring, conveying cardiotonic activity; and sugar moieties,

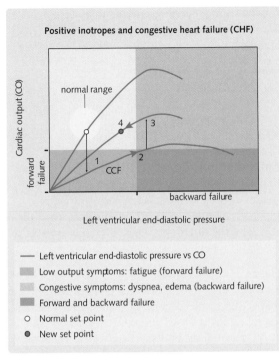

Positive inotropes and congestive heart failure (CHF)

normal range

4 3

1 2

CCF

backward failure

Left ventricular end-diastolic pressure

Cardiac output (CO)

forward failure

— Left ventricular end-diastolic pressure vs CO

▨ Low output symptoms: fatigue (forward failure)

▨ Congestive symptoms: dyspnea, edema (backward failure)

▨ Forward and backward failure

○ Normal set point

● New set point

Fig. 7.9 The Frank–Starling curve, positive inotropes, and congestive heart failure (CHF). Normal cardiac output is determined by the pressure in the left ventricle at end-diastole. In CHF, the set point for cardiac output is reduced and cardiac output falls (1). Compensatory neurohumoral responses become activated which increase end-diastolic pressure and improve cardiac output; however, this can give rise to backward failure (2). Positive inotropic agents increase cardiac output (3). The improved cardiac output reduces the drive for a high end-diastolic pressure, and decompensation occurs to a new set point.

able to modulate potency and pharmacokinetic distribution.

Although the positive inotropic actions of cardiac glycosides shift the Frank–Starling ventricular function curve to a more favorable position (Fig. 7.9), thus improving the symptoms of CHF, there is no evidence that they have a beneficial effect on the long-term prognosis of patients with CHF.

Mechanism of action: Cardiac glycosides act by inhibiting the membrane Na^+/K^+ ATPase pump (see Fig. 7.6). This increases intracellular Na^+ concentration, thus reducing the sodium gradient across the membrane and decreasing the amount of calcium pumped out of the cell by the Na^+/Ca^{2+} exchanger during diastole. Consequently, the intracellular calcium concentration rises,

leading to an increase in the force of cardiac contraction and maintaining normal blood pressure.

In addition, cardiac glycosides alter the electrical activity of the heart, both directly and indirectly. At therapeutic doses, they decrease the heart rate, slow atrioventricular (AV) conductance, and shorten the atrial action potential by stimulating vagal activity (vagotonic). This is useful in atrial fibrillation. At toxic doses, they indirectly (reflexly) increase the sympathetic activity of the heart and cause arrhythmias, including heart block. The direct effects are mainly due to loss of intracellular potassium, and they are most pronounced at high doses. The resting membrane potential is reduced, causing enhanced automaticity, slowed cardiac conduction, and increased AVN refractory period.

The increased cytosolic calcium concentration may reach toxic levels, thereby saturating the sarcoplasmic reticulum sequestration mechanism and causing oscillations in calcium owing to calcium-induced calcium release. This results in oscillatory after-potentials (ectopic beats) and subsequent arrhythmias.

In addition, cardiac glycosides have a direct effect on α-adrenoceptors, causing vasoconstriction and a consequent increase in peripheral vascular resistance, which is further enhanced by a centrally mediated increase in sympathetic tone.

Route of administration: Oral.

Indications: Heart failure and supraventricular arrhythmias.

Contraindications: Heart block, hypokalemia associated with the use of diuretics (the lack of competition from potassium potentiates the binding to and the effects of cardiac glycosides on the Na^+/K^+ ATPase pump).

Adverse effects: Arrhythmias, anorexia, nausea and vomiting, visual disturbances, and abdominal pain and diarrhea.

Therapeutic notes: The cardiac glycosides have a very narrow therapeutic window; toxicity, therefore, is relatively common. If this occurs, the drug should be withdrawn, and, if necessary, potassium supplements and antiarrhythmic drugs (e.g., lidocaine) should be administered. For severe intoxication, antibodies specific to cardiac glycosides (Digibind®) are available.

133

Phosphodiesterase inhibitors

Examples of phosphodiesterase (PDE) inhibitors include inamrinone and milrinone. These have been developed as a result of the many adverse effects and problems associated with cardiac glycosides. There is no evidence that they improve the mortality rate.

Mechanism of action: The type III PDE (PDE–3) isoenzyme is found in myocardial and vascular smooth muscle.

Phosphodiesterase is responsible for the degradation of cAMP; therefore, inhibiting this enzyme raises cAMP levels, and this causes an increase in myocardial contractility and vasodilatation (see Fig. 7.6). Cardiac output is increased, and pulmonary wedge pressure and total peripheral resistance are reduced, without much change in heart rate or blood pressure.

Route of administration: Intravenous.

Indications: PDE inhibitors are given for severe acute heart failure that is resistant to other drugs.

Adverse effects: Nausea and vomiting, arrhythmias, liver dysfunction, abdominal pain, and hypersensitivity.

Beta-adrenoceptor agonists

Examples of β-adrenoceptor agonists include dobutamine and dopamine. They are used intravenously in CHF emergencies (see Fig. 7.6).

Drugs with proven mortality benefits in cardiac failure should be remembered. They are β-adrenoceptor antagonists, ACE inhibitors, nitrates with hydralazine, and spironolactone.

Diuretics

The diuretics used in CCF are thiazides, loop diuretics, and spironolactone.

Diuretics inhibit sodium and water retention by the kidneys, and so reduce edema due to heart failure. Venous pressure and consequently cardiac preload are reduced, increasing the efficiency of the heart as a pump (Chapter 9). Spironolactone appears to have a beneficial effect in heart failure at doses lower than it would be expected to function as a diuretic.

Angiotensin-converting-enzyme inhibitors

For details of angiotensin-converting-enzyme (ACE) inhibitors see below.

Nitrates

See antianginal drugs.

Vasodilating drugs

Hydralazine is discussed below.

Antiarrhythmic drugs

Antiarrhythmic drugs are classified according to a system devised by Vaughan Williams in 1970 and later modified by Harrison. A summary of the effects of the different classes of drug is given in Fig 7.10.

Class I

All class I drugs block the voltage-dependent sodium channels in a dose-dependent manner. Their action resembles that of local anesthetics (Chapter 5).

All class I drugs prolong the effective refractory period (terminate re-entry), and they convert unidirectional block to bidirectional block (prevent re-entry).

Class Ia

Examples of class Ia drugs include quinidine, procainamide, and disopyramide.

Class Ia drugs affect atrial muscle, ventricular muscle, the bundle of His, the Purkinje fibers, and the AVN.

Mechanism of action: Class Ia drugs block voltage-dependent sodium channels in their open (activated) or refractory (inactivated) state (Figs. 7.3 and 7.4). Their effects are to slow phase 0 (increasing the effective refractory period), slow phase 4 (reducing automaticity), and to prolong action potential duration.

Route of administration: Oral, intravenous.

Indications: Ventricular and supraventricular arrhythmias.

Contraindications: Heart block, sinus node dysfunction, cardiogenic shock, and severe uncompensated heart failure. Procainamide should not be given to patients with systemic lupus erythematosus.

Adverse effects: Arrhythmias, nausea and vomiting, hypersensitivity, thrombocytopenia, and agranulocytosis. Procainamide can cause a lupus-like syndrome, and disopyramide causes hypotension.

Effects of antiarrhythmic drugs					
Class	Example	Myocardial contractility	AV conduction	AP duration	Effective refractory period
Ia	Procainamide	↓	↓↓	↑	↑
Ib	Lidocaine	–	–	↓	↑↑
Ic	Flecainide	↓↓	↓↓	–	–
II	Propranolol	↓↓	–/↓	–	–
III	Amiodarone	–	↑	↑↑↑	↑↑↑
Iv	Verapamil	↓↓↓	↓↓	↓↓	–

Fig. 7.10 Effects of the antiarrhythmic drugs (AP, action potential; AV, atrioventricular). The number of arrows indicates the degree of the effect caused.

Class Ib

Examples of class Ib drugs include lidocaine, mexiletine, and phenytoin.

Mechanism of action: Class Ib drugs exert their effects in several ways (see Fig. 7.3). These include:

- Blocking voltage-dependent sodium channels in their refractory (inactivated) state (i.e., when depolarized, as occurs in ischemia).
- Binding to open channels during phase 0, and dissociating by the next beat if the rhythm is normal, but abolishing premature beats.
- Decreasing action potential duration.
- Increasing the effective refractory period.

Route of administration: Lidocaine is administered intravenously, and mexiletine and phenytoin either orally or intravenously.

Indications: Ventricular arrhythmias following myocardial infarction. Phenytoin is used in epilepsy (Chapter 6).

Contraindications: Class Ib drugs should not be given to patients with sinoatrial disorders, AV block, or porphyria.

Adverse effects: Hypotension, bradycardia, drowsiness and confusion, convulsions, and paraesthesia (pins and needles).

Lidocaine may cause dizziness and respiratory depression; mexiletine may cause nausea and vomiting, constipation, arrhythmias, and hepatitis; and phenytoin may cause nausea and vomiting, and peripheral neuropathy.

Class Ic

Flecainide is the only drug used from class Ic.

Mechanism of action: Flecainide blocks sodium channels in a fashion similar to the class Ia and Ib drugs, but it shows no preference for refractory channels. Class Ic drugs, therefore, result in a general reduction in the excitability of the myocardium.

Route of administration: Oral, intravenous.

Indications: Ventricular tachyarrhythmias.

Contraindications: Heart failure, history of myocardial infarction.

Adverse effects: Dizziness, visual disturbances, arrhythmias.

Class II

Examples of class II drugs include propranolol, atenolol, and metoprolol (see Figs. 7.4 and 7.6).

Class II drugs are β-adrenoceptor antagonists (atenolol and metoprolol are β_1 selective). They have been shown to reduce sudden death after myocardial infarction by 50% (although this is believed to be due to prevention of cardiac rupture as opposed to prevention of ventricular fibrillation).

Class III

Examples of Class III drugs include bretylium, amiodarone, sotalol, and ibutilide.

Mechanism of action: All Class III drugs used clinically are potassium channel blockers. They prolong cardiac action potential duration (increased QT interval on the ECG), and they prolong the effective refractory period (see Fig. 7.3).

Amiodarone also blocks sodium and calcium channels (i.e., slows phase 0 and 3) and blocks α- and β-adrenoceptors. Sotalol is a β-adrenoceptor antagonist with class III activity.

Route of administration: Bretylium is administered intravenously; amiodarone and sotalol are administered orally or intravenously.

Indications: Class III drugs are given for ventricular and supraventricular arrhythmias.

Contraindications: Bretylium should not be given to patients with pheochromocytoma; amiodarone should not be given to those with AV block, sinus bradycardia, or thyroid dysfunction.

For contraindications regarding sotalol, see under β-blockers.

Adverse effects: Class III drugs can cause arrhythmias, especially *torsade de pointes*.

Bretylium may cause hypotension, nausea and vomiting; amiodarone may cause thyroid dysfunction, liver damage, pulmonary fibrosis (potentially fatal), photosensitivity, and neuropathy.

For adverse effects regarding sotalol, see under β-blockers.

Class IV

Examples of class IV drugs include verapamil and diltiazem (see Figs 7.3 and 7.6).

Class IV drugs are calcium antagonists (calcium channel blockers) that shorten phase 2 of the action potential, thus decreasing action potential duration. They are particularly effective in nodal cells, where calcium spikes initiate conduction.

Details of the drugs are given in the section on antianginal drugs.

Other antiarrhythmics

The cardiac glycosides and adenosine are agents used in arrhythmias, but they do not fit into the four classes described.

Adenosine

Adenosine is produced endogenously, and it acts upon many tissues, including the lungs, afferent nerves, and platelets.

Mechanism of action: Adenosine acts at A_1 receptors in cardiac conducting tissue, and it causes myocyte hyperpolarization. This acts to slow the rate of rise of an action potential, which brings about delay in conduction.

Route of administration: Intravenous.

Indications: Paroxysmal supraventricular tachycardia. Aid diagnosis of broad and narrow complex supraventricular tachycardia.

Contraindications: Second- or third-degree heart block, sick sinus syndrome.

Adverse effects: Transient facial flushing, chest pain, dyspnea, and bronchospasm. Side effects are very short lived, often lasting less than 30 seconds.

Epinephrine

Epinephrine is a sympathomimetic agent used in cardiac arrest and in the management of anaphylaxis. Epinephrine is discussed below.

The drugs used in stable angina pectoris are β-adrenoceptor antagonists, nitrates, calcium antagonists, antiplatelets, and potassium channel activators.

Antianginal drugs

Acute attacks of angina are treated with sublingual nitrates or, in the hospital setting, with an opioid (Chapter 6).

Stable angina is treated with long-acting nitrates, antiplatelets, β-adrenoceptor antagonists, calcium antagonists, or potassium-channel activators.

Unstable angina is a medical emergency, and it requires hospital admission. Unstable angina is treated with:

- Antiplatelets (aspirin, clopidogrel, dipyridamole, and the glycoprotein IIb/IIIa inhibitors).
- Heparin/low-molecular weight heparin.
- Standard antianginal drug regimen.

Organic nitrates

The organic nitrates glyceryl trinitrate (GTN), isosorbide mononitrate (ISMN), and isosorbide dinitrate (ISDN) can relieve angina within minutes.

Mechanism of action: Most nitrates are prodrugs, decomposing to form nitric oxide (NO), which activates guanylyl cyclase, thereby increasing the levels of cyclic guanosine monophosphate (cGMP). Protein kinase G is activated, and contractile proteins are phosphorylated. Dilatation of the systemic veins decreases preload and, consequently, the oxygen demand of the heart, while dilatation of the coronary arteries increases blood flow and oxygen delivery to the myocardium.

Route of administration: Sublingual, oral (modified release), or from transdermal patches. GTN can be given by intravenous infusion.

Indications: Organic nitrates are given for the prophylaxis and treatment of angina and in left ventricular failure.

Contraindications: Organic nitrates should not be given to patients with hypersensitivity to nitrates or those with hypotension and hypovolemia.

Adverse effects: Postural hypotension, tachycardia, headache, flushing, and dizziness.

Therapeutic notes: To avoid nitrate tolerance, a drug-free period of approximately 8 hours is needed.

Beta-adrenoceptor antagonists (β-blockers)

Examples of β-blockers include propranolol, atenolol, bisoprolol, and metoprolol.

Beta-adrenoceptors are found in many tissues, although the β_1-adrenoceptor is found predominantly in the heart, and the β_2-adrenoceptor is found mainly in the smooth muscle of the vasculature and bronchioles Some overlap does exist.

Different β-blockers have different affinity for the two types of adrenoceptor. Propranolol is nonselective, having equal affinity for both the β_1- and β_2-adrenoceptors. Atenolol, bisoprolol, and metoprolol have greater affinity for the β_1-adrenoceptor, and are, therefore, more "cardiac-selective." Some β-blockers even appear to have partial agonistic effects at β-adrenoceptors as well a antagonistic effects.

Mechanism of action: The aim of using β-adrenoceptor antagonists in cardiac disease is to block β-adrenoceptors in the heart. This has the effect of causing a fall in heart rate (slowing of phase 4; see Fig. 7.4), in systolic blood pressure, in cardiac contractile activity, and in myocardial oxygen demand.

Route of administration: Oral, intravenous.

Indications: Angina, post-myocardial infarction, arrhythmias, hypertension, thyrotoxicosis, glaucoma, and anxiety.

Contraindications: Nonselective β-blockers (e.g., propranolol) must not be given to asthmatic patients. At high doses β_1-adrenoceptor antagonists lose their selectivity, and they should be used with caution in those with asthma. Other contraindications for β-blockers include bradycardia, hypotension, AV block, and CHF.

Adverse effects: Bronchospasm, fatigue and insomnia, dizziness, cold extremities (β_2-adrenoceptor effect), bradycardia, heart block, hypotension, and decreased glucose tolerance in diabetic patients.

Calcium-channel blockers

Examples of calcium-channel blockers include verapamil, diltiazem, and nifedipine.

Mechanism of action: Verapamil and diltiazem block L-type calcium channels found in the heart and in the vascular smooth muscle, thereby reducing calcium entry into cardiac and vascular cells (see Figs. 7.3, 7.6, and 7.12). This decrease in intracellular calcium reduces cardiac contractility and causes vasodilatation, which results in several effects: reduced preload due to the reduced venous pressure, reduced afterload due to the reduced arteriolar pressure, increased coronary blood flow, reduced cardiac contractility and thus reduced myocardial oxygen consumption, and a decreased heart rate. High doses of these drugs affect AV nodal conduction.

Nifedipine blocks L-type calcium channels in vascular cells. It does not affect cells, with minimal effects on cardiac contractility, or AVN conduction, and its beneficial effects are due to increased coronary flow and peripheral vasodilatation.

Route of administration: Oral.

Indications: Calcium-channel blockers are used for the prophylaxis and treatment of angina and hypertension. Verapamil and diltiazem are given for supraventricular arrhythmias, and nifedipine for Raynaud's syndrome (peripheral vasoconstriction).

Contraindications: Calcium-channel blockers should not be given to patients in cardiogenic shock.

Nifedipine is contraindicated in advanced aortic stenosis; verapamil and diltiazem should not be given to patients in severe heart failure (owing to their negative inotropic action), to those taking β-blockers (risk of AV block and impaired cardiac output), and those with severe bradycardia.

Adverse effects: Verapamil and diltiazem may cause hypotension, rash, bradycardia, CHF, heart block, and constipation. Nifedipine may cause hypotension, rash, reflex tachycardia, peripheral edema, flushing, and dizziness.

There are three classes of calcium-channel blockers. Two of them act mostly upon the heart (verapamil and diltiazem), and the other acts mostly upon peripheral vascular tone (nifedipine). Concurrent use of a β-adrenoceptor antagonist and a calcium-channel blocker can result in profound bradycardia.

Classes of drugs to treat angina, cardiac failure, and arrhythmias		
Angina	**Heart failure**	**Arrhythmias**
Organic nitrates	Cardiac glycosides	Na^+ channel blockers (Class I)
β_1-adrenoceptor antagonists	Phosphodiesterase inhibitors	β_1-adrenoceptor antagonists (Class II)
Ca^{2+} antagonists	β_1-adrenoceptor agonists	K^+ channel blockers (Class III)
Antiplatelets	Diuretics	Ca^{2+} antagonists (Class IV)
Potassium-channel activators	ACE inhibitors	Cardiac glycosides
	Nitrates	Adenosine
	Vasodilating drugs	

Fig. 7.11 Classes of drugs used to treat angina, cardiac failure, and arrhythmias.

Fig. 7.11 summarizes the main drug classes used in angina, cardiac failure, and arrhythmias.

The overall aims of symptom management in angina are: to dilate coronary arteries to allow maximal myocardial perfusion; to decrease the heart rate to minimize oxygen demands of the myocardium, and lengthen diastole when cardiac perfusion occurs; and to prevent platelets from aggregating and forming platelet plugs. In addition to this, reversible risk factors need to be addressed to limit the progression of the disease.

Circulation

Control of vascular tone
Alpha-adrenoceptor activation

Alpha-adrenoceptor activation (Fig. 7.12) causes contraction of vascular smooth muscle through the activation of phospholipase C (PLC). The resulting increased level of IP_3 causes the release of calcium from the endoplasmic reticulum, thus increasing the calcium level. Calcium then binds to calmodulin, thus activating myosin light-chain kinase (MLCK) and allowing contraction.

Beta₂-adrenoceptor activation

Beta₂-adrenoceptor activation (see Fig. 7.12) causes relaxation of vascular smooth muscle through the activation of adenylyl cyclase. The resulting increased level of cAMP activates protein kinase A, which phosphorylates and inactivates MLCK.

M₃ receptor activation

M_3 receptor activation causes relaxation of vascular smooth muscle through the release of nitric oxide (NO) (see Fig. 7.12). Guanylyl cyclase is activated by NO, thus increasing the levels of cGMP and activating protein kinase G. Protein kinase G inhibits contraction by phosphorylating contractile proteins.

Renin–angiotensin system

A decrease in plasma volume results in the activation of the renin–angiotensin system (RAS), which is summarized in Fig. 7.13 (see also Chapter 9).

Angiotensin-converting enzyme (ACE) catalyses the production of angiotensin II. Angiotensin II causes:

- Potent vasoconstriction (40 times as potent as norepinephrine).
- Release of norepinephrines.
- Stimulation of the secretion of aldosterone.

ACE also catalyses the inactivation of bradykinin, which is an endogenous vasodilator.

Aldosterone is a steroid that induces the synthesis of sodium channels and Na^+/K^+

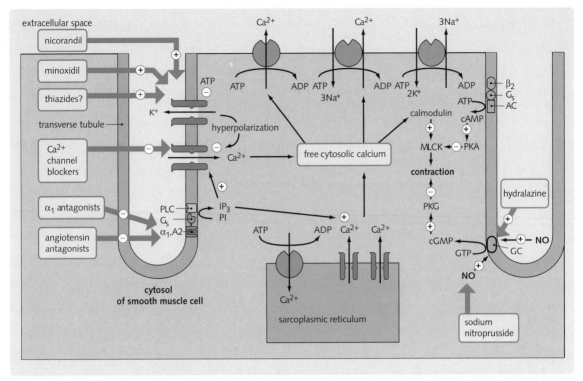

Fig. 7.12 Drugs affecting vascular tone (AC, adenyl cyclase; α_1, α_1-adrenoceptor; A2, angiotensin II; β_2, β_2-adrenoceptor; GC, guanylyl cyclase; GS, stimulatory G-protein; IP$_3$, inositol triphosphate; MLCK, myosin light-chain kinase; NO, nitric oxide; PLC, phospholipase C; PI, phosphatidylinositol; PKA, protein kinase A; PKG, protein kinase G).

ATPase pumps in the luminal membrane of the cortical collecting ducts. This results in a greater amount of sodium and, consequently, water being reabsorbed, thus increasing the blood volume and pressure.

Certain renal diseases and renal artery occlusion will cause activation of the RAS and result in the development of hypertension.

Hypertension

Normal blood pressure is generally regarded as 120/80 mmHg (systolic pressure/diastolic pressure). Hypertension is defined as a diastolic arterial pressure greater than 90 mmHg or a systolic arterial pressure greater than 140 mmHg. The condition can be fatal if left untreated, as it greatly increases the risk of thrombosis, stroke, and renal failure.

Three factors determine blood pressure. These are blood volume, cardiac output, and peripheral vascular resistance.

"Primary" or "essential" hypertension accounts for 90–95% of all cases of hypertension. This has no known cause, but it is associated with:
- Age (40+).
- Obesity.
- Physical inactivity.
- Smoking and alcohol consumption.
- Genetic predisposition.

"Secondary" hypertension accounts for the remaining 5–10% of cases of hypertension. The cause is usually one of the following:
- Renal disease, which activates the RAS.
- Endocrine disease (e.g., pheochromocytoma, steroid-secreting tumor of the adrenal cortex, epinephrine-secreting tumor of the adrenal medulla).

Treatment of hypertension

The treatment of hypertension is aimed at various targets; these are summarized in Fig. 7.14.

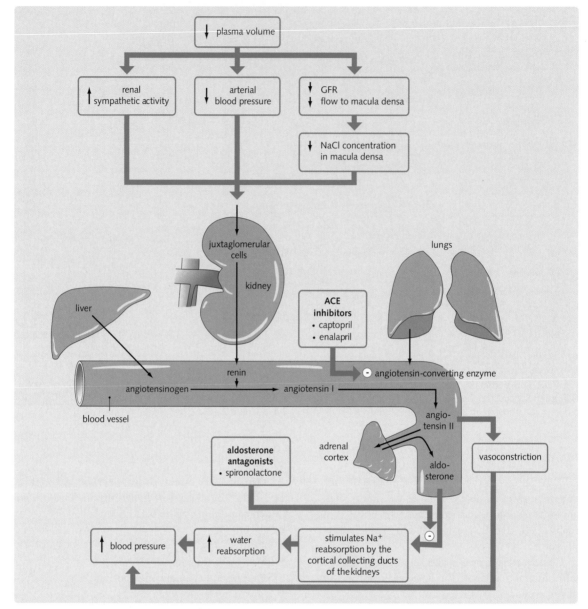

Fig. 7.13 Renin–angiotensin system and angiotensin-converting enzyme (ACE) inhibitors (GFR, glomerular filtration rate).

Vasodilators

Angiotensin-converting enzyme inhibitors

Captopril, enalapril, lisinopril, and ramipril are examples of ACE inhibitors.

Mechanism of action: ACE inhibitors cause inhibition of ACE with consequent reduced angiotensin II and aldosterone levels (see Fig. 7.13), and increased bradykinin levels. This causes vasodilatation with a consequent reduction in peripheral resistance, little change in heart rate and cardiac output, and reduced sodium retention.

Route of administration: Oral.

Indications: Hypertension, heart failure, and renal dysfunction (especially in diabetic patients to slow progression of diabetic or reduced renal functional nephropathy).

Contraindications: Pregnancy, renovascular disease, aortic stenosis.

Adverse effects: Characteristic cough, hypotension, dizziness and headache, diarrhea, and muscle cramps.

Advantages and disadvantages of drugs used in hypertension with respect to associated conditions					
	Diuretic	β-Blocker	ACE inhibitor/angiotesin II receptor antagonist	Calcium channel blockers	α-Blocker
Diabetes	Care[a]	Care[a]	yes	yes	yes
Gout	No	yes	yes	yes	yes
Dyslipidaemia	Care[b]	Care[b]	yes	yes	yes
Ischaemic heart disease	yes	yes	yes	Care[d]	yes
Heart failure	yes	Care[c]	yes	yes	yes
Asthma	yes	No	yes	yes	yes
Peripheral vascular disease	yes	Care	Care[e]	yes	yes
Renal artery stenosis	yes	Care	No	yes	yes
Pregnancy	Caution	Not in late pregnancy	No	No	Caution

[a] Diuretics may aggravate diabetes: β-blockers worsen glucose intolerance and mask symptoms of hypoglycemia.
[b] Both diuretics and β-blockers disturb the lipid profile.
[c] There is some evidence for beneficial effects of some β-blockers when used cautiously in heart failure.
[d] Verapamil and diltiazem may exacerbate heart failure, although amlodipine appears to be safe.
[e] Patients with peripheral vascular disease may also have renal artery stenosis; therefore, ACE inhibitors should be used cautiously.

Fig. 7.14 Advantages and disadvantages of drugs used in hypertension with respect to associated conditions (from Clinical Medicine, 4th ed., by P Kumar and M Clark. W.B. Saunders, 1998).

Therapeutic noters: First-dose hypotension is relatively common, and so these drugs should ideally be given just before bed.

Angiotensin-II (AT$_I$) receptor antagonists

Losartan and valsartan are examples of angiotensin-II (AT$_I$) receptor antagonists.

Mechanism of action: Angiotensin-II receptor antagonists cause inhibition at the angiotensin II (AT$_I$) receptor (see Fig. 7.12), resulting in vasodilatation with a consequent reduction in peripheral resistance.

Route of administration: Oral.

Indications: Hypertension.

Contraindications: Pregnancy, breastfeeding. Caution in renal artery stenosis and aortic stenosis.

Adverse effects: Cough (less common than with ACE inhibitors), orthostatic hypotension, dizziness, headache and fatigue, hyperkalemia, and rash.

Calcium antagonists

Nifedipine has more effect upon vascular tone than diltiazem or verapamil, which are more cardio selective (see Fig. 7.12).

Alpha$_1$-adrenoceptor antagonists

Prazosin and doxazosin are examples of α$_1$-adrenoceptor antagonists.

Mechanism of action: Alpha$_1$-adrenoceptor antagonists cause inhibition of α$_1$-adrenoceptor-mediated vasoconstriction—consequently reducing peripheral resistance and venous pressure (see Fig. 7.12). They also lower plasma low-density lipoprotein (LDL) cholesterol levels, very-low-density lipoprotein (VLDL) levels, and triglyceride (TGA) levels; and they increase high-density lipoprotein (HDL) cholesterol levels—thus reducing the risk of coronary artery disease.

Route of administration: Oral.

Indications: Hypertension (especially in patients with CHF), prostate hyperplasia (reduced bladder and prostate resistance), and coronary artery disease.

Contraindications: Prazosin should not be given to people with CCF due to aortic stenosis.

Adverse effects: Postural hypotension, dizziness, headache and fatigue, weakness, palpitations, and nausea.

Hydralazine

Hydralazine is a second- or third-line drug for the treatment of mild to moderate hypertension.

Mechanism of action: Hydralazine effects are unclear, although it appears to interfere with the action of IP_3 in vascular smooth muscle, thereby reducing peripheral resistance and blood pressure (see Fig. 7.12).

Route of administration: Oral, intravenous.

Indications: Moderate to severe hypertension. Also used in conjunction with β-blockers and thiazides in hypertensive emergencies and in hypertensive pregnant women.

Contraindications: Idiopathic systemic lupus erythematosus, severe tachycardia.

Adverse effects: Tachycardia, fluid retention, nausea and vomiting, and headache.

Minoxidil

Owing to its adverse effects, minoxidil is a drug of last resort in the long-term treatment of hypertension.

Mechanism of action: Minoxidil activates vascular smooth muscle ATP-sensitive potassium channels, resulting in hyperpolarization of the cell membrane and consequent reduced calcium entry through L-type channels (see Fig. 7.12). The overall effect is inhibition of smooth muscle contraction and subsequent vasodilatation.

Route of administration: Oral for hypertension; topical cream for baldness.

Indications: Severe hypertension. Baldness.

Contraindications: Pheochromocytoma or porphyria.

Adverse effects: Hirsutism (limits use in women), sodium and water retention, tachycardia, and cardiotoxicity.

Therapeutic effects: Although unrelated chemically, the drug diazoxide acts in a similar fashion to minoxidil and activates potassium channels, resulting in vasodilatation.

Sodium nitroprusside

Mechanism of action: Sodium nitroprusside is a prodrug that spontaneously decomposes into NO inside smooth muscle cells. NO activates guanylyl cyclase, thus increasing intracellular cGMP levels, and causing vasodilatation (see Fig. 7.12).

Route of administration: Intravenous.

Indications: Sodium nitroprusside is given by intravenous titration in hypertensive crises, for controlled hypotension in surgery, and in heart failure.

Contraindications: Sodium nitroprusside should not be given to patients with severe hepatic impairment, vitamin B_{12} deficiency, or Leber's optic atrophy.

Adverse effects: Headache and dizziness, nausea, abdominal pain, palpitations, and retrosternal discomfort.

Therapeutic notes: Sodium nitroprusside is broken down in the body to thiocyanate, which has a half-life of only a few minutes, although prolonged exposure to nitroprusside and thiocyanate can result in thiocyanate toxicity (weakness, nausea, and inhibition of thyroid function).

The more common adverse effects of the vasodilating drugs are hypotension and headache, both of which directly result from reducing peripheral vascular resistance.

Diuretic drugs

Diuretics used in hypertension include thiazides, loop diuretics, and potassium-sparing diuretics.

See Chapter 9 for details of each of these drugs.

Mechanism of action: The antihypertensive action of diuretic drugs does not seem to correlate with their diuretic activity: loop diuretics are powerful diuretics but only moderate antihypertensives; thiazides are moderate diuretics but powerful antihypertensives.

It has recently been suggested that the antihypertensive effects of diuretics (especially the thiazides) are not necessarily a result of their diuretic effect but rather may be due to activation of ATP-regulated potassium channels in resistance arterioles, with a mechanism of action similar to that of minoxidil. This causes hyperpolarization and, consequently, inhibition of calcium entry into vascular smooth muscle cells with consequent vasodilatation and reduced peripheral vascular resistance (see Fig. 7.12).

Centrally acting antihypertensive drugs

Clonidine, methyldopa, and guanabenz are examples of centrally acting antihypertensive drugs. These agents are second- or third-line drugs in the treatment of hypertension.

Mechanism of action: Centrally acting antihypertensive drugs are α_2-adrenoceptor agonists. The activation of presynaptic α_2-adrenoceptors causes inhibition of noradrenaline release and consequent vasodilatation. The activation of postsynaptic α_2-adrenoceptors causes vasoconstriction, although presynaptic effects dominate.

Centrally acting antihypertensive drugs reduce the activity of the vasomotor center in the brain, causing reduced sympathetic activity and subsequent vasodilatation. They also reduce heart rate and cardiac output.

Route of administration: Oral. Clonidine can be given by intravenous infusion.

Indications: Hypertensive patients when first-line antihypertensive agents are ineffective or contraindicated. Methyldopa is safe for hypertension in pregnancy, asthmatic patients, and those with heart failure.

Contraindications: Methyldopa should not be given to people with depression, liver disease, or phaeochromocytoma.

Adverse effects: Dry mouth, sedation, orthostatic hypotension, male sexual dysfunction, and galactorrhea. Methyldopa can cause diffuse parenchymal liver injury, fever, and, rarely, hemolytic anemia. Clonidine can cause a withdrawal hypertensive crisis on stopping treatment.

Pheochromocytoma

Pheochromocytoma is a rare endocrine tumor, most commonly of the adrenal gland. These tumors can secrete epinephrine and various intermediates in its biosynthesis. These vasoactive compounds result in the clinical signs and symptoms of pheochromocytomas, which include facial flushing, sweating, breathlessness, anxiety, tachycardia, and paroxysmal hypertension.

Medical management of pheochromocytoma-induced hypertension relies on the powerful α-adrenoceptor antagonist phenoxybenzamine.

Alpha-adrenoceptor blockade reduces peripheral vascular resistance and lowers blood pressure. The use of β-adrenoceptor antagonists is dangerous, as tumor-secreted sympathomimetics act unopposed on α-adrenoceptors, increasing both peripheral vascular resistance and blood pressure.

Phenoxybenzamine

Mechanism of action: Phenoxybenzamine antagonizes α-adrenoceptors in the vascular smooth muscles, resulting in vasodilatation.

Route of administration: Oral, intravenous.

Indications: Hypertensives episodes in pheochromocytoma.

Contraindications: History of cerebrovascular events, post-myocardial infarction.

Adverse effects: Postural hypotension, tachycardia, nasal congestion.

Therapeutic notes: Phentolamine is another powerful α-1 selective adrenoceptor antagonist that can be used in pheochromocytoma, although it has a much shorter half-life and is commonly used prior to and during surgery to excise the tumor.

Vasoconstrictors and the management of shock
Shock

Shock is a state of circulatory collapse, characterized by an arterial blood pressure unable to maintain adequate tissue perfusion. Shock is a life-threatening condition.

The body responds inappropriately to shock, releasing mediators such as histamine, prostaglandins, bradykinin, and 5-hydroxytryptamine (5-HT, serotonin), which cause capillary dilatation and increased capillary permeability. This further reduces blood pressure and cardiac output.

Signs of shock include:
• Very low arterial blood pressure.
• A weak, rapid pulse.
• Cold, pale, sweaty skin.
• Rapid breathing.
• Dry mouth.
• Reduced urine output.
• Anxiousness.

Causes of shock include:
• Hemorrhage.
• Burns.

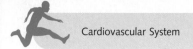

- Dehydration.
- Severe vomiting or diarrhea.
- Bacterial septicemia.
- Myocardial infarction.
- Pulmonary embolism.

Types of shock include:
- Hypovolemic, which is caused by a reduction in the circulating blood volume.
- Cardiogenic, reduced cardiac output due to "pump failure."
- Septic, which is caused by massive vasodilation.
- Anaphylactic, a severe allergic reaction, in which there is a massive generalized release of vasodilating mediators.
- Spinal, disruption of neuronal control upon vascular tone and cardiac output.

Management of shock
The medical management of shock ultimately depends upon its underlying cause. For example, if a child is shocked due to chronic diarrhea and vomiting, fluid and electrolyte replacement is most appropriate management.

The following drugs are useful in restoring blood pressure and tissue perfusion, but on the whole they do not address the underlying cause of the different types of shock.

Sympathomimetic amines
Examples of sympathomimetic amines include epinephrine, norepinephrine, phenylephrine, and ephedrine.

Sympathomimetic amines raise blood pressure at the expense of vital organs such as the kidneys, and they raise peripheral resistance, which is already high in patients with shock.

Mechanism of action: Epinephrine and norepinephrine are agonists at both α- and β-adrenoceptor, and phenylephrine is an α$_1$-adrenoceptor agonist. Ephedrine is a β-adrenoceptor agonist and causes norepinephrine release. These drugs work either by activating α-adrenoceptors which then activate phospholipase C, causing vasoconstriction and a consequent increase in arterial blood pressure, or by activating β-adrenoceptors, which then activate adenylyl cyclase, causing an increased heart rate, increased cardiac contractility, and vasodilatation.

Route of administration: Parenterally, commonly intravenously.

Indications: Shock, acute hypotension, and reversal of hypotension caused by spinal or epidural anesthesia. Epinephrine is used in cardiac arrest and anaphylaxis.

Contraindications: Sympathomimetic amines should not be given to people who are pregnant or have hypertension.

Adverse effects: Tachycardia, anxiety, insomnia, arrhythmias, dry mouth, and cold extremities.

Therapeutic notes: In a cardiac arrest, epinephrine is used at a concentration of 1 mg per 10 mL (1:10 000) intravenously, whereas in anaphylaxis adrenaline is used at a concentration of 1 mg per 1 mL (1:1000) intramuscularly.

Dopamine and dobutamine
Mechanism of action: Dopamine is a precursor of norepinephrine. It activates dopamine receptors and α- and β-adrenoceptors. When administered by intravenous infusion, dopamine acts on:
- Dopamine receptors, causing vasodilatation in the kidneys at low doses.
- Alpha$_1$-adrenoceptors, causing vasoconstriction in other vasculature.
- Beta$_1$-adrenoceptors, causing positive inotropic and chronotropic effects.

Dobutamine has no effect upon dopaminergic receptors but does activate β$_1$-adrenoceptors.

If renal perfusion is not impaired, dobutamine and dopamine are a more appropriate means of treating shock than α-adrenoceptor agonists. This form of treatment maintains renal perfusion and inhibits the activation of the RAS.

Route of administration: Intravenous.

Indications: CHF (emergencies only), cardiogenic shock, septic shock, hypovolemic shock, cardiomyopathy, and cardiac surgery.

Contraindications: Tachyarrhythmias; dopamine is contraindicated in people with pheochromocytoma.

Adverse effects: Tachycardia and hypertension; dopamine causes nausea and vomiting, and hypotension.

Therapeutic notes: Although low doses of dopamine cause vasodilatation, high doses cause vasoconstriction and may exacerbate heart failure.

Vasopressin and desmopressin
Vasopressin (antidiuretic hormone [ADH]) and desmopressin are examples of antidiuretic peptides.

Vasopressin is short acting ($t_{1/2} = 10$ minutes) while desmopressin is longer acting ($t_{1/2} = 75$ minutes).

Mechanism of action: Antidiuretic peptides activate V_1 receptors on smooth muscle cells, which stimulate phospholipase C, causing contraction. They also activate V_2 receptors on the tubular cells of the kidneys, which stimulate adenylyl cyclase and thereby increase the permeability of these cells to water, and reduce sodium and water excretion. Vasopressin has a much greater affinity for V_2 receptors than V_1 receptors.

Route of administration: Oral, intravenous, intranasal.

Indications: Pituitary diabetes insipidus. The antidiuretic peptides are no longer used in the management of shock, although their pharmacology is both academically interesting and a potential target for future drugs.

Contraindications: Vascular disease, chronic nephritis.

Adverse effects: Fluid retention, nausea, pallor, abdominal cramps, and belching. They may induce anginal attacks (due to coronary vasoconstriction).

Corticosteroids

The use of corticosteroids in septic shock remains controversial, although they are also given by intravenous injection in the treatment of anaphylactic shock as an adjunct to epinephrine (Chapter 11).

It is possible to distinguish between the types of shock clinically:
• Hypovolemic—low JVP; cool, clammy peripheries; confusion/restlessness.
• Cardiogenic—raised JVP; cool, clammy peripheries; anxiousness/agitation.
• Septic—warm, sweaty peripheries; pyrexia; nausea.
• Anaphylactic—warm peripheries, urticaria, nausea.
• Spinal—history of trauma or spinal anesthesia.

Tachycardia, hypotension, and tachypnea will feature in all types of shock.

Lipoprotein circulation and atherosclerosis

Lipoproteins provide a means of transporting lipids (cholesterol, triglycerides, and phospholipids), which are insoluble in the blood, around the body.

Four classes of lipoproteins exist. These differ in size, density, constituent lipids, and type of surface protein (apoprotein). They are:
• High-density lipoproteins (HDL).
• Low-density lipoproteins (LDL).
• Very-low-density lipoproteins (VLDL).
• Chylomicrons.

Lipid transport in the blood is via two pathways, exogenous and endogenous, which are summarized in Fig. 7.15.

In the exogenous pathway (numbers refer to those in Fig. 7.15):
• Diet-derived lipid breakdown leads to the formation of chylomicrons.
• Lipoprotein lipase (LPL), found in the endothelium of extrahepatic tissues, hydrolyses the triglycerides in chylomicrons to glycerol and free fatty acids (FFAs), for use by the tissues.
• The chylomicron remnant is taken up by the liver.
• The liver secretes cholesterol and bile acids into the gut, creating an enterohepatic circulation.

In the endogenous pathway (numbers refer to those in Fig. 7.15):
• The liver secretes VLDLs, the components of which may be derived either endogenously or from the diet.
• Lipoprotein lipase (LPL), found in the endothelium of extrahepatic tissues, hydrolyses triglycerides in the VLDLs to glycerol and FFAs, for use by the tissues, and leaves LDL.
• LDL is then taken up by the liver and extrahepatic tissues.
• HDL is secreted by the liver into the plasma, where it is modified by lecithin cholesterol acyltransferase (LCAT) and uptake of cholesterol from the tissues. Lecithin cholesterol acyltransferase (LCAT) transfers cholesterol esters to LDLs and VLDLs.

Hyperlipidemias

Hyperlipidemias are characterized by markedly elevated plasma triglycerides, cholesterol, and

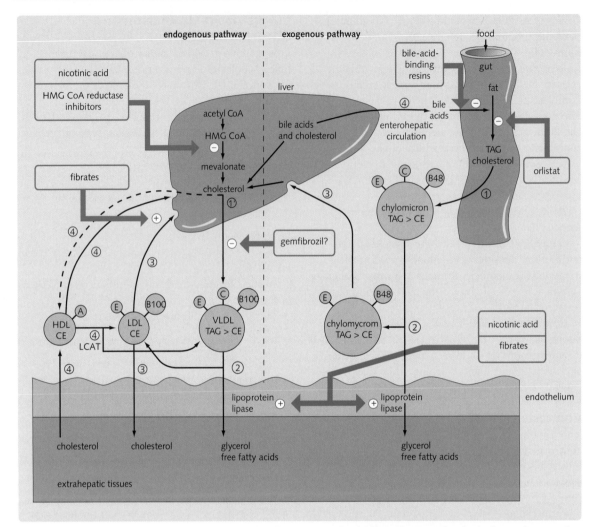

Fig. 7.15 Endogenous and exogenous pathways of lipid transport (CE, cholesterol ester; HDL, high-density lipoprotein; LCAT, lecithin cholesterol acyltransferase; TAG, triacylglycerol; VLDL, very-low-density lipoproteins; numbers refer to steps in pathways, see text).

lipoprotein concentrations. Cholesterol is deposited in various tissues. Deposition in arterial plaques results in atherosclerosis, which leads to heart attacks, strokes, and peripheral vascular disease. Deposition in tendons and skin results in xanthomas.

Primary
Primary hyperlipidemias are genetic, and numerous types exist.

Secondary
Secondary hyperlipidemias are the consequences of other conditions such as:
- Diabetes.
- Liver disease.

- Nephrotic syndrome.
- Renal failure.
- Alcoholism.
- Hypothyroidism.
- Estrogen administration.

Treatment (lipid-lowering drugs)
HMG CoA reductase inhibitors ("statins")
Atorvastatin, pravastatin, fluvastatin, lovastatin, rosuvastatin, and simvastatin are examples of 3-hydroxy–3-methylglutaryl coenzyme A (HMG CoA) reductase inhibitors. These drugs have been shown to reduce blood cholesterol by up to 35% in some patients.

HMG CoA reductase inhibitors can reduce the risk of dying from a coronary event by up to nearly half.

Mechanism of action: Statins reversibly inhibit the enzyme HMG CoA reductase, which catalyses the rate-limiting step in the synthesis of cholesterol: HMG CoA → mevalonic acid → cholesterol (see Fig. 7.15). The decrease in cholesterol synthesis also increases the number of LDL receptors, thus decreasing LDL levels.

Route of administration: Oral.

Indications: Hyperlipidemia resistant to dietary control, as part of secondary prevention in patients with serum cholesterol greater than 5.5 mmol/L (although this value will vary depending upon local policy).

Contraindications: Pregnancy, breastfeeding, liver disease.

Adverse effects: Reversible myositis, constipation or diarrhea, abdominal pain and flatulence, nausea and headache, fatigue and insomnia, and rash.

Fibrates

Fibrates include fenofibrate and gemfibrozil. These are broad-spectrum lipid-modulating agents that are ineffective in patients with elevated cholesterol but normal triglyceride concentrations.

Mechanism of action: Fibrates work in several ways, as follows: stimulation of lipoprotein lipase (see Fig. 7.15), thus reducing the triglyceride content of VLDLs and chylomicrons; stimulation of hepatic LDL clearance, by increasing hepatic LDL uptake (see Fig. 7.15); reduction of plasma triglyceride, LDL, and VLDL concentrations; and increase of HDL-cholesterol concentration. Gemfibrozil decreases lipolysis and may decrease VLDL secretion.

Route of administration: Oral.

Indications: Hyperlipidemia unresponsive to dietary control.

Contraindications: Gallbladder disease, severe renal or hepatic impairment, hypoalbuminemia, pregnancy, breastfeeding.

Adverse effects: Side effects of fibrates include:
- Myositis-like syndrome (especially if renal function is impaired).
- Gastrointestinal disturbances.
- Dermatitis, pruritus, rash, and urticaria.
- Impotence.
- Headache, dizziness, blurred vision.

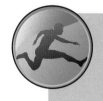 Changing a patient's diet alone can lower serum cholesterol, and this should be the first-line treatment option in mild to moderate hyperlipidemia.

Nicotinic acid (niacin)

The side effects of nicotinic acid limit its use in the treatment of hyperlipidemias. Nicotinic acid has been shown to reduce the incidence of coronary artery disease.

Mechanism of action: Nicotinic acid has the following effects: it inhibits cholesterol synthesis (see Fig. 7.15), thereby decreasing VLDL and thus LDL production; it stimulates lipoprotein lipase, thus reducing the triglyceride content of VLDLs and chylomicrons; it increases HDL-cholesterol; it increases the levels of tissue plasminogen activator; and it decreases the levels of plasma fibrinogen.

Route of administration: Oral.

Indications: Hyperlipidemias unresponsive to other measures.

Contraindications: Pregnancy, breastfeeding.

Adverse effects: Flushing, dizziness, headache, palpitations, nausea and vomiting, and pruritus.

Bile-acid-binding resins

Cholestyramine, colestipol, and colesevelam have been shown to decrease the rate of mortality from coronary artery disease.

Mechanism of action: Basic anion-exchange resins act by binding bile acids in the intestine (see Fig. 7.15), thus preventing their reabsorption and promoting hepatic conversion of cholesterol into bile acids. This increases hepatic LDL receptor activity, thus increasing the breakdown of LDL-cholesterol. Plasma LDL-cholesterol is, therefore, lowered.

Route of administration: Oral.

Indications: Bile-acid-binding resins are especially useful when elevated cholesterol results from a high LDL concentration.

Cholestyramine is used in the primary prevention of coronary heart disease in men aged 35–59 years with primary hypercholesterolemia. It also relieves pruritus associated with partial biliary obstruction and primary biliary cirrhosis.

Contraindications: Complete biliary obstruction.

Adverse effects: Bile-acid-binding resins are not absorbed; therefore, they have very few systemic side effects. Side effects include nausea and vomiting, constipation, heartburn, abdominal pain and flatulence, and aggravation of hypertriglyceridemia. They may interfere with the absorption of fat-soluble vitamins and certain drugs.

Colesevelam has the fewest side effects of these drugs, with fewer GI symptoms and less interference with the oral absorption of other drugs.

Therapeutic notes: To avoid interference with their absorption, other drugs should not be taken within 1 hour before or 3–4 hours after cholestyramine, colesevelam, or colestipol administration.

Other lipid-lowering drugs

Fish oils rich in ω–3 marine triglycerides can be useful in the treatment of severe hypertriglyceridemia, although they may sometimes worsen hypercholesterolemia. Their role in clinical practice remains to be thoroughly ascertained.

Ispaghula husk is taken orally, and it is presumed to act by binding bile acids, preventing their reabsorption. It is potentially useful in patients with hypercholesterolemia, but not hypertriglyceridemia.

Hemostasis and thrombosis

Principles of hemostasis

Hemostasis is the eradication of bleeding from damaged blood vessels.

If hemostasis is defective or unable to cope with blood loss from larger vessels, blood may accumulate in the tissues. This accumulated blood is called a hematoma.

The three stages involved in hemostasis are blood vessel constriction, formation of a platelet plug, and formation of a clot.

Blood vessel constriction

The first response to a severed blood vessel is contraction of the smooth muscle of the vessel. This is mediated by the release of thromboxane A_2 and other substances from platelets.

Blood vessel constriction slows the flow of blood through the vessel, thus reducing the pressure, and pushes opposing surfaces of the vessel together. In very small vessels, this results in permanent closure of the vessel, but in most cases blood vessel constriction is insufficient for this to occur.

Platelet plug formation

Exposure to the collagen underlying the vessel endothelium, as occurs during vessel injury, allows platelets to adhere to the collagen by binding to von Willebrand's factors. These factors, secreted by the platelets and endothelium, bind to the exposed collagen; platelets then bind to this complex.

Release of ADP, 5-HT, thromboxane A_2, and other substances by the platelets causes the latter to aggregate, while fibrin acts to bind them together.

The synthesis and release of prostacyclin by the intact endothelium inhibit platelet aggregation, and this acts to limit the extent of the platelet plug.

Intact endothelial cells also produce NO, a potent vasodilator and inhibitor of platelet aggregation.

Clot formation

Blood coagulation is the conversion of liquid blood into a solid gel, known as a clot. A clot consists of a meshwork of fibrin within which blood cells are trapped. It functions to reinforce the platelet plug.

Fibrin is formed from its precursor fibrinogen, through the action of an enzyme called thrombin.

The formation of thrombin occurs via two distinct pathways, the intrinsic and the extrinsic pathways, which together are known as the coagulation cascade. Both pathways involve the conversion of inactive factors into active enzymes, which then go on to catalyze the conversion of other factors into enzymes, and so on (Fig. 7.16).

The extrinsic pathway is so called because the component needed for its initiation is contained outside the blood. Tissue factor binds factor VII on exposure of blood to subendothelial cells and converts it to its active form, VIIa. This enzyme then catalyzes the activation of factors X and IX.

The intrinsic pathway is so called because its components are contained in the blood. It merges with the extrinsic pathway at the step prior to thrombin activation.

The thrombin formed stimulates the activation of factors XI, VIII, and V, and thus acts as a form of positive feedback.

Three naturally occurring anticoagulants limit the extent of clot formation. These are:

• Tissue factor pathway inhibitor, which binds to the tissue factor–VIIa complex and inhibits its actions.
• Protein C, which is activated by thrombin, and inactivates factors VII and V.

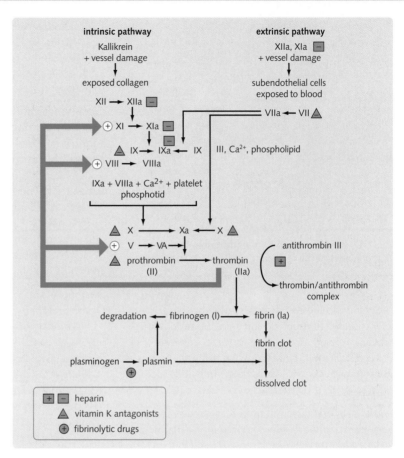

Fig. 7.16 Effects of heparin, vitamin K, and fibrinolytic drugs on the coagulation cascade (Factor III, factor/tissue thromboplastin).

- Antithrombin III, which is activated by heparin and inactivates thrombin and other factors.

Fibrinolysis

The fibrinolytic or thrombolytic system functions to dissolve a clot once repair of the vessel is under way.

Plasmin digests fibrin. It is formed from plasminogen through the action of plasminogen activators, the best example of which is tissue plasminogen activator (t-PA).

Thrombosis

Thrombosis is the pathologic formation of a clot known as a thrombus, which may cause occlusion within blood vessels or the heart, and result in death. Thrombosis causes:

- Arterial occlusion, which may lead to myocardial infarction, stroke, and peripheral ischemia.
- Venous occlusion, which may lead to deep venous thrombosis and pulmonary embolism.

Arterial thrombi form because of endothelial injury, which is in turn the result of underlying arterial wall pathology, such as atherosclerosis.

Venous and atrial thrombi tend to form as a result of blood stasis, allowing the build-up of platelets and fibrin. People with hypercoagulability, because of a lack of one or more of the naturally occurring anticoagulants, are particularly susceptible.

Arterial thrombi consist mainly of platelets, whereas venous thrombi consist mainly of fibrin.

Management of disorders of hemostasis
Bleeding disorders

Hereditary bleeding disorders are rare. Hemophilia is a genetic disorder in which excessive bleeding occurs, owing to the absence of factor VIII (hemophilia A) or IX (hemophilia B). Von Willebrand's disease is characterized by abnormal bruising and mucosal bleeding.

149

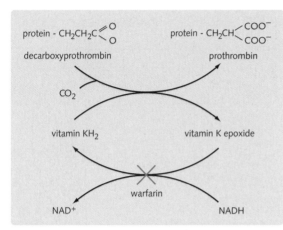

Fig. 7.17 Role of vitamin K in prothrombin formation. Warfarin inhibits the reduction of vitamin K epoxide.

Acquired bleeding disorders may be due to liver disease, vitamin K deficiency, or anticoagulant drugs.

Caution should be taken when using the following drugs in patients with thromboembolic disease.

Vitamin K
Mechanism of action: Vitamin K is needed for the post-transcriptional γ-carboxylation of glutamic acid residues of prothrombin (factor II) and clotting factors VII, IX, and X by the liver (Fig. 7.17). Vitamin K is also necessary for normal calcification of bone.

Route of administration: Oral, intramuscular, intravenous.

Indications: Vitamin K is used as an antidote to the effects of oral anticoagulants and in patients with biliary obstruction or liver disease, where vitamin K deficiency may be a problem. It is also used after prolonged treatment with antibiotics that inhibit the formation of vitamin K by intestinal bacteria, and as prophylaxis against hypoprothrombinemia in the newborn.

Adverse effects: Side effects of vitamin K include hemolytic anemia and hyperbilirubinemia in the newborn.

Protamine
Mechanism of action: Protamine is a strongly basic protein, which forms an inactive complex with heparin, and as such is used in patients in whom heparin treatment has resulted in hemorrhage. High doses of protamine appear to have anticoagulant effects through an unknown mechanism.

Route of administration: Intravenous.

Indications: Hemorrhage secondary to heparinization.

Adverse effects: Nausea, vomiting, flushing, hypotension.

Clotting factors
Deficient clotting factors can be replaced by the administration of fresh plasma. Factors VIII and IX are available as freeze-dried concentrates.

Mechanism of action: All clotting factors are necessary for normal blood coagulation.

Route of administration: Intravenous.

Indications: Hemophilia; antidote to the effects of oral anticoagulants.

Adverse effects: Allergic reactions, including fevers and chills.

Desmopressin
Desmopressin is a synthetic analog of vasopressin.

Mechanism of action: Desmopressin causes the release of factor VII. Desmopressin is also used in diabetes insipidus, as it has anti-diuretic effects.

Route of administration: Parenteral.

Indications: Desmopressin is given for mild factor VIII deficiency, and in the treatment of diabetes insipidus.

Adverse effects: Fluid retention, hyponatremia, headache, nausea, and vomiting.

> The liver is important in coagulation, as it is the site at which many of the clotting factors are produced. It also produces bile salts necessary for the absorption of vitamin K, which is needed by the liver to produce prothrombin and clotting factors VII, IX, and X.

Anticoagulants
Vitamin K antagonists
Warfarin is an example of vitamin K antagonists.

Mechanism of action: Vitamin K antagonists block the reduction of vitamin K epoxide, which is necessary for its action as a cofactor in the synthesis of factors II, VII, IX, and X (see Fig. 7.16).

Route of administration: Oral.

Indications: Prophylaxis and treatment of deep vein thrombosis and pulmonary embolism; the prophylaxis of embolization in atrial fibrillation and rheumatic disease, and in patients with prosthetic heart valves.

Contraindications: Cerebral thrombosis, peripheral arterial occlusion, peptic ulcers, hypertension, pregnancy.

Adverse effects: Hemorrhage. Warfarin is subject to many potential DDIs, which can dangerously elevate or decrease warfarin levels.

Therapeutic notes: The onset of action of vitamin K antagonists takes several hours, owing to the time needed for the degradation of factors that have already been carboxylated ($t_{1/2}$: VII = 6 hours, IX = 24 hours, X = 40 hours, II = 60 hours).

Heparin and the low-molecular-weight heparins

Mechanism of action: Heparin activates antithrombin III, which limits blood clotting by inactivating thrombin and factor X. Heparin also inhibits platelet aggregation, possibly as a result of inhibiting thrombin. Low-molecular weight heparins are simply fragments of heparin which exhibit very similar activity to heparin.

Route of administration: Intravenous, subcutaneous.

Indications: Treatment of deep vein thrombosis and pulmonary embolism; prophylaxis against postoperative deep vein thrombosis and pulmonary embolism in high-risk patients; myocardial infarction.

Contraindications: Heparin should not be given to patients with hemophilia, thrombocytopenia, or peptic ulcers.

Adverse effects: Hemorrhage (treated by stopping therapy or administering a heparin antagonist such as protamine sulphate), skin necrosis, thrombocytopenia, hypersensitivity reactions.

Therapeutic regimen: Heparin is given intravenously by intravenous infusion or every 12 hours by the subcutaneous route. Low-molecular-weight heparins are given as a once daily subcutaneous injection.

Therapeutic notes: Heparin has an immediate onset and, therefore, can be used in emergencies. Low-molecular-weight heparins (e.g., enoxaparin) have a lower incidence of thrombocytopenia than heparin.

Hirudins

Mechanism of action: Derived from the medical leech, hirudin, or rather its recombinant derivatives, desirudin and lepirudin, inactivate thrombin.

Route of administration: Subcutaneous, intravenous.

Indications: Desirudin is used in patients with type II (immune) heparin-induced thrombocytopenia. Desirudin is used for prophylaxis of deep vein thrombosis in patients undergoing hip and knee replacement.

Contraindications: Active bleeding, renal or hepatic impairment.

Adverse effects: Hemorrhage, hypersensitivity reactions.

Antiplatelet agents
Aspirin

Aspirin is acetylsalicylic acid and originally derived from the willow tree.

Mechanism of action: Aspirin blocks the synthesis of thromboxane A_2 from arachidonic acid in platelets by acetylating and thus inhibiting the enzyme cyclooxygenase. Thromboxane A_2 stimulates phospholipase C, thus increasing calcium levels and causing platelet aggregation. Aspirin also blocks the synthesis of prostacyclin from endothelial cells, which inhibits platelet aggregation. However, this effect is short lived because endothelial cells, unlike platelets, can synthesize new cyclooxygenase (Fig. 7.18).

Route of administration: Oral.

Indications: Prevention and treatment of myocardial infarction and ischemic stroke.

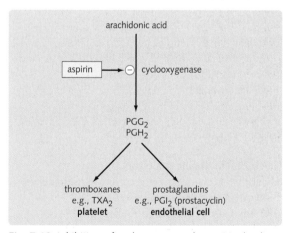

Fig. 7.18 Inhibition of cyclooxygenase by aspirin, leading to a reduction in the formation of thromboxane and prostacyclin (PG, prostaglandin; PGI_2, prostacyclin; TXA_2, thromboxane A_2).

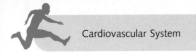

Aspirin is also used as an analgesic and an anti-inflammatory agent (Chapter 4).

Contraindications: Children under 12 years of age (at risk of Reye's syndrome). Breastfeeding, hemophilia, peptic ulcers, or known hypersensitivity reactions.

Adverse effects: Bronchospasm, gastrointestinal hemorrhage.

Therapeutic regimen: Aspirin at 75–162.5 mg PO daily after myocardial infarction has been shown to decrease mortality significantly. Given on alternate days, aspirin may reduce the incidence of primary myocardial infarction.

Dipyridamole

Mechanism of action: Dipyridamole causes inhibition of the phosphodiesterase enzyme that hydrolyses cAMP. Increased cAMP levels result in decreased calcium levels and inhibition of platelet aggregation.

Route of administration: Oral.

Indications: Dipyridamole is used in conjunction with warfarin and other oral anticoagulants in the prophylaxis against thrombosis associated with prosthetic heart valves.

Adverse effects: Hypotension, nausea, diarrhea, and headache.

Clopidogrel

Mechanism of action: Clopidogrel inhibits activation of the glycoprotein IIb/IIIa receptor on the surface of platelets, which is required for aggregation to occur.

Route of administration: Oral.

Indications: Secondary prevention of cardiovascular and cerebrovascular events.

Adverse effects: Hemorrhage, abdominal discomfort, nausea, and vomiting.

Therapeutic notes: If a patient is truly allergic to aspirin, clopidogrel can be used in its place.

Ticlopidine acts in a similar fashion to clopidogrel but is associated with neutropenia.

Glycoprotein IIb/IIIa inhibitors

Abciximab is the main drug currently in this class.

Mechanism of action: Abciximab is an antibody fragment directed toward the glycoprotein IIb/IIIa (GPIIb/IIIa) receptor of platelets. Binding and inactivation of the GPIIb/IIIa receptor prevent platelet aggregation.

Route of administration: Intravenous.

Indications: Prevention of ischemic cardiac complications in patients undergoing percutaneous coronary intervention; short-term prevention of myocardial infarction in patients with unstable angina.

Contraindications: Active bleeding.

Adverse effects: Hemorrhage, nausea, vomiting, hypotension.

Therapeutic notes: Tirofiban and eptifibatide also act by inhibiting the GPIIb/IIIa receptor, although are peptide fragments. As peptides, these agents are potentially antigenic, and they should be used only once.

Fibrinolytic agents
Streptokinase

Mechanism of action: Streptokinase forms a complex with and activates plasminogen into plasmin, a fibrinolytic enzyme.

Route of administration: Intravenous.

Indications: Life-threatening venous thrombosis, pulmonary embolism, arterial thromboembolism, and acute myocardial infarction.

Contraindications: Recent hemorrhage, trauma, surgery, bleeding diathesis, aortic dissection, coma, history of cerebrovascular disease.

Adverse effects: Nausea, vomiting, and bleeding.

Therapeutic regimen: Streptokinase is commonly used in conjunction with antiplatelet and anticoagulant drugs.

Streptokinase is derived from hemolytic streptococci and is therefore antigenic. Repeated administration of streptokinase can result in an anaphylaxis-like reaction. If repeated fibrinolytic therapy is needed, the nonantigenic tissue-type plasminogen activators should be employed.

Tissue-type plasminogen activators (t-PAs)

Alteplase and reteplase are examples of t-PAs.

Mechanism of action: t-PAs are tissue-type plasminogen activators.

Route of administration: Intravenous.

Indications: Myocardial infarction, pulmonary embolism.

Contraindications: As for streptokinase.

Adverse effects: Nausea, vomiting, and bleeding.

While the administration of a fibrinolytic drug may improve the life expectancy of someone suffering from an acute myocardial infarction, it can also have disastrous effects. There are stringent criteria for administering or not administering fibrinolytic drugs. Learn these from a medical textbook.

Antifibrinolytic agents

Tranexamic acid and aminocaproic acid

Mechanism of action: Tranexamic acid is antifibrinolytic, inhibiting plasminogen activation and thereby preventing fibrinolysis.

Route of administration: Oral, intravenous.

Indications: Tranexamic acid agents are used for gastrointestinal hemorrhage and conditions in which there is hemorrhage or risk of hemorrhage (e.g., hemophilia, menorrhagia, and dental extraction).

Contraindications: Thromboembolic disease.

Adverse effects: Nausea, vomiting, and diarrhea. Thromboembolic events are rare.

Aprotinin

Mechanism of action: Aprotinin inhibits the proteolytic enzymes plasmin and kallikrein, thus inhibiting fibrinolysis.

Route of administration: Intravenous.

Indications: Aprotinin is used when there is a risk of blood loss after open heart surgery and for hyperplasminemia.

Adverse effects: Allergy and localized thrombophlebitis.

The blood and fluid replacement

Anemia

Anemia is a common problem throughout the world. In the young, it is commonly due to nutritional deficiencies (vitamin B_{12}, folate, and iron); in fertile women, menstrual loss accounts for most cases; and in the elderly, malignancy and renal failure are the more common causes.

Treatment

Iron

Ferrous sulphate, ferrous fumarate, and ferrous gluconate are the more common iron salt preparations.

Mechanism of action: Dietary supplementation of iron increases serum iron and stored iron in the liver and bone. Adequate iron is necessary for normal erythropoiesis as well as for numerous iron-containing proteins.

Route of administration: Oral. Parenteral preparations of iron exist, but they are seldom used.

Indications: Iron-deficiency anemia.

Contraindications: Caution in pregnancy.

Adverse effects: Gastrointestinal irritation, nausea, epigastric pain, altered bowel habits.

Adverse effects: Iron overdose or chronic iron overload can be harmful and either acquired or inherited in the form of hemochromatosis. The iron-chelating agent deferoxamine can be given parenterally, which allows iron to be excreted in the urine.

Vitamin B_{12}

Hydroxocobalamin and cyanocobalamin are vitamin B_{12} drug preparations.

Mechanism of action: Vitamin B_{12} is required for DNA synthesis and effective erythropoiesis.

Route of administration: Intramuscular, oral.

Indications: Pernicious anemia, other macrocytic megaloblastic anemias.

Contraindications: None.

Adverse effects: Itching, fever, chills, flushing, nausea.

Therapeutic notes: Initial treatment requires regular weekly injections, but once serum vitamin B_{12} is normalized, injections should be given at 3-month intervals.

Folate

Folic acid is the form in which folate is administered.

Mechanism of action: Folate is required for DNA synthesis and effective erythropoiesis.

Route of administration: Oral.

Indications: Macrocytic megaloblastic anemias, prevention of neural tube defects in pregnancy.

Contraindications: None.

Adverse effects: None.

Therapeutic notes: Since the introduction of folate acid supplements for pregnant women, the rate of neural tube defects in newborn babies has fallen markedly.

Erythropoietin

Epoetin is a recombinant erythropoietin.

Erythropoietin is synthesized in the kidney in response to a fall in the oxygen tension of the blood passing through it.

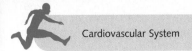

Mechanism of action: Erythropoietin acts upon the bone marrow to stimulate stem cells to divide to produce cells of the red-cell lineage.

Route of administration: Parenteral.

Indications: Anemia of chronic renal failure, anemia following cancer chemotherapy, prior to autologous blood donation.

Contraindications: Uncontrolled hypertension.

Adverse effects: Dose-dependent increase in blood pressure and platelet count, influenza-like symptoms.

Therapeutic notes: Erythropoietin is often featured in the news, as an increased hemoglobin concentration most probably improves an athlete's performance, making this drug a potential drug of abuse in sports.

Myeloproliferative disorders

The pharmacologic management of the meloproliferative disorders is outside the scope of this text, although it relies on cytotoxic drugs. Information about these agents should be learned from a hematology or general medical textbook.

Fluid replacement

Fluid replacement should ideally be achieved orally, although this is often not practical. Intravenous administration of fluids is commonplace in hospitals.

Intravenous fluids are given for many reasons. In trauma, they are used to replace blood loss; in septicemia, they are used to raise blood pressure and tissue perfusion; in the unconscious, they are used to replace water and electrolytes lost in the urine and via insensible routes.

There are many types of intravenous fluid. The more common fluids given intravenously are blood, the crystalloids (sodium chloride [normal saline] and dextrose saline), and the colloids (dextrans and gelatin). Each has its role to play in the management of various conditions. Supplements can be added to intravenous fluids to provide the patient with all their requirements.

The art of fluid replacement and fluid management is best learned from an anesthetics or general medical textbook.

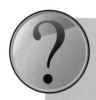

- What mechanisms are involved in controlling heart rate?
- What are the differences between nodal and nonnodal cells within the heart?
- What are the more common causes of cardiac failure, and associated signs and symptoms?
- What is meant by the term arrhythmia? What processes may result in arrhythmias?
- What are the principal drugs used in cardiac failure, their mechanism of action, and potential adverse effects?
- How do the anti-arrhythmic drugs act in principle? List the classes of anti-arrhythmics and name an example of each.
- What are the more common antianginal drugs, their mechanism of action, and potential adverse effects?
- What mechanisms are involved in controlling vascular tone?
- Draw a flow diagram of the renin–angiotensin system.
- Indicate on this flow diagram where ACE inhibitors, ATII receptor antagonists, and aldosterone antagonists act.
- What are the drugs which have vasodilating actions, and their mechanism of action and potential adverse effects?
- What is shock? What are the main classes of drugs used in its management and their mechanisms of action?
- What are the categories of drugs used in the management of hyperlipidemia? What are their mechanism of action and adverse effects?
- What are the steps in hemostasis? List any common disorders of hemostasis.
- What is thrombosis, and what are the potential complications of this process?
- What are the classes of drugs used in bleeding disorders, their mechanisms of action, and adverse effects?
- What are the drugs used to prevent thrombosis, their mechanisms of action, and adverse effects?
- What is fibrinolysis? What are the agents used as fibrinolytics, their importance in clinical practice, their mechanisms of action, and potential adverse effects?
- What is anemia? What are its more common causes and the drugs used to treat these causes?
- When should fluid replacement be via the intravenous route rather than the oral route? What are some of the intravenous fluids commonly given in hospitals?

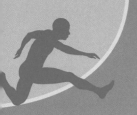

Reversible airways disease

Asthma

Asthma is a respiratory disease characterized by recurrent reversible obstruction to airflow in the bronchiolar airways. Asthma may be allergic (extrinsic) or nonallergic (intrinsic), although in practice this distinction offers little help.

Allergic asthma

Allergic asthma is the most common form of asthma. Allergic asthma occurs in people sensitive to allergens—antigenic substances in inspired air. Affected individuals have high circulating levels of immunoglobulin E (IgE) and are usually atopic (i.e., genetically prone to allergies). Allergic disorders are discussed in Chapter 4.

Nonallergic asthma

Nonallergic asthma is an intrinsic type of asthma, and it may not be attributable to any allergic reaction. It tends to develop later in life, although on closer questioning a history of childhood asthma-like symptoms often becomes apparent.

Severe asthma (status asthmaticus)

Severe asthma, or status asthmaticus, is a life-threatening acute deterioration of otherwise stable asthma. It is a potentially fatal condition that must be dealt with as an emergency, and it requires hospital admission. The signs, symptoms, and management of status asthmaticus should be learned and remembered.

Pathogenesis of asthma

Asthma is characterized by episodes of wheezing and breathlessness caused by bronchospasm, mucosal edema, and excess mucus formation. In asthma, smooth muscle that surrounds the bronchi is hyperresponsive to stimuli, and underlying inflammatory changes are present in the airways. Asthmatic stimuli include inhaled allergens (e.g., pollen, animal dander), occupational allergens, and drugs or nonspecific stimuli such as cold air, exercise, stress, and pollution.

Stimuli cause asthmatic changes through several complex pathways (Fig. 8.1). The possible mechanisms of these pathways include the following:

- Immune reactions (type 1 hypersensitivity) and release of inflammatory mediators: The cross-linking of IgE by allergens causes mast-cell degranulation, and release of histamine and powerful eosinophil and neutrophil chemotactic factors. The eosinophils, neutrophils, and other inflammatory cells release inflammatory mediators that cause a bronchial inflammatory reaction, tissue damage, and an increase in bronchial hyperresponsiveness. Bronchial inflammatory mediators include leukotrienes, prostaglandins, thromboxane, platelet-activating factor, and eosinophilic major basic protein.
- An imbalance in airway smooth muscle tone involving the parasympathetic nerves (vagus), nonadrenergic noncholinergic (NANC) nerves, and circulating adrenaline that act under normal circumstances to control airway diameter.
- Abnormal calcium flux across cell membranes, increasing smooth muscle contraction, and mast-cell degranulation.
- Leaky tight junctions between bronchial epithelial cells allowing allergen access.

In many patients, the asthmatic attack consists of two phases—an immediate-phase response and a late-phase response.

A good understanding of the pathology involved in asthma is imperative to understanding the mechanism of action of the drugs used to treat this common condition.

Immediate-phase response

An immediate-phase response occurs on exposure to the eliciting stimulus. The response consists mainly of bronchospasm. Bronchodilators are effective in this early phase.

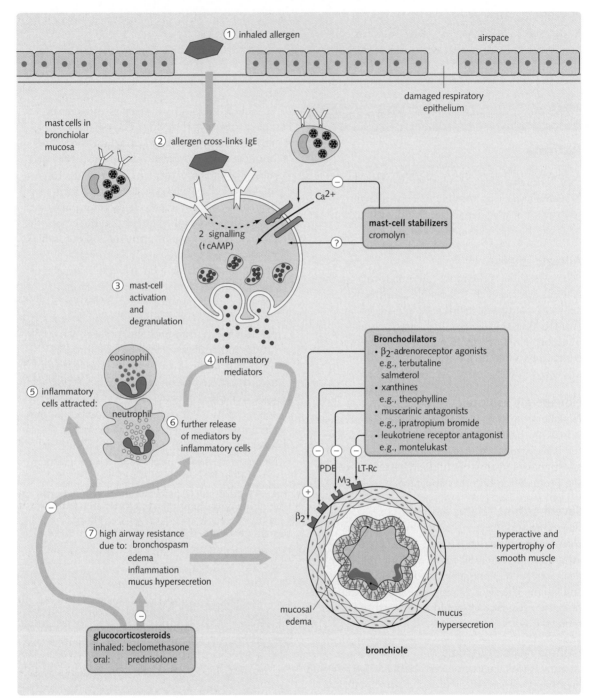

Fig. 8.1 Pathogenesis and drug action in asthma (PDE, phosphodiesterase; LT-Rc, leukotriene receptor). Allergens interact with respiratory mucosa (1), and trigger IgE-mediated mast-cell response (2). Activation of mast cells causes them to degranulate (3) and release various pro-inflammatory mediators (4), which attract and recruit further inflammatory cells (5). These cells also secrete mediators, which amplify the inflammatory response (6). The over-all effect is narrowing of small airways (7) by bronchospasm, edema, and increased secretions.

Late-phase response

Several hours later, the late-phase response occurs. This consists of bronchospasm, vasodilatation, edema, and mucus secretion caused by inflammatory mediators released from eosinophils, platelets, and other cells, and neuropeptides released by axon reflexes. Anti-inflammatory drug action is necessary for the prevention and/or treatment of this phase (see Fig. 8.1).

Chronic obstructive pulmonary disease

Chronic obstructive pulmonary disease (COPD) occurs mainly in long-standing smokers and comprises elements of chronic bronchitis and emphysema. Most patients with COPD get some symptom relief from bronchodilators and anti-inflammatory agents in a fashion similar to the asthmatics, yet the response of their airways to these drugs is much less marked, and there are no proven benefits upon life expectancy. Long-term oxygen therapy is also used in patients with COPD.

Management of reversible airways disease

Anti-asthmatic drugs include symptomatic bronchodilators (these are most effective in the immediate-phase response), and prophylactic or anti-inflammatory agents, which prevent and/or resolve the late-phase response. The stepwise management of asthma is summarized in Fig. 8.2.

Bronchodilators
Beta$_2$-adrenoceptor agonists

Examples of β_2-adrenoceptor agonists include albuterol, terbutaline, and salmeterol.

Mechanism of action: Airway smooth muscle does not have a sympathetic nervous supply, but it does contain β_2-adrenoceptors that respond to circulating adrenaline. The stimulation of β_2-adrenoceptors leads to a rise in intracellular cAMP levels and subsequent smooth muscle relaxation and bronchodilation.

Beta$_2$-adrenoceptor agonists may also help prevent the activation of mast cells, as a minor effect.

Modern selective β_2-adrenoceptor agonists are potent bronchodilators and have very few β_1-stimulating properties (i.e., they produce less cardiac tachycardia).

Route of administration: Inhaled. Oral administration is reserved for children and people unable to use inhalers; intravenous administration for status asthmaticus.

Indications: β_2-adrenoceptor agonists are used to relieve bronchospasm. They may be used alone in mild, occasional asthma, but they are more commonly used in conjunction with other drugs, (e.g., corticosteroids).

Contraindications: Caution in hyperthyroidism, cardiovascular disease, and arrhythmias.

Adverse effects: Fine tremor, tachycardia, and hypokalemia after high doses.

Therapeutic notes: β_2-adrenoceptor agonists treat the symptoms of asthma but not the underlying disease process. Salmeterol is a long-acting drug that can be administered twice daily. It is not suitable for relief of an acute attack.

Anticholinergics

Ipratropium bromide and tiotropium are examples of anticholinergic (antimuscarinic) drugs.

Mechanism of action: Parasympathetic vagal fibers provide a bronchoconstrictor tone to the smooth muscle of the airways. They are activated by reflex on stimulation of sensory (irritant) receptors in the airway walls.

Muscarinic antagonists act by blocking muscarinic receptors, especially the M$_3$ subtype, which responds to this parasympathetic bronchoconstrictor tone.

Route of administration: Inhaled.

Indications: Anticholinergics are used as adjuncts to β_2-adrenoceptor agonists in the treatment of asthma and are widely used in the treatment of COPD.

Contraindications: Glaucoma, prostatic hypertrophy, or pregnancy.

Adverse effects: Dry mouth may occur. Systemic anticholinergic effects are very rare.

Xanthines

Theophylline is an example of a xanthine.

Mechanism of action: The xanthines appear to increase cAMP levels in the bronchial smooth muscle cells by inhibiting phosphodiesterase, an enzyme which catalyses the hydrolysis of cAMP to AMP. Increased cAMP relaxes smooth muscle, causing bronchodilation.

Route of administration: Oral. Aminophylline is the intravenous xanthine used in severe asthma attacks.

Indications: Xanthines are used in asthmatic children unable to use inhalers and adults with

Stepwise approach for managing asthma in adults and children older than 5 years of age	
Classify Severity: Clinical features before treatment or adequate Control	**Medications required to maintain long-term control:** Daily Medications
Step 1: Mild Intermittent	■ No daily medication needed. ■ Severe exacerbations may occur, separated by long periods of lung function and no symptoms. A course of systemic corticosteroids is recommend.
Step 2: Mild Persistent	■ **Preferred treatment** – **Low-dose inhaled corticosteroids** ■ Alternative treatment (listed alphabetically): cromolyn, leukotriene modifier, nedocromil OR sustained-release theophylline to serum concentration of 5-15 mcg/mL.
Step 3: Moderate Persistent	■ **Preferred treatment** – **Low-to-medium-dose inhaled corticosteroids or long-acting beta$_2$-agonists.** ■ Alternative treatment (listed alphabetically): – Increase inhaled corticosteroids within medium-dose range OR – Low-to-medium dose inhaled corticosteroids and either leukotriene modifier or theophylline. - If needed (particularly in patients with recurring severe exacerbations): ■ **Preferred treatment** – **Increase inhaled corticosteroids within medium-dose range and add long-acting beta$_2$ agonists.** ■ Alternative treatment: Increase inhaled corticosteroids within medium-dose range and add either leukotriene modifier or theophylline.

Step 4: Severe Persistent	■ **Preferred treatment**
	  – **High dose inhaled corticosteroids or long-acting beta$_2$-agonists.**
	  AND
	  – **Lond-acting inhaled beta$_2$ agonists**
	  AND, If needed,
	  Corticosteroid tablets or syurp long term. (Make attempts to
	  – reduce systemic corticosteroids and maintain with high-dose inhaled corticosteroids.)

Quick Relief : All Patients	■ 2–4 puffs **short-acting inhaled beta$_2$ agonist** as needed
Step down :	Review treatment every 1 to 6 months; a gradual stepwise reduction in treatment may be possible.
Step up :	If control is not maintained, consider step up. First review patient medication technique, adherence, and enviromental control.

Fig. 8.2 Staged management of asthma in adults and children over the age of 5 years. Therapy should be started based on clinical symptoms and worked upward until control of symptoms is achieved. Once symptoms have been controlled, it may be possible to step down (adapted from the NAEEP Expert Panel Report, Guidelines for the Diagnosis and Management of Asthma—Update on Selected Topics 2002. NIH publication no. 02–5075, May 2003. U.S. Department of Health and Human Services, Public Health Service, National Institutes of Health, National Heart, Lung and Blood Institute).

predominantly nocturnal symptoms. They are administered intravenously in status asthmaticus.

Contraindications: Cardiac disease, hypertension, hepatic impairment. Xanthines interact with many other drugs and must be prescribed with caution.

Adverse effects: Nausea, vomiting, tremor, insomnia, and tachycardia.

Therapeutic notes: Oral xanthines are formulated as sustained-release preparations. Xanthines often cause adverse effects, having a narrow therapeutic window, but they are useful as oral drugs in preventing attacks for up to 12 hours.

Leukotriene receptor antagonists

Montelukast and zafirlukast are examples of leukotriene receptor antagonists.

Mechanism of action: The leukotriene receptor antagonists are believed to act at leukotriene receptors in the bronchiolar muscle, antagonizing endogenous leukotrienes, thus preventing bronchoconstriction.

Leukotrienes are thought to be partly responsible for airway narrowing that is sometimes observed with the use of nonsteroidal anti-inflammatory drugs in asthmatics (NSAIDs; Chapter 4). The NSAIDs inhibit cyclooxygenase and divert arachidonic acid breakdown via the lipoxygenase pathway, liberating leukotrienes among other mediators.

Route of administration: Oral.

Indications: Prophylaxis of asthma.

Contraindications: Elderly, pregnancy, and Churg–Strauss syndrome.

Adverse effects: Gastrointestinal disturbance, dry mouth, and headache.

Therapeutic notes: The leukotriene receptor antagonists are less effective than corticosteroids and are used as adjuncts with other asthma medications.

 In an asthmatic emergency, when thinking what drugs to use, do not forget oxygen.

Prophylactic and anti-inflammatory drugs
Mast-cell stabilizers

Cromolyn sodium and nedocromil sodium are examples of mast-cell stabilizers.

Mechanism of action: The exact modes of action of mast-cell stabilizers are unclear. These drugs appear to stabilize antigen-sensitized mast cells by reducing calcium influx and subsequent release of inflammatory mediators.

Route of administration: Inhaled.

Indications: Mast-cell stabilizers are useful in young patients (<20 years old) with marked allergic disease and moderate asthma.

Adverse effects: Cough, transient bronchospasm, and throat irritation.

Therapeutic notes: Mast-cell stabilizers have a prophylactic action; they must be taken regularly for several weeks before any beneficial effects are noted. These drugs are, therefore, of no use in acute asthma attacks.

Anti-inflammatory glucocorticoids

Anti-inflammatory glucocorticoids include beclomethasone, fluticasone, budesonide, and prednisolone.

Mechanism of action: Corticosteroids depress the inflammatory response in bronchial mucosa and so diminish bronchial hyperresponsiveness. The specific effects include:

- Reduced mucosal edema and mucus production.
- Decreased local generation of prostaglandins and leukotrienes, with less inflammatory-cell activation.
- Adrenoceptor upregulation.
- Long-term reduced T-cell cytokine production and reduced eosinophil and mast-cell infiltration of bronchial mucosa.

For the intracellular events involved in corticosteroid action, see Chapter 11.

Route of administration: Corticosteroids are usually delivered by metered-dose inhaler. Both oral and intravenous administrations are reserved for severe asthma and status asthmaticus.

Indications: Corticosteroids are used in patients with more than minimal symptoms—often in combination with β_2-agonists or drugs that block allergies (see Fig. 8.2).

Contraindications: Caution in growing children and in those with systemic and localized respiratory/ENT infections.

Adverse effects: Dysphonia, oral thrush, and systemic penetration in high dosage. If given orally, cushingoid effects may occur (Chapter 11).

Therapeutic notes: The initial treatment of severe or refractory asthma may require oral corticosteroids. If possible, maintenance should be achieved with inhaled corticosteroids via a metered dose to minimize side effects. Inhaled corticosteroids are usually effective in 3–7 days, but they must be taken regularly.

Use of inhalers, nebulizers, and oxygen

In the treatment of asthma, inhalers and nebulizers are used to deliver drugs directly to the airways. This allows higher drug concentrations to be achieved locally, while minimizing systemic effects. Whatever

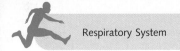

device is used, less than 15% of the dose is deposited on the bronchial mucosa.

Inhalers

There are several types of inhaler—metered-dose, breath-activated spray, and breath-activated powder. They vary in cost, delivery efficiency, and ease of use.

Spacer devices, used in conjunction with inhalers, improve drug delivery, and they are easy to use. Spacers are particularly effective in children.

Nebulizers

Nebulizers convert a solution of drug into an aerosol for inhalation. They are more efficient than inhalers, and they are used to deliver higher doses of drug. They are useful in status asthmaticus and for the acute hospital treatment of severe asthma.

The long-term use of nebulizers is limited by cost, convenience, and the danger of patient over-reliance.

Oxygen

High-flow oxygen should be given to all patients in respiratory distress unless they suffer from COPD and have a "hypoxic drive." In this situation, oxygen can be administered, but at a lower concentration.

Oxygen increases alveolar oxygen tension and decreases the work of breathing necessary to maintain arterial oxygen tension.

Respiratory stimulants and pulmonary surfactants

Respiratory stimulants

Respiratory stimulants, or analeptic drugs, have a very limited place in the treatment of ventilatory failure in patients with chronic obstructive airways disease. They have largely been replaced by the use of ventilatory support.

Doxapram is an example of a respiratory stimulant.

Mechanism of action: Doxapram is used to improve both rate and depth of breathing.

Doxapram is a central stimulant drug that acts on both carotid chemoreceptors and the respiratory center in the brainstem to increase respiration.

Route of administration: Intravenous.

Indications: Acute respiratory failure.

Adverse effects: Perineal warmth, dizziness, sweating, increase in blood pressure and heart rate.

Therapeutic notes: Apart from naloxone and flumazenil, the respiratory stimulants are seldom employed in clinical practice.

Pulmonary surfactants

Pulmonary surfactants are used in the management of respiratory distress syndrome, which is most common among premature babies. Pulmonary surfactants act to decrease the surface tension of the alveoli, and they allow ventilation to occur more easily. They are usually administered via endotracheal tubes directly into the pulmonary tree.

Antitussives, mucolytics, and decongestants

Antitussives

Antitussives are drugs that inhibit the cough reflex.

Cough is usually a valuable protective reflex mechanism for clearing foreign material and secretions from the airways. In some conditions, however, such as inflammation or neoplasia, the cough reflex may become inappropriately stimulated, and, in such cases, antitussive drugs may be used.

Antitussives either reduce sensory receptor activation or work by an ill-defined mechanism, depressing a "cough center" in the brainstem.

Drugs that reduce receptor activation
Menthol vapor and topical local anesthetics
Benzocaine is an example of a topical local anesthetic.

Mechanism of action: Menthol vapor and topical local anesthetics reduce the sensitivity of peripheral sensory "cough receptors" in the pharynx and larynx to irritation.

Route of administration: Topical as a spray, lozenge, or vapor.

Indications: Menthol vapor and topical local anesthetics are used for unwanted cough.

Drugs that reduce the sensitivity of the "cough center"
Opioids (Chapter 4)
Opioids reduce the sensitivity of the "cough center." Examples of these drugs include codeine and dextromethorphan.

Mechanism of action: Although not clearly understood, opioids seem to work via agonist action on opiate receptors, depressing a "cough center" in the brainstem.

Route of administration: Oral.

Indications: Opioids are used for inappropriate coughing.

Adverse effects: There are generally few side effects of opioids at antitussive doses. Codeine can cause constipation and inhibition of mucociliary clearance.

Mucolytics

Mucolytics are drugs that reduce the viscosity of bronchial secretions. They are sometimes used when excess bronchial secretions need to be cleared.

Acetylcysteine

Mechanism of action: Acetylcysteine reduces the viscosity of bronchial secretions by cleaving disulfide bonds cross-linking mucus glycoprotein molecules.

Route of administration: Oral.

Indications: Acetylcysteine may be of benefit in some chronic obstructive airways disease, although evidence supporting its use does not exist.

Therapeutic notes: A novel drug with mucolytic properties is dornase alfa, a genetically engineered enzyme which cleaves extracellular DNA and is used in cystic fibrosis, being administered by inhalation.

Decongestants

Nasal decongestion can occur acutely or be a chronic disorder.

Decongestion relies on administration of agents that ultimately have sympathomimetic effects. This results in vasoconstriction of the mucosal blood vessels of the nose and a reduction in edema and secretions.

Pseudoephedrine is the most commonly used decongestant

Mechanism of action: Ephedrine's sympathomimetic activity results in vasoconstriction of nasal blood vessels, limiting edema and nasal secretions.

Route of administration: Topical or oral.

Indications: Nasal congestion.

Contraindications: Caution in children.

Adverse effects: Local irritation, nausea, headache. Rebound nasal congestion on withdrawal.

Therapeutic notes: Oral preparations are less effective than topical, and they are contraindicated in diabetes, hypertension, and hyperthyroidism.

Allergic disorders and drug therapy

Allergic disorders

Allergic reactions occur when the immune system mounts an inappropriate response to an innocuous foreign substance.

Most common allergic disorders are caused by IgE-mediated type I immediate hypersensitivity reactions that occur in a previously sensitized person re-exposed to the sensitizing antigen. Type I immediate hypersensitivity reactions are also known as atopic disorders.

Patients with atopic disorders have an inherited predisposition to develop IgE antibodies to allergens that are innocuous and non-antigenic in normal people. These specific IgE antibodies become bound to high-affinity IgE receptors (FcεRI) on the surface of tissue mast cells and blood basophils. The cross-linking of this cell-surface-bound IgE by antigens (allergens), on subsequent exposure, induces degranulation and release of mediators such as histamine, leukotrienes, and prostaglandins (Fig. 8.3).

The released vasoactive and inflammatory mediators produce many local and systemic effects, including vasodilatation, increased vascular permeability, smooth muscle contraction, edema, glandular hypersecretion, and inflammatory cell infiltration.

Depending on the site of this reaction and release of mediators, a variety of disorders can result (Fig. 8.4).

Drug therapy of allergic disorders

The most effective therapy in hypersensitivity reactions is avoidance of the offending antigen or environment. When this is not possible, drug therapy can be of use (Fig. 8.5).

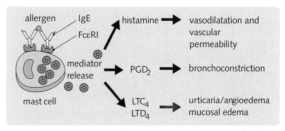

Fig. 8.3 Mechanism of type 1 hypersensitivity (allergic) reaction (FcεRI, cell surface IgE receptor; LT, leukotriene; PG, prostaglandin). (Redrawn from Page et al., 2002.)

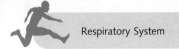

Type I hypersensitivity/allergic disorders

Disorder	Site of reaction	Response	Common allergens
Anaphylaxis	Circulation	Edema, circulatory collapse, death	Venoms Drugs
Allergic rhinitis/ hay fever	Nasal passages Conjunctiva	Irritation, edema, mucosal hypersecretion	Pollen Dust
Asthma	Bronchioles	Bronchoconstriction, mucosal secretion, airway inflammation	Pollen Dust
Food allergy	GIT	Vomiting, diarrhea, urticaria (hives)	Seafood Milk etc.
Wheal and flare	Skin	Vasodilatation and edema	Insect venom

Fig. 8.4 Type I hypersensitivity/ allergic disorders (GIT, gastrointestinal tract).

Drug therapy in allergic disorders

Disorder	Drugs used	Chapter	Mechanism of action
Anaphylaxis	Epinephrine	5 & 7	Vasoconstriction (α_1) Bronchodilation(β_2)
	Antihistamines	6 & 8	Pro-inflammatory mediator antagonism
	Glucocorticoids	7 & 11	Anti-inflammatory
Allergic rhinitis/ hay fever	Antihistamines	6 & 8	Pro-inflammatory mediator antagonism
	Mast-cell stabilizers	8	Inhibition of mast-cell degranulation
	Glucocorticoids	7 & 11	Anti-inflammatory
	Sympathomimetic vasoconstrictors	5, 7 & 8	Decongestion of nasal mucosa
Asthma	See pp 158–162	8	See Fig. 8.1
Food allergies	Antihistamines	8	Pro-inflammatory mediator antagonism
Wheal and flare	Antihistamines	8	Pro-inflammatory mediator antagonism

Fig. 8.5 Drug therapy in allergic disorders.

Histamine and antihistamines

Histamine is a basic amine that is stored in mast cells (fixed in the tissues) and in circulating basophils; it is also found in the stomach and central nervous system (CNS).

The effects of histamine are mediated by three different receptor types found on target cells (Fig. 8.6).

As the major chemical mediator released during an allergic reaction, histamine produces a number of effects, mainly via action on H_1 receptors. Therefore, H_1 antagonists (antihistamines) are of potential benefit in the treatment of allergic disorders.

H_1 Receptor antagonists: antihistamines

There are two types of antihistamines. These are:
- "Old" sedative types (e.g., diphenhydramine and promethazine).
- "New" nonsedative types (e.g., cetirizine and loratadine).

Mechanism of action: Antihistamines work by antagonism of histamine H_1 receptors (see Fig. 8.6).

In the periphery, their action can inhibit allergic reactions where histamine is the main mediator involved.

The "old-style" antihistamines are able to cross the blood–brain barrier where both specific and nonspecific actions in the CNS produce sedation and antiemetic effects.

Indications: The main use of antihistamines is in the treatment of seasonal allergic rhinitis ("hay fever"). They are also used for the treatment and prevention of allergic skin reactions such as urticarial rashes, pruritus, and insect bites and in the emergency treatment of anaphylactic shock.

The "old-style" antihistamines can also be used as mild hypnotics (Chapter 6) and to suppress nausea in motion sickness, owing to their actions on the CNS.

Histamine receptors	
Histamine receptor	Effect
H$_1$	Responsible for most of the actions of histamine in a type I hypersensitivity reaction: • capillary and venous dilatation (producing "flare" or systemic hypotension) • increased vascular permeability (producing "wheal" or edema) • contraction of smooth muscle (producing bronchial and gastrointestinal contraction)
H$_2$	Regulation of gastric acid secretion: • H$_2$-receptors respond to histamine secreted from the enterochromaffin-like cells that are adjacent to the parietal cell (see Chapter 10).
H$_3$	Involved in neurotransmission: • exact physiologic role not clear (presynaptic inhibition of neurotransmitter release in the CNS and autonomic nervous system? role in itch and pain perception?)

Fig. 8.6 Effects at histamine receptors.

Route of administration: Oral, topical, transnasal. Intravenous diphenhydramine can be used in anaphylaxis.

Adverse effects: "Old-style" antihistamines produce quite pronounced sedation or fatigue as well as antimuscarinic effects such as dry mouth. The newer agents do not do this.

Rare hazardous arrhythmias have been associated with some of the "non-sedating" class of antihistamines (e.g., terfenadine), especially at high plasma levels or when used in combination with imidazole antifungal agents or macrolide antibiotics (Chapter 12).

Hypersensitivity reactions, especially to topically applied antihistamines, may occur.

Mast-cell stabilizers, the anti-inflammatory glucocorticoids, and sympathomimetic decongestants are all used in allergy, and these have already been described.

Remember that an allergic reaction can occur locally, systemically, or both.

- What is asthma?
- What are the pathologic processes that occur at the cellular level in an asthmatic reaction? How do they produce the signs and symptoms of asthma?
- What are the broad categories of drugs used to treat reversible airways disease, their mechanism of action, routes of administration, and adverse effects?
- What are the components of the stepwise management of asthma in adults?
- What is chronic obstructive airways disease? How can it be treated?
- What are the roles and uses of inhalers, nebulizers, and oxygen in the therapy of asthma?
- What drugs might make the symptoms of asthma worse? What are the mechanisms behind this?
- In what clinical setting might a respiratory stimulant be used? Give an example of a respiratory stimulant and an indication for its use. What are its mechanisms of action and potential adverse effects?
- What is an allergic disorder? Name two examples of allergic disorders, and explain why they occur.
- What commonly used drugs are employed in the therapy of allergy? What are their routes of administration, mechanisms of action, and adverse effects?

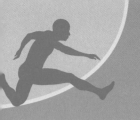

9. Kidney and Urinary System

Kidney

Principles of renal function

Despite making up only 1% of total body weight, the kidneys receive approximately 25% of the cardiac output.

The volume of plasma filtered by the kidneys is termed the glomerular filtration rate (GFR) and is equal to approximately 180 L/day for a person weighing 70 kg. This means that the entire plasma volume is filtered about 60 times a day.

Functions of the kidney

The kidney has several functions. These include:
- Regulation of body water content.
- Regulation of body mineral content and composition.
- Regulation of body pH.
- Excretion of metabolic waste products (e.g., urea, uric acid, and creatinine).
- Excretion of foreign material (e.g., drugs).
- Secretion of renin, erythropoietin, and 1, 25-dihydroxyvitamin D_3.
- Gluconeogenesis.

The nephron

Each kidney is made up of approximately one million functional units, known as nephrons (Fig. 9.1).

Each nephron consists of:
- A renal corpuscle, which comprises a glomerulus and a Bowman's capsule.
- A tubule, which comprises a proximal tubule, loop of Henle, distal convoluted tubule, and collecting duct system.

Blood supply

Blood reaches each kidney via the renal artery, which divides into numerous branches before forming the afferent arterioles. These afferent arterioles enter the glomerular capillaries (the glomeruli) and leave as the efferent arterioles.

The efferent arteriole leaving most nephrons immediately branches into a set of capillaries known as the peritubular capillaries. These branch extensively and form a network of capillaries surrounding the tubules in the cortex into which reabsorption from the tubule occurs and from which various substances are secreted into the tubule.

Glomerular filtration

During glomerular filtration, the fluid fraction of blood in the glomerulus, is forced through the capillary endothelium, a basement membrane, and the epithelium of the Bowman's capsule to enter a fluid-filled space known as Bowman's space.

Approximately 20% of the plasma entering the glomerulus is filtered. The filtered fluid is known as the glomerular filtrate, and it consists of protein-free plasma.

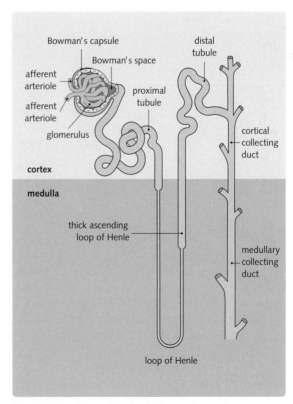

Fig. 9.1 Structure of the juxtaglomerular nephron (redrawn from Page et al., 2002).

Tubular function

The tubules are involved in reabsorption and secretion.

Important components of plasma tend to be reabsorbed more or less completely; for example, sodium and glucose are 99–100% reabsorbed. Waste products are only partially reabsorbed; for example, approximately 45% of urea is reabsorbed.

The tubules secrete hydrogen and potassium ions as well as organic species such as creatinine and drugs such as penicillin.

Sodium and water reabsorption

Approximately 99% of filtered water and sodium is reabsorbed, but none is secreted.

Sodium is pumped out of tubular cells into the interstitium by the Na^+/K^+ ATPase in their basolateral membrane. This forms a concentration gradient of sodium: high concentration within the filtrate of the tubule lumen, and low concentration within the cytoplasm of the tubular cells. This gradient forms the basis of most reabsorption and

secretion processes that subsequently occur. Sodium reabsorption from the lumen varies according to the section of the tubule (Figs. 9.2 to 9.5).

Water is reabsorbed by passive diffusion, following the movement of sodium ions, and through specific water channels (aquaporins) in the collecting tubules, which greatly increases the reabsorption of water.

Proximal tubule

The Bowman's capsule extends into the proximal tubule, which is made up of an initial convoluted section and a straight section. The proximal tubule is the site into which many drugs are secreted. It is permeable to water and ions.

Approximately two thirds of the filtrate volume is reabsorbed back into the blood in the proximal tubule.

Sodium movement into the cell is coupled with that of glucose and amino acids, whereas chloride movement is by passive diffusion (see Fig. 9.2). Reabsorption of bicarbonate also takes place in the proximal tubule.

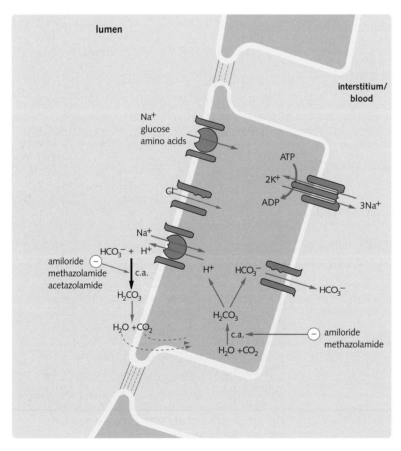

Fig. 9.2 The proximal tubule is one of the sites of bicarbonate (HCO_3^-) reabsorption. Carbonic acid (H_2CO_3) is formed in the cytoplasm from the action of carbonic anhydrase (c.a.) on carbon dioxide (CO_2) and water. H_2CO_3 immediately dissociates into HCO_3^-, which moves down its concentration gradient across the basolateral membrane, and H^+, which is secreted into the lumen in exchange for Na^+. In the lumen, H^+ combines with filtered HCO_3^- to form H_2CO_3 and subsequently CO_2 and water, which are able to diffuse back into the cell.

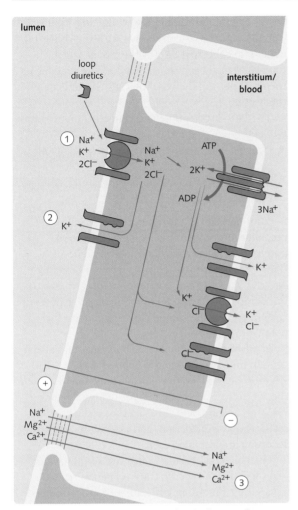

Fig. 9.3 Transport mechanism in the thick ascending loop of Henle. Loop diuretics block the $Na^+/K^+/2Cl^-$ cotransporter (1), thereby increasing the excretion of Na^+ and Cl^-. These drugs also decrease the potential difference across the tubule cell, which arises from the recycling of K^+ (2), and this leads to increased excretion of Ca^{2+} and Mg^{2+} by inhibiting paracellular diffusion (3) (redrawn from Page et al., 2002).

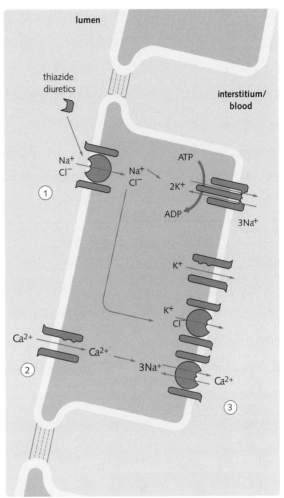

Fig. 9.4 Transport mechanisms in the early distal tubule. Thiazide diuretics increase the excretion of Na^+ and Cl^- by inhibiting the Na^+/Cl^- cotransporter (1). The reabsorption of Ca^{2+} (2) is increased by these drugs by a mechanism that may involve stimulation of Na^+/Ca^{2+} countertransport (3) due to an increase in the concentration gradient for Na^+ across the basolateral membrane (redrawn from Page et al., 2002).

Loop of Henle

The loop of Henle is shaped like a hairpin; it consists of a descending limb, a thin ascending limb, and a thick ascending limb.

Twenty-five per cent of filtered sodium is reabsorbed in the thick ascending limb (see Fig. 9.3), but this portion of the tubule is impermeable to water. Increase in the solute load (sodium) in the interstitium between the ascending loop and the collecting tubules sets up an osmotic gradient, which subsequently permits water reabsorption from the collecting tubules—the countercurrent multiplier system.

Juxtaglomerular apparatus

Where the afferent and efferent arterioles enter the glomerulus, a group of specialized cells, the macula densa, are situated in what is named the juxtaglomerular apparatus. These cells secrete renin, which is fundamental in the renin–angiotensin system. The renin–angiotensin system is involved directly in vascular tone and in the release of aldosterone (Chapter 7).

169

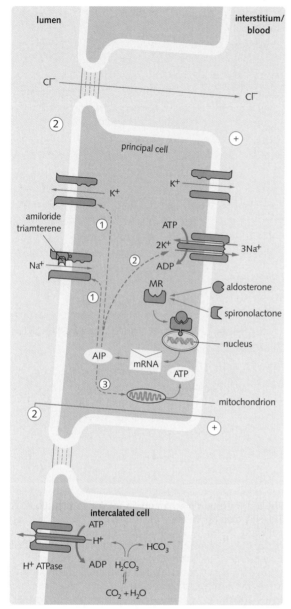

Distal convoluted tubule and collecting tubule

The distal tubule is continuous with the collecting duct. The collecting duct is the site at which the tubules of many nephrons merge before draining into the renal pelvis. The renal pelvis is continuous with the ureter.

The late distal tubule and collecting duct contain two cell types (see Fig. 9.5):

- Principal cells, which incorporate sodium and potassium channels.
- Intercalated cells, which incorporate H^+ ATPases that secrete hydrogen ions.

Sodium movement into the principal cells exceeds potassium movement out, so that a negative potential difference is established. Sodium is transported across the basolateral membrane by Na^+/K^+ ATPase, and potassium is moved into the cell before being forced out by the negative potential.

This part of the tubule is the major site for potassium secretion.

The late distal tubule and collecting duct also contain mineralocorticoid receptors. When aldosterone binds to these, it produces an increase in the synthesis of sodium and potassium channels, Na^+/K^+ ATPase, and ATP, so that sodium reabsorption is increased, and potassium and proton secretion are also increased.

The collecting tubule is also the site for water reabsorption via specific water channels named aquaporins. Fine-tuning the amount of water needed to be reabsorbed is controlled by the hypothalamus, which governs how much antidiuretic hormone (ADH or vasopressin) is released from the pituitary gland. Release of ADH results in more aquaporins being inserted into the luminal membrane and more water being reabsorbed (Chapter 7).

Several different sodium channels exist in the renal tubule, which is why the various diuretic drugs act at different sites along its course and have different molecular actions and clinical side effects.

Fig. 9.5 Transport mechanisms in the late distal tubule and collecting duct. Amiloride and triamterene block the luminal Na^+ channels, which reduces the lumen-negative potential difference across the principal cell and decreases the driving force for K^+ secretion from the principal cell and H^+ secretion from the intercalated cell. The net effect is increased Na^+ excretion and decreased K^+ and H^+ excretion. Aldosterone binds to a cytoplasmic mineralocorticoid receptor (MR), stimulating the production of aldosterone-induced proteins (AIP), which (1) activate and increase the synthesis of Na^+ and K^+ channels, (2) increase the synthesis of Na^+/K^+ ATPase, and (3) increase mitochondrial production of adenosine triphosphate (ATP). The effect of aldosterone is to decrease Na^+ excretion and increase K^+ and H^+ excretion in urine, whereas spironolactone, an aldosterone antagonist, has the opposite effects (redrawn from Page et al., 2002).

Atrial natriuretic peptide, derived from the atria of the heart in response to fluid-overload, is believed to act upon the distal nephron causing a water and solute diuresis. This remains a further potential target for future therapeutic manipulation.

Edema

Underlying causes

Edema occurs when the rate of fluid formation exceeds that of fluid reabsorption from the interstitial fluid into the capillaries.

Edema has many causes. The more common causes for systemic edema are congestive cardiac failure and hypoalbuminemia (including liver failure and the nephrotic syndrome).

Loss of fluid from the intravascular space into the interstitial compartment results in an apparent hypovolemic state. Poor perfusion of the kidneys activates the renin–angiotensin system, which causes sodium and water retention. This exacerbates the problem of edema.

Treatment with diuretics

Diuretics are drugs that work on the kidneys to increase urine volume by reducing salt and water reabsorption from the tubules. They are prescribed in the treatment of edema, where there is an increase in interstitial fluid volume leading to tissue swelling.

Drugs used in the management of renal failure are discussed in Chapter 11.

Loop diuretics

Furosemide, bumetanide, and torsemide are examples of loop diuretics.

Loop diuretics cause the excretion of 15–25% of filtered sodium as opposed to the normal 1% or less. This can result in a profound diuresis.

Site of action: Loop diuretics act at the thick ascending segment of the loop of Henle.

Mechanism of action: Loop diuretics inhibit the $Na^+/K^+/2Cl^-$ cotransporter (symporter) in the luminal membrane (see Fig. 9.3). This increases the amount of sodium reaching the collecting duct and thereby increases potassium and proton secretion. Calcium and magnesium reabsorption is also inhibited, owing to the decrease in potential difference across the cell normally generated from the recycling of potassium.

Loop diuretics additionally have a venodilator action, which often brings about relief of clinical symptoms prior to the onset of diuresis.

Route of administration: Oral, intravenous, or intramuscular. Intravenous route is used in emergencies, as therapeutic effect is much quicker (about 30 minutes compared with 4–6 hours for an oral dose).

Indications: Acute pulmonary edema, oliguria due to acute renal failure, and resistant chronic heart failure (CHF) and hypertension.

Contraindications: Loop diuretics should not be given to those with severe renal impairment. They should be given only with extreme caution to patients receiving:

- Cardiac glycosides, as the hypokalemia caused by loop diuretics potentiates the action of cardiac glycosides and consequently increases the risk of cardiac glycoside-induced arrhythmias.
- Aminoglycoside antibiotics, as these interact with loop diuretics and increase the risk of ototoxicity and potential hearing loss.

Adverse effects: Hypokalemia, hyponatremia, hyperuricemia, hypotension, and hypovolemia. Metabolic alkalosis may occur because of increased proton secretion and consequent excretion. Hypocalcemia and hypomagnesemia are also possible.

Most diuretics block sodium reabsorption from the renal tubule. High solute load in the tubule results in an osmotic diuresis.

Thiazide and related diuretics

Bendroflumethiazide, chlorthalidone, metolazone, and indapamide are examples of thiazide or related diuretics.

Thiazides produce a moderately potent diuresis, causing the excretion of 5–10% of filtered sodium.

Site of action: Thiazide diuretics act on the early distal tubule.

Mechanism of action: Thiazide diuretics inhibit the Na^+/Cl^- cotransporter in the luminal membrane (see Fig. 9.4). Like loop diuretics, they increase the secretion of potassium and protons into the collecting

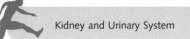

ducts, but, in contrast, they decrease calcium excretion by a mechanism possibly involving the stimulation of a sodium/calcium exchange across the basolateral membrane; this is due to reduced tubular cell sodium concentration.

Route of administration: Oral, peak effect at 4–6 hours.

Indications: Hypertension, and edema secondary to CHF, liver disease, or nephrotic syndrome. Occasionally used for prophylaxis of calcium-containing renal stones.

Contraindications: Hypokalemia, hyponatremia, or hypercalcemia. Caution when prescribing to those taking cardiac glycosides or to those with diabetes mellitus (thiazides may cause hyperglycemia).

Adverse effects: Hypokalemia, hyperuricemia, hyponatremia, hypermagnesemia, hypercalcemia, and metabolic alkalosis.

Potassium-sparing diuretics

Spironolactone, amiloride, and triamterene are all potassium-sparing diuretics.

Potassium-sparing diuretics produce mild diuresis, and they cause the excretion of 2–3% of filtered sodium.

Site of action: Potassium-sparing diuretics work at the late distal tubule and collecting duct.

Mechanism of action: There are two classes of potassium-sparing diuretics (see Fig. 9.5):

• Sodium-channel blockers (e.g., amiloride and triamterene). These drugs block sodium reabsorption by the principal cells, thus reducing the potential difference across the cell and reducing potassium secretion. Secretion of proton from the intercalated cells is also decreased.

• Aldosterone antagonists (e.g., spironolactone, eplerenone). Spironolactone is a competitive antagonist at aldosterone receptors and thus reduces sodium reabsorption and, therefore, potassium and proton secretion. The degree of diuresis depends on aldosterone levels.

Route of administration: Oral.

Indications: In conjunction with other diuretics (thiazides, loop diuretics) in managing heart failure or hypertension to maintain normal serum potassium levels.

Aldosterone antagonists are used in the treatment of hyperaldosteronism, which can be primary (Conn's syndrome) or secondary (as a result of CHF, liver disease, or nephrotic syndrome).

Contraindications: Potassium-sparing diuretics interact with angiotensin-converting enzyme inhibitors, increasing the risk of hyperkalemia. They should not be given to patients with renal failure.

Adverse effects: Gastrointestinal disturbances, hyperkalemia, and hyponatremia. Aldosterone antagonists have a wide range of adverse effects, including gynecomastia, menstrual disorders, and male sexual dysfunction.

Therapeutic notes: Low-dose spironolactone has beneficial effects in CHF. Several preparations exist which combine a potassium-sparing diuretic with either a thiazide or a loop diuretic.

Osmotic diuretics

Mannitol is an osmotic diuretic.

Site of action: Osmotic diuretics exert their effects in tubular segments that are water permeable: proximal tubule, descending loop of Henle, and the collecting ducts.

Mechanism of action: Osmotic diuretics are freely filtered at the glomerulus but only partially, if at all, reabsorbed. Passive water reabsorption is reduced by the presence of this nonreabsorbable solute within the tubule lumen. The net effect is increased water loss, with a relatively smaller loss of sodium.

Route of administration: Mannitol is administered intravenously.

Indications: Osmotic diuretics are used mainly for raised intracranial and, rarely, raised intraocular pressure (glaucoma).

Contraindications: Congestive heart failure, pulmonary edema.

Adverse effects: Chills and fever.

Therapeutic notes: Osmotic diuretics are seldom used in heart failure, as expansion of blood volume can be greater than the degree of diuresis produced.

Carbonic anhydrase inhibitors

Carbonic anhydrase inhibitors are no longer used as diuretics, being employed now solely in the management of glaucoma (Chapter 12) and to treat symptoms of "mountain sickness."

Urinary system

Urinary retention

Acute urinary retention is treated with urethral catheterization. Chronic urinary retention is usually painless, and management depends upon the underlying cause. In men, the most common cause of chronic urinary retention is benign prostatic hyperplasia (BPH). Surgery is the definitive treatment, though many patients can be treated medically. The three classes of drugs that can be employed to treat bladder outflow obstruction secondary to BPH are α_1-selective blockers, parasympathomimetics, and antiandrogens.

Alpha-blockers
Doxazosin and prazosin are examples of α_1-selective blockers, which act by relaxing the smooth muscle at the urethra opening of the bladder, and so increasing the flow of urine. Since the α_1-selective blockers are also used as vasodilators in cardiovascular disease (Chapter 7), hypotension can be a side effect, although they are otherwise well tolerated.

Parasympathomimetics
Carbachol and bethanechol are parasympathomimetics, which act by increasing detrusor muscle contraction. Their effect is most marked when there is bladder outlet obstruction, and they have no role in the relief of acute urinary retention. Side effects include sweating, bradycardia, and intestinal colic. They are now used infrequently, being superseded by catheterization.

Antiandrogens
Finasteride is a specific inhibitor of the enzyme 5α-reductase, which converts testosterone to the more potent androgen dihydrotestosterone. This inhibition loads to a reduction in prostate size and improvement of urinary flow. The antiandrogens are described in Chapter 11.

Urinary incontinence
Urinary incontinence by definition is the inability to prevent the discharge of urine. The three main types of urinary incontinence are true incontinence, stress incontinence, and urge incontinence.

Urge incontinence is the only type that is practically amenable to pharmacologic intervention, mostly with antimuscarinic drugs.

Antimuscarinics
Oxybutynin is the most widely used antimuscarinic for urge incontinence.

Mechanism of action: Oxybutynin relaxes the detrusor muscle of the bladder.

Route of administration: Oral.

Indications: Urinary frequency, urgency, and urge incontinence.

Contraindications: Intestinal obstruction, significant bladder outflow obstruction, and glaucoma.

Adverse effects: Dry mouth, constipation, blurred vision, nausea, and vomiting.

Therapeutic notes: The main side effects are typically the anticholinergic ones, and they are commonly dose related.

Erectile dysfunction
Erectile dysfunction (impotence) is a very common problem worldwide, and it has numerous causes.

The penis is innervated by autonomic (involuntary) and somatic (voluntary) nerves. Parasympathetic innervation brings about erection, and sympathetic innervation is responsible for ejaculation. Nonadrenergic, noncholinergic neurotransmission (NANC) also appears to promote erection.

Nitric oxide is believed to be the principal mediator of inducing and sustaining an erection. This highly reactive species activates the guanylyl cyclase enzyme, which subsequently generates cyclic guanosine monophosphate (cGMP).

The synthesis of cGMP in turn activates a protein kinase, which phosphorylates ion channels in the plasma membrane and causes hyperpolarization of the smooth muscle cell. Intracellular calcium ions are consequently sequestered into the endoplasmic reticulum, and further calcium influx into the cell is inhibited by the closure of calcium channels. The overall effect of a fall in intracellular calcium is a relaxation of the smooth muscle and increased blood flow to the penis.

While nitric oxide has a very short half-life and is molecularly unstable, cGMP is broken down by a specific group of enzymes, the phosphodiesterases, which subsequently results in the penis returning to its flaccid state. Phosphodiesterase type 5 is thought to be the principal species within the penis, and clearly a target for therapeutic manipulation.

Phosphodiesterase inhibitors
Sildenafil is a selective inhibitor of phosphodiesterase type 5.

Mechanism of action: Inhibition of phosphodiesterase-mediated degradation of cGMP. Higher intracellular levels of cGMP result in continual relaxation of penile smooth muscle and maintenance of an erection.

Route of administration: Oral.

Indications: Erectile dysfunction.

Contraindications: Concurrent treatment with nitrates. Conditions in which vasodilatation or sexual activity is inadvisable.

Adverse effects: Dyspepsia, headache, flushing, and visual disturbances.

Therapeutic notes: Nonselective inhibition of phosphodiesterase type 6 in the retina is responsible for occasional color disturbances in some patients' vision. Erection will not occur unless there is sexual stimulation.

Prostaglandin E₁

Alprostadil is a synthetic prostaglandin E_1 analog, and, like prostaglandin E_1, it has a similar effect to nitric oxide upon penile smooth muscle. Alprostadil can be administered by direct injection into the corpus cavernosum of the penis or applied into the urethra. The most common and most serious side effect is priapism, and any erection lasting longer than 4 hours should be reported.

Phosphodiesterase enzymes degrade the cyclic nucleotides cAMP and cGMP. Inhibitors of the phosphodiesterases, such as sildenafil, and the less specific xanthines such as theophylline, result in accumulation of these mediators, which brings about the physiologic effects of these drugs.

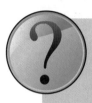

- What is the fraction of the cardiac output that the kidneys receive? What is meant by the term glomerular filtration rate?
- What are the main functions of the kidney?
- What are the differences between glomerular filtration, tubular secretion, and tubular reabsorption? Which constituents of blood are filtered, and which are not?
- What is diuresis? What is a diuretic? What are the classes of diuretic drugs used in clinical practice and an example of each?
- What is edema? What are its more common causes?
- How do loop diuretics work?
- Why should potassium-sparing diuretics be used with caution in renal failure? Explain the pathophysiology.
- What pharmacologic treatments are there for the management of urinary outflow obstruction secondary to benign prostatic hyperplasia?
- Antimuscarinic (anticholinergic) drugs are used for urinary incontinence. What are the side effects of anticholinergic drugs?
- What is the mechanism of action of the phosphodiesterase inhibitors in the management of erectile dysfunction?

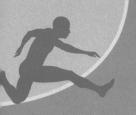

10. Gastrointestinal System

Stomach

Peptic ulceration

The gastric epithelium secretes several substances—hydrochloric acid (HCl) from the parietal cells, digestive enzymes from the peptic cells, and mucus from the mucus-secreting cells. The acid and enzymes convert food into a thick, semiliquid paste called chyme, while mucus protects the stomach from its own corrosive secretions.

Peptic ulceration results from a breach in the mucosa lining the alimentary tract caused by acid and enzyme attack (Fig. 10.1). Unprotected mucosa rapidly undergoes autodigestion, leading to a range of damage—inflammation or gastritis, necrosis, hemorrhage, and even perforation as the erosion deepens.

Gastric and duodenal ulcers differ in their location, epidemiology, incidence, and etiology, but they present with similar symptoms and are treated on similar principles. Peptic ulcer disease is chronic, recurrent, and common, affecting at least 10% of the population in developed countries. *Helicobacter pylori* plays a role in the pathogenesis of a significant proportion of peptic ulcer disease.

Protective factors

The mucosal defenses against acid/enzyme attack consist of:

- The mucus barrier (approximately 500 μm thick), a mucus matrix into which bicarbonate ions are secreted, producing a buffering gradient.
- The surface epithelium, which requires prostaglandins E_2 and I_2, synthesized by the gastric mucosa. These are thought to exert a cytoprotective action by increasing mucosal blood flow.

Weakened mucosal defense	Normal	Increased attack
weakened defenses vulnerable to being breached by normal acid/enzyme levels	acid/enzyme attack is adequately balanced by mucosal and other defences	increased attack breaks down the defenses that would normally be adequate
e.g., • Helicobacter pylori infection. • loss of normal mucosal defenses, e.g., NSAIDs (see Chapter 10)	e.g., • healthy state	e.g., • hyperacidity (Zollinger–Ellison syndrome)

Fig. 10.1 Peptic ulceration (NSAIDs, nonsteroidal anti-inflammatory drugs). (Adapted from General and Systematic Pathology, 2nd ed., by JCE Underwood [ed.]. Churchill Livingstone, 1996.)

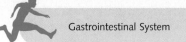

Sir Francis Avery-Jones said: "An ulcer represents the adverse outcome of a conflict between the aggressive forces in the stomach or duodenum (acid/enzymes) and the defense mechanisms (mucus–bicarbonate barrier/surface epithelium)." This concept can be used as a way to rationalize your thinking of the causes and, therefore, appropriate treatment of peptic ulcers.

Acid secretion

The regulation of acid secretion by parietal cells is especially important in peptic ulceration, and it constitutes a major target for drug action (Fig. 10.2). Acid is secreted from gastric parietal cells by a unique proton pump that catalyses the exchange of intracellular protons for extracellular potassium. The secretion of HCl is controlled by the activation of three main receptors on the basolateral membrane of the parietal cell. These are:

- Gastrin receptors, which respond to gastrin secreted by the G cells of the stomach antrum.
- Histamine (H_2) receptors, which respond to histamine secreted from the enterochromaffin-like paracrine cells that are adjacent to the parietal cell.
- Muscarinic (M_1, M_3) receptors on the parietal cell, which respond to acetylcholine (ACh) released from neurons innervating the parietal cell.

Although the parietal cells possess muscarinic and gastrin receptors, both ACh and gastrin mainly exert their acid secretory effect indirectly, by stimulating nearby enterochromaffin-like cells to release histamine. Histamine then acts locally on the parietal cells, where activation of the H_2 receptor results in the stimulation of adenylyl cyclase and the subsequent secretion of acid. Excessive production of gastrin from a rare tumor, a gastrinoma, can result in excess acid production, and in peptic ulceration, a condition known as Zollinger–Ellison syndrome.

Gastroesophageal reflux disease

Stomach contents are normally prevented from re-entering the esophagus by the lower esophageal sphincter (LES). Loss of tone of the LES and a rise in intra-abdominal pressure are the most common causes of gastroesophageal reflux disease (GERD), of which heartburn is the major symptom.

Conservative treatment options include weight loss and raising the head of the patient's bed. Precipitating factors should be avoided, as should excess smoking and alcohol. The drugs used in GERD are the same as for other acid-related disorders (Fig. 10.3).

Prevention and treatment of acid-related disease

Drugs that are effective in the treatment of peptic ulcers either reduce/neutralize gastric acid secretion or increase mucosal resistance to acid-pepsin attack. Peptic ulcers thus treated will heal rapidly, but recurrence is common unless *H. pylori* is eliminated.

Reduction of acid secretion
Proton pump inhibitors

Omeprazole and lansoprazole are examples of proton pump inhibitors (PPIs).

Mechanism of action: PPIs cause irreversible inhibition of H^+/K^+ ATPase that is responsible for proton secretion from parietal cells (see Fig. 10.2). They are inactive prodrugs and are converted at acidic pH to sulfonamide, which combines covalently, and therefore irreversibly, with sulfhydryl groups on H^+/K^+ ATPase. This inhibition is highly specific and localized.

Route of administration: Oral. Some PPIs can be given intravenously.

Indications: Short-term treatment of peptic ulcers, eradication of *H. pylori*, severe GERD, confirmed esophagitis, Zollinger–Ellison syndrome.

Contraindications: No important contraindications are reported with PPIs.

Adverse effects: Gastrointestinal upset, nausea, and headaches. There might be a risk of gastric atrophy with long-term treatment.

Histamine H_2 receptor antagonists

Examples of H_2 receptor antagonists include cimetidine, ranitidine, and famotidine.

Mechanism of action: H_2 receptor antagonists competitively block the action of histamine on the parietal cell by their antagonism of H_2 receptors (see Fig. 10.2).

Route of administration: Oral. Some antihistamines can be given intravenously.

Indications: H_2 receptor antagonists are the first-line treatment of peptic ulcer disease and GERD.

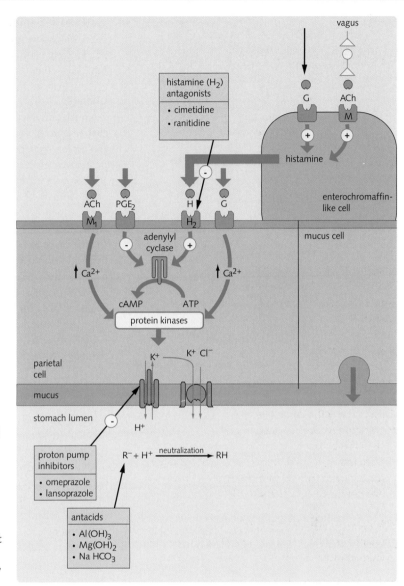

Fig. 10.2 Acid secretion from parietal cells is reduced by muscarinic antagonists, histamine (H_2) antagonists, and the proton pump inhibitors. Gastrin (G) and acetylcholine (Ach) stimulate the parietal cell directly to increase acid secretion and also stimulate enterochromaffin-like cells to secrete histamine, which then acts upon the H_2 receptors of the parietal cell. Antacids raise the luminal pH by neutralizing hydrogen ions. Mucosal strengtheners adhere to and protect ulcer craters, and they may kill *H. pylori* (redrawn from Page et al., 2002).

Contraindications: Cimetidine should be avoided by patients stabilized on warfarin, phenytoin, and theophylline. Ranitidine is associated with fewer DDIs than cimetidine.

Adverse effects: Dizziness, fatigue, gynecomastia, and rash.

Therapeutic notes: H_2 receptor antagonists do not reduce acid production to the same extent as PPIs, but they do relieve the pain of ulcer and promote healing. The drugs are administered at nighttime, when acid buffering by food is at its lowest. The usual regimen is twice daily for 4–8 weeks. Cimetidine inhibits the P450 enzyme system, reducing the metabolism of drugs such as warfarin, phenytoin, theophylline, and methylenedioxymethamphetamine (MDMA; "ecstasy") and thus potentiating their pharmacologic effect.

Mucosal strengtheners
Misoprostol
Mechanism of action: Misoprostol is a synthetic analog of prostaglandin E. It imitates the action of endogenous prostaglandins (PGE$_2$ and PGI$_2$) in maintaining the

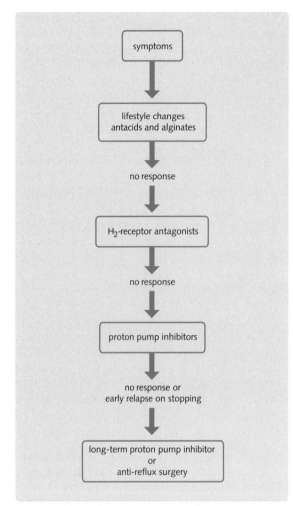

Fig. 10.3 Treatment of gastroesophageal reflux disease: a stepwise approach (adapted from Davidson's Principles and Practice of Medicine, 18th ed., by C Haslett [ed.]. Churchill Livingstone).

integrity of the gastroduodenal mucosal barrier, and it promotes healing (see Fig. 10.2).

Route of administration: Oral.

Indications: Ulcer healing and ulcer prophylaxis with nonsteroidal anti-inflammatory drug (NSAID) use.

Contraindications: Misoprostol should not be given to people with hypotension or to women who are pregnant or breastfeeding.

Adverse effects: Diarrhea and abdominal pain.

Therapeutic notes: Misoprostol is most effective at correcting the deficit caused by NSAIDs that inhibit cyclooxygenase–1 and reduce prostaglandin

synthesis (Chapter 4). Misoprostol can prevent NSAID-associated ulcers; therefore, it is particularly useful in the elderly from whom NSAIDs cannot be withdrawn.

Chelates

Bismuth and sucralfate appear to help protect the gastric mucosa by several means, including inhibiting the action of pepsin, promoting synthesis of protective prostaglandins, and stimulating the secretion of bicarbonate. They are administered orally and are generally well tolerated.

Antacids

Examples of antacids include aluminium hydroxide, magnesium hydroxide, and sodium bicarbonate.

Mechanism of action: Antacids consist of alkaline Al^{3+}, Mg^{2+}, and Na^+ salts that are used to raise the luminal pH of the stomach. They neutralize acid and, as a result, may reduce the damaging effects of pepsin, which is pH dependent (see Fig. 10.2). Additionally, Al^{3+} and Mg^{2+} salts bind and inactivate pepsin.

Route of administration: Oral.

Indications: Symptomatic relief of ulcers, nonulcer dyspepsia, and GERD.

Contraindications: Aluminium hydroxide and magnesium hydroxide should not be given to people with hypophosphatemia. Sodium bicarbonate should be avoided in patients on a salt-restricted diet (in those with heart failure and in hepatic and renal impairment).

Adverse effects: Constipation and diarrhea.

Therapeutic notes: Antacids are still useful for the relief of symptoms of ulceration; frequent high dosing can promote ulcer healing, but this is rarely practical.

Helicobacter pylori eradication regimens

H. pylori plays a significant role in the pathogenesis of peptic ulcer disease. It does not cause ulcers in everyone it infects (50–80% of the population), but of those who develop ulcers, 90% can be found to have an *H. pylori* infection in their antrum.

Treatment of peptic ulcer disease should include eradication of *H. pylori*. The rate of recurrence of duodenal ulcer after healing can be as high as 80% within 1 year when *H. pylori* eradication is not part of the treatment, but less than 5% when *H. pylori* is eradicated.

The ideal treatment for *H. pylori* eradication is not yet clear. Current regimens under evaluation include:
- The classic triple therapy: 1 or 2 weeks' treatment with omeprazole, metronidazole, and amoxicillin or clarithromycin. This eliminates *H. pylori* in 90% of patients, but adverse effects, compliance, and resistance can be problematic.
- Dual therapy: omeprazole is given in combination with a single antibiotic, usually either amoxicillin or clarithromycin. This regimen is less effective at *H. pylori* eradication, and it is not recommended.

Peptic ulcer disease is very common and potentially life threatening. Always check with patients if they have an ulcer or suffer with ulcer-like symptoms before prescribing NSAIDs.

Nausea and vomiting

Nausea is an unpleasant feeling in the upper abdomen and throat, which usually precedes vomiting, although for many patients nausea is experienced without vomiting. Nausea alone can be as distressing as the act of vomiting itself. The more common causes of nausea and vomiting are shown in Fig. 10.4.

The act of vomiting is coordinated in the vomiting center within the brainstem. This center receives neuronal input from several sources, although fibers from the chemoreceptor trigger zone (CTZ) of the fourth ventricle appear fundamental in bringing about emesis. The CTZ lies outside the blood–brain barrier, and it is sensitive to many stimuli, such as drugs and endogenous and potentially exogenous

Causes of nausea and vomiting
• Gastrointestinal irritation • Motion sickness • Vestibular disease • Hormone disturbance • Drugs and radiation • Exogenous toxins • Pain • Psychogenic factors • Intracranial pathology

Fig. 10.4 Common causes of nausea and vomiting.

chemical mediators. The CTZ contains numerous dopamine receptors, which partially explains why antiparkinsonian drugs (dopaminergic drugs) often induce nausea and vomiting, while some antidopaminergic drugs are used as antiemetics.

Treatment
Antiemetic drugs
H$_1$ receptor antagonists
Cyclizine, diphenhydramine, and hydroxyzine are antiemetic antihistamines.

Mechanism of action: These antihistamines have little effect on nausea and vomiting induced by substances acting directly upon the CTZ, though they appear to be effective antiemetics in motion sickness and vestibulocochlear disease.

Route of administration: Oral and parenteral preparations are available for these drugs..

Indications: Motion sickness, vestibular disorders, vertigo.

Adverse effects: Drowsiness, dry mouth, blurred vision.

Therapeutic notes: Antihistamines have significant antimuscarinic activity, and they should be used with caution in prostatic hypertrophy, urinary retention, and glaucoma.

Phenothiazines
Prochlorperazine is the most widely used antiemetic drug in this class, although the phenothiazines are also used for their antipsychotic properties (Chapter 6). Promethazine is a phenothiazine with H$_1$ blocking activity.

Mechanism of action: Numerous effects. Block dopamine, histamine, and muscarinic receptors.

Route of administration: Oral, rectal, and intramuscular.

Indications: Nausea and vomiting, vertigo, psychosis (Chapter 6).

Contraindications: May exacerbate existing parkinsonian symptoms.

Adverse effects: Sedation, postural hypotension, increased prolactin levels, extrapyramidal effects.

Dopamine antagonists
Domperidone and metoclopramide are examples of the antiemetic dopamine antagonists.

Mechanism of action: Domperidone and metoclopramide block dopamine (especially D$_2$) receptors, and they act on the CTZ. Their central antiemetic effect is enhanced, as they also promote gastric emptying and small intestine peristalsis.

Route of administration: Metoclopramide—oral, intramuscular, intravenous. Domperidone—oral, rectal.

Indications: Nausea and vomiting, functional dyspepsia.

Contraindications: Metoclopramide is not routinely given to patients under the age of 20, as there is an increased risk of extrapyramidal side effects in the young.

Adverse effects: Extrapyramidal effects, hyperprolactinemia.

5-HT$_3$ receptor antagonists

Ondansetron is an example of a 5-HT$_3$ receptor antagonist.

Mechanism of action: Antagonism of the 5-HT$_3$ (serotonin) receptor in the CTZ is believed to be responsible for the antiemetic effects of this class of drugs.

Route of administration: Oral, rectal, intramuscular, intravenous.

Indications: Nausea and vomiting, especially associated with administration of cytotoxic drugs.

Adverse effects: Constipation, headache.

Other antiemetics

The synthetic cannabinoid dronabinol has antiemetic properties where there is direct stimulation of the CTZ. Hyoscine is a muscarinic-receptor antagonist, and like the antihistamines it is most effective in the treatment of motion sickness. Betahistine dihydrochloride is used in Ménière's disease, although its prime effects are assumed to be upon the vestibulocochlear nerve.

Nausea is one of the most distressing symptoms for the patient, and while antiemetic drugs only control symptoms, prescribing them really does bring about immediate relief.

Intestines

Intestinal motility

Normal motility, or peristalsis, of the intestinal tract acts to mix bowel contents thoroughly and to propel them in a caudal direction. Regulation of normal intestinal motility is under neuronal and hormonal control.

Neuronal control

Two principal intramural plexi form the enteric nervous system:

- The myenteric plexus (Auerbach's plexus), located between the outer longitudinal and middle circular muscle layers.
- The submucous plexus (Meissner's plexus), on the luminal side of the circular muscle layer.

Together, these autonomic ganglionated plexi control the functioning of the gastrointestinal tract through complex local reflex connections between sensory neurons, smooth muscle, mucosa, and blood vessels.

Extrinsic parasympathetic fibers from the vagus are excitatory, while extrinsic sympathetic fibers are inhibitory.

The enteric autonomic nervous system is a major target in the pharmacologic therapy of gastrointestinal disorders.

Hormonal control

The activity of the gastrointestinal tract is influenced both by endocrine (e.g., gastrin) and paracrine (e.g., histamine, secretin, cholecystokinin, vasoactive intestinal peptide) secretions. Other than in the context of local control of acid secretion in the stomach, an understanding of these other hormones is not of immediate relevance to an understanding of the pharmacologic therapy of gastrointestinal disorders.

Drugs that affect intestinal motility

Four classes of drug are used clinically for their effects on gastrointestinal motility (Fig. 10.5):

- Motility stimulants.
- Antispasmodics.
- Laxatives (purgatives).
- Antidiarrheals.

Motility stimulants

Agents that increase the motility of the gastrointestinal tract without a laxative effect are used for motility disorders such as GERD and gastric stasis (slow stomach emptying), or for diagnostic techniques such as duodenal intubation. Domperidone and metoclopramide, in addition to their antiemetic effects, both act to increase gastric and intestinal motility, though their mechanism of action for the latter remains unclear. Erythromycin increases gastric motility through activation of motilin receptors.

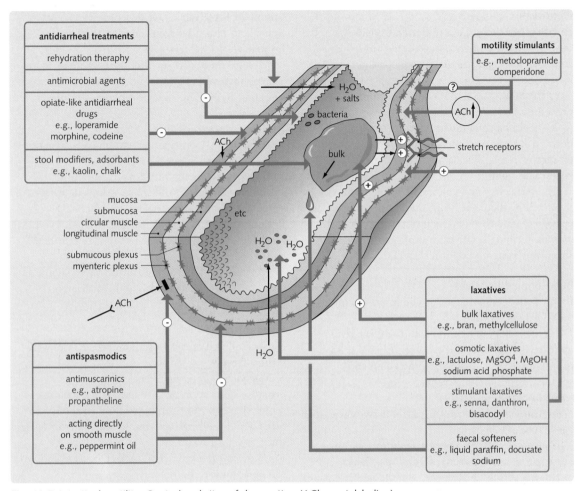

Fig. 10.5 Intestinal motility: Control and sites of drug action (ACh, acetylcholine).

Antispasmodics

The smooth muscle relaxant properties of antispasmodic drugs may be useful as adjunctive treatment in nonulcer dyspepsia, irritable bowel syndrome, and diverticular disease.

The two classes of antispasmodic drug are antimuscarinics and drugs acting directly on smooth muscle.

Antimuscarinics

Examples of antimuscarinics include atropine and propantheline.

Mechanism of action: Antimuscarinics act by inhibiting parasympathetic activity, causing relaxation of gastrointestinal smooth muscle.

Route of administration: Oral.

Indications: Nonulcer dyspepsia, irritable bowel syndrome, and diverticular disease.

Contraindications: Antimuscarinics tend to relax the lower esophageal sphincter and should be avoided in GERD. Other contraindications include angle-closure glaucoma, myasthenia gravis, paralytic ileus, and prostatic enlargement.

Adverse effects: Anticholinergic effects—dry mouth, blurred vision, dry skin, tachycardia, urinary retention.

Irritable bowel syndrome is extremely common in all age groups and in both sexes, and it is often self-limiting over time. Sinister pathology should be excluded, and the patient reassured. Dietary modification and antispasmodics form the mainstay of treatment.

Laxatives

Laxatives are drugs used to hasten transit time in the gut and encourage defecation. Laxatives are used to relieve constipation (an infrequent or difficult passage of stool) and to clear the bowel prior to medical and surgical procedures.

It should be remembered that individual bowel habit can vary considerably—the passage of stools twice a day to once every 3 days is normal.

The frequency and volume of stool are best regulated by diet, but drugs may be necessary. The passage of food through the intestine can be hastened by bulk-forming laxatives, osmotic laxatives, stimulant laxatives, or fecal softeners.

Bulk-forming laxatives

Bran, methylcellulose, and psyllium are examples of bulk-forming laxatives.

Mechanism of action: Bulk-forming laxatives increase the volume of the nonabsorbable solid residue in the gut, distending the colon and stimulating peristaltic activity.

Route of administration: Oral.

Indications: Constipation, particularly when small hard stools are present.

Contraindications: Dysphagia, intestinal obstruction, colonic atony, fecal impaction.

Adverse effects: Flatulence, abdominal distention, and gastrointestinal obstruction.

Therapeutic notes: Adequate fluid intake should be encouraged, and clinical effects may take several days to develop.

Osmotic laxatives

Examples of osmotic laxatives include lactulose and saline purgatives.

Mechanism of action: Osmotic laxatives are poorly absorbed compounds that increase the water content of the bowel by osmosis. Lactulose is a semisynthetic disaccharide that is not absorbed from the gastrointestinal tract. Similarly, magnesium and sodium salts are poorly absorbed and osmotically active.

Route of administration: Oral.

Indications: Constipation, hepatic encephalopathy.

Contraindications: Intestinal obstruction.

Adverse effects: Flatulence, cramps, and abdominal discomfort.

Stimulant laxatives

Senna and bisacodyl are examples of stimulant laxatives.

Mechanism of action: Stimulant laxatives increase gastrointestinal peristalsis and water and electrolyte secretion by the mucosa, possibly by stimulating enteric nerves.

Route of administration: Oral.

Indications: Constipation and bowel evacuation prior to medical/surgical procedures.

Contraindications: Intestinal obstruction.

Adverse effects: In the short term, side effects of stimulant laxatives include intestinal cramp. Prolonged use can lead to damage to the nerve plexi, resulting in the deterioration of intestinal function and atonic colon.

Therapeutic notes: Stimulant laxatives should be given for short periods only, and danthron is indicated for use only in the terminally ill.

Fecal softeners

Mineral oil and docusate sodium are examples of fecal softeners.

Mechanism of action: Fecal softeners promote defecation by softening (e.g., docusate sodium) and/or lubricating (e.g., mineral oil) feces to aid their passage through the gastrointestinal tract.

Route of administration: Oral. Docusate sodium can be administered rectally.

Indications: Constipation, fecal impaction, hemorrhoids, and anal fissures.

Contraindications: Should not be given to children less than 3 years old.

Adverse effects: The prolonged use of mineral oil may impair the absorption of fat-soluble vitamins A and D and cause "paraffinomas."

Therapeutic notes: The prolonged use of fecal softeners is not recommended.

Antidiarrheal drugs

Diarrhea is the passage of frequent, liquid stools. Causes of diarrhea include infections, toxins, drugs, chronic disease, and anxiety.

Acute secretory diarrhea usually results from an infection. It is extremely common, and it causes much preventable mortality, especially in children under 2 years of age in developing countries. The vigor with which diarrhea should be treated depends very much on the cause and the clinical evaluation of patient risk.

There are four approaches to the treatment of severe acute diarrhea:

- Maintenance of fluid and electrolyte balance through oral rehydration therapy (ORT).
- Use of antimicrobial drugs.
- Use of opioid-like antimotility drugs.
- Use of stool modifiers/adsorbents.

Oral rehydration therapy

ORT should be the first priority in the treatment of acute diarrhea of all causes, and it can be life saving.

ORT solutions are isotonic or slightly hypotonic. They vary in composition, but a standard formula would contain NaCl, KCl, sodium citrate, and glucose in appropriate concentrations.

Intravenous rehydration therapy is needed if dehydration is severe.

Antimicrobial drugs

Antibiotic treatment of diarrhea is useful only when a pathogen has been identified or is highly suspected. Acute infectious diarrhea is usually self-limiting. Antibiotic therapy itself carries certain risks, including spreading antibiotic resistance among enteropathogenic bacteria and destroying normal commensal gut flora, allowing overgrowth of the bacterium *Clostridium difficile*, which can result in pseudomembranous colitis—a potentially fatal condition.

Antibiotic treatment is indicated in:

- Severe cholera or *Salmonella typhimurium* infection—ciprofloxacin.
- *Shigella* species infections—ciprofloxacin.
- *Campylobacter jejuni*—erythromycin or ciprofloxacin.

Antibiotics are discussed in detail in Chapter 3.

Opioid-like antimotility drugs

Examples of opiate-like antimotility drugs include loperamide and diphenoxylate.

Mechanism of action: Opioid-like antimotility drugs act on μ-opiate receptors in the myenteric plexus, which increases the tone and rhythmic contraction of the intestine, but lessens propulsive activity. Loperamide and diphenoxylate also have an antisecretory action.

Route of administration: Oral.

Indications: Opioid-like antimotility drugs have a limited role as an adjunct to fluid and electrolyte replacement in acute diarrhea. They are also used as adjunctive therapy in some chronic diarrheal conditions.

Contraindications: Opioid-like antimotility drugs should not be given to people with diarrheal conditions such as acute ulcerative colitis or antibiotic-associated colitis. They are not recommended for children.

Adverse effects: Nausea, vomiting, abdominal cramps, constipation, and drowsiness.

Therapeutic notes: Loperamide does not enter the CNS and is the most appropriate opioid for local effects on the gut.

Stool modifiers/adsorbents

Examples of stool modifiers/adsorbents include kaolin, chalk, charcoal, and methylcellulose.

Mechanism of action: It has been suggested that stool modifiers/adsorbents act by absorbing toxins or by coating and protecting the intestinal mucosa, although there is no evidence to support this.

Route of administration: Oral.

Indications: There is little evidence to recommend adsorbents at all.

Contraindications: Adsorbents are not recommended for acute diarrheas.

Adverse effects: Stool modifiers/adsorbents may reduce the absorption of other drugs.

Therapeutic notes: Adsorbents are popular "remedies" for the treatment of diarrhea, although there is little evidence of their benefits.

Diarrhea can be life threatening, especially in children. Management in most cases relies on fluid replacement prior to treating the underlying cause.

Inflammatory bowel disease

The inflammatory bowel diseases fall into two categories that share a number of common features. Symptoms often relapse and remit, and their etiology remains unclear. Crohn's disease can affect the entire gut, and inflammation occurs throughout the full thickness of the bowel wall, while ulcerative colitis affects only the large bowel, and inflammation is limited to bowel mucosa.

Treatment

Treatment of these conditions is not only pharmacologic, but it also depends on psychological support, correction of nutritional deficiencies, and often surgical resection.

Drug treatment is aimed at controlling inflammation and bringing about remission, and the mainstays of drug treatment for these diseases are glucocorticoids, aminosalicylates, immunosuppressives, cytotoxics, and antibiotics.

Glucocorticoids

Examples of glucocorticoids include prednisolone, budesonide, and prednisone.

Mechanism of action: Glucocorticoids have an anti-inflammatory effect (Chapter 11).

Route of administration: In localized disease, glucocorticoids may be administered rectally as enemas, suppositories, or foams. In extensive or severe disease, oral or intravenous therapy may be required.

Indications: Glucocorticoids are given for acute relapses of inflammatory bowel disease.

Contraindications: Bowel obstruction or perforation, or for prolonged periods.

Adverse effects: Cushingoid side effects may occur with long-term glucocorticoid use (Chapter 11).

Therapeutic notes: Budesonide is locally acting and poorly absorbed, so it has few systemic side effects.

Aminosalicylates

Sulfasalazine, mesalazine, and olsalazine are examples of aminosalicylates.

Mechanism of action: Sulfasalazine is broken down in the gut to the active component— 5-aminosalicylate (5-ASA)—and sulfapyridine, which acts as a vehicle to transport the drug to the colon. Mesalazine is 5-ASA, and olsalazine is two molecules of 5-ASA. The mechanism of action of the active molecule 5-ASA is unknown, although it is postulated to act by scavenging free radicals or interfering with cytokine networks.

Route of administration: Oral, rectal.

Indications: Maintenance therapy of inflammatory bowel conditions.

Contraindications: Aminosalicylates should not be given to people with salicylate hypersensitivity or renal impairment.

Adverse effects: Sulfapyridine is responsible for the majority of this drug's side effects: nausea, vomiting, headache, and rashes. Blood disorders and oligospermia have been reported.

Immunosuppressives, cytotoxics, and antibiotics

When steroids are needed to control symptoms but side effects are troublesome or potentially so, the immunosuppressant azathioprine (Chapter 4) is used as an adjunct to other therapies. In addition, cytotoxic drugs such as methotrexate (Chapter 2), anticytokine antibodies, and the antibiotic metronidazole (Chapter 3) have all been employed to modulate the disease process with varying degrees of success.

Obesity

Obesity is becoming increasingly common in the west, and it is associated with many diseases, such as cardiovascular disease, diabetes mellitus, gallstones, and osteoarthritis.

Treatment

Dietary restriction and an exercise program should be explored prior to surgical or pharmacologic intervention. The most widely used anti-obesity drugs act directly upon the gastrointestinal tract.

Drugs acting on the gastrointestinal tract

Orlistat and methylcellulose are examples of such anti-obesity drugs.

Mechanism of action: Orlistat is a pancreatic lipase inhibitor, which reduces the breakdown and subsequent absorption of fat from the gut. Methylcellulose is believed to act as a bulk-forming agent and to reduce food intake by promoting early satiety (fullness).

Route of administration: Oral.

Adverse effects: Orlistat often results in oily, frequent stools, flatulence, and abdominal and rectal pain. Methylcellulose may produce flatulence and abdominal distention.

Other anti-obesity drugs

The centrally acting appetite suppressant phentermine is licensed, but limitations on its use yield marginal weight loss, so it is seldom prescribed. Numerous other drugs are being evaluated for their anti-obesity properties, including the endogenous mammalian peptide leptin, which appears to induce satiety and counteract the properties of another transmitter, neuropeptide Y, which is believed to promote feeding.

Anal disorders

Hemorrhoids, anal fissures, and pruritus are commonly encountered problems. Bland ointments are the best treatment option, with careful attention to cleanliness. When necessary, topical preparations containing local anesthetic (Chapter 5) or corticosteroids (Chapter 11) may provide symptomatic relief. Perianal thrush can be treated with nystatin (Chapter 3). Hemorrhoids are often treated by injection with a sclerosant, commonly oily phenol.

Stoma care is simple, although it requires a thoughtful, practical approach and empathy with the patient.

Pancreas and gallbladder

Pancreatic supplements

Pancreatic exocrine secretions contain important enzymes that break down proteins (trypsin, chymotrypsin), starch (amylase), and fats (lipase). These are essential for efficient digestion.

Pancreatin, an extract of pancreas containing protease, lipase, and amylase, is given by mouth to compensate for reduced or absent exocrine secretions in cystic fibrosis and following pancreatectomy, total gastrectomy, or chronic pancreatitis. Pancreatin is inactivated by gastric acid, and so precautions must be taken to optimize delivery of the pancreatin to the duodenum. Pancreatin preparations are best taken with food; histamine H_2 antagonists (e.g., cimetidine) may be taken an hour before ingestion of the pancreatin in order to reduce gastric acid secretion, although acid-resistant (enterically coated) formulations are now available.

Gallbladder

Bile is secreted by the liver and stored in the gallbladder. Bile contains cholesterol, phospholipids,

Even though pancreatin contains peptides, which would normally be degraded in the stomach, these tablets are coated in an acid-resistant layer. The enzymes and proenzymes within them have endogenous resistance to both acid and proteases, and they become active in the small intestine.

and bile salts. Bile salts are important for keeping cholesterol in solution. The formation of "stones" in the bile is relatively common (cholelithiasis), and this can result in blockage of the draining duct, with subsequent infection and inflammation (cholecystitis).

Surgical removal of the gallbladder (cholecystectomy) has largely replaced the use of drugs in the management of symptomatic gall tones, although drugs are suitable for patients not treatable by other means.

The dissolution of small cholesterol stones is carried out by prolonged oral administration of the bile acid ursodeoxycholic acid.

Ursodeoxycholic acid

The bile salt ursodeoxycholic acid is administered orally and handled by the body in the same fashion as endogenous bile salt. It works by decreasing both the secretion of cholesterol into the bile and its absorption from the intestine.

The net effect is a reduced cholesterol concentration in the bile and a tendency for the dissolution of existing stones.

Cholestyramine

This orally administered anion-exchange resin binds bile acids in the gut, preventing their reabsorption and enterohepatic recirculation. It is used in the treatment of pruritus associated with partial biliary obstruction and primary biliary cirrhosis, and in hypercholesterolemia.

- Describe how the pathophysiology of peptic ulceration involves disturbance of the balance between the aggressive forces (acid/enzymes) and the defense mechanisms (mucus–bicarbonate barrier/surface epithelium) of the stomach and duodenum.
- Describe the factors that control acid production and maintain mucosal defenses.
- Relate these first two points to the principles by which the pharmacologic treatments work.
- Name examples of each of the different classes of drug.
- Discuss the significance of *Helicobacter pylori* in peptic ulceration.
- Describe the treatment options for the eradication of *Helicobacter pylori*.
- List some common causes for both nausea and vomiting, and outline the physiology of the two.
- Identify the more common antiemetic drugs and explain how they act.
- Briefly describe the endogenous control of intestinal motility.
- Name the common diseases that affect the intestines that require medical treatment.
- Describe functional bowel disease, and list the classes of drugs used in its management.
- Describe what a laxative drug is, and name the various classes of agents that have laxative properties.
- Outline the immediate therapeutic management of a child presenting with chronic diarrhea.
- Identify the infectious agents which are likely to result in diarrhea.
- Explain how the opioid-like drugs affect diarrhea. Name their side effects.
- List the main groups of drugs used to treat chronic inflammatory bowel disease.
- Explain the routes of administration for glucocorticoids to treat inflammatory bowel disease, and explain how they act.
- List the adverse effects of long-term steroid use.
- Describe the drugs available to treat obesity, and briefly summarize how they act.
- Explain why pancreatic supplementation is important in cystic fibrosis, and identify the consequences for patients who do not take pancreatic supplementation.

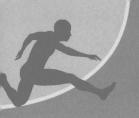

11. Endocrine and Reproductive Systems

Thyroid gland

Principles of thyroid function
Production of thyroid hormones

The thyroid gland secretes three hormones, triiodothyronine (T_3), thyroxine (T_4), and calcitonin, although T_3 and T_4 are regarded as the "true" thyroid hormones. Reference to thyroid hormones will relate to these two. Calcitonin will be discussed at the end of this chapter.

The principal effects of the thyroid hormones are determination of basal metabolic rate, and influence of growth through stimulation of growth hormone synthesis and action. Other effects are summarized in Fig. 11.1.

The follicular cells of the thyroid gland synthesize and glycosylate thyroglobulin before secreting it into their lumen. Iodination of the tyrosine residues on this molecule is catalyzed by thyroid peroxidase, and this results in the formation of monoiodotyrosine (MIT) or diiodotyrosine (DIT). The coupling of MIT with DIT produces T_3, and the coupling of two DIT molecules produces T_4. Coupling is also catalyzed by thyroid peroxidase.

The thyroglobulin, now known as colloid, is endocytosed into the follicular cells, where it is broken down to release T_3, T_4, MIT, and DIT. T_3 and T_4 are secreted into the plasma; MIT and DIT are metabolized within the cells, and their iodide is recycled (Fig. 11.2).

The iodine required for the synthesis of T_3 and T_4 comes mainly from the diet in the form of iodide. Through the action of a thyrotropin-dependent pump, iodide is concentrated in the follicular cells, where it is converted into iodine by thyroid peroxidase.

Control of thyroid hormone secretion

The production of thyroid hormones is slow but constant, and control of their plasma levels is determined by varying their rate of secretion (Fig. 11.3).

The hypothalamus contains thyroid hormone receptors that are able to detect and respond to decreased levels of T_3 and T_4 by causing the release of thyrotropin-releasing hormone (TRH).

TRH reaches the anterior pituitary via the portal circulation, and it stimulates TRH receptors on thyrotroph cells, which in turn secrete thyroid-stimulating hormone (TSH).

TSH reaches the thyroid gland through the systemic circulation, where it stimulates thyroid hormone secretion. Both T_3 and T_4 bind to proteins in the plasma (mostly thyroxine binding globulin), and less than 1% of total thyroid hormones are free. It is the free thyroid hormones that exert their physiological effects. T_3 is about five times more biologically active than T_4, and T_4 is converted in some peripheral tissues to T_3.

T_3 and T_4 exert negative feedback upon the hypothalamus and pituitary.

Physiological effects of thyroid hormones
• Fetal development (physical and cognitive)
• Metabolic rate
• Body temperature
• Cardiac rate and contractility
• Peripheral vasodilatation
• Red cell mass and circulatory volume
• Respiratory drive
• Peripheral nerves (reflexes)
• Hepatic metabolic enzymes
• Bone turnover
• Skin and soft tissue effects

Fig. 11.1 Physiologic effects of thyroid hormones (from Page et al., 2002).

Most modern laboratory thyroid function tests measure just TSH, though levels of free and total T_3 and T_4 can be measured as well as thyroxine-binding globulin.

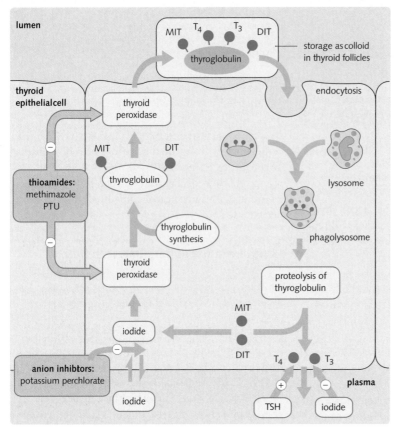

Fig. 11.2 Synthesis of thyroid hormones and the site of action of some antithyroid drugs (DIT, diiodotyrosine; MIT, monoiodotyrosine; PTU, propylthiouracil; T_3, triiodothyronine; T_4, thyroxine; TSH, thyroid-stimulating hormone). (Redrawn from Page et al., 2002.)

Thyroid dysfunction
Hypothyroidism

Hypothyroidism—thyroid insufficiency—is relatively common in adults, and it is associated with tiredness and lethargy, weight gain, intolerance to cold, dry skin, bradycardia, and mental impairment.

Children with hypothyroidism manifest delayed bone growth, whereas a deficiency *in utero* also results in mentally retarded infants; this condition is known as cretinism.

Hashimoto's thyroiditis is an autoimmune disease resulting in fibrosis of the thyroid gland. It is the most common cause of hypothyroidism, and, like most autoimmune diseases, it is more prevalent in women.

Myxedema is also immunologic in origin, and it represents the most severe form of hypothyroidism—sometimes causing coma.

Thyroid hormone resistance and reduced TSH secretion will also produce the symptoms of hypothyroidism.

The causes of hypothyroidism are summarized in Fig. 11.4.

Hyperthyroidism

Hyperthyroidism—thyroid excess—results either from the overproduction of endogenous hormone or exposure to excess exogenous hormone.

Symptoms include increased basal metabolic rate (BMR) with consequent weight loss, increased appetite, increased body temperature, and sweating as well as nervousness, tremor, tachycardia, and classic ophthalmic signs.

Graves' disease (diffuse toxic goiter) is the most common cause of hyperthyroidism. It is an autoimmune disease caused by the activation of TSH receptors by antibodies. This results in an enlargement of the gland and, therefore, excess hormone production.

Toxic nodular goiter is the second most common cause of hyperthyroidism. It is due to either a single adenoma (hyperfunctioning adenoma) or multiple adenomas (multinodular goiter).

The causes of hyperthyroidism are summarized in Fig. 11.5.

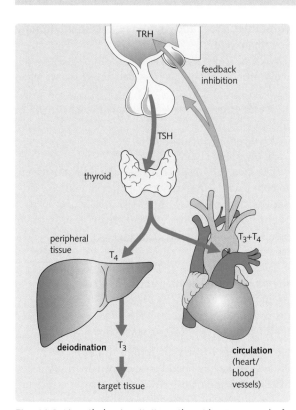

Fig. 11.3 Hypothalamic–pituitary–thyroid axis; control of thyroid hormone synthesis (T_3, triiodothyronine; T_4, thyroxine; TSH, thyroid-stimulating hormone; TRH, thyrotropin-releasing hormone). (Redrawn from Page et al., 2002.)

Causes of hypothyroidism	
Primary	Chronic lymphocytic thyroiditis (Hashimoto's disease)
	Subacute thyroiditis
	Painless thyroiditis (postpartum thyroiditis)
	Radioactive iodine ingestion
	Post thyroidectomy
	Iodine deficiency or excess
	Inborn errors of thyroid hormone synthesis
Secondary	Pituitary disease
Target tissues	Thyroid hormone resistance

Fig. 11.4 Causes of hypothyroidism. (From Page et al., 2002.)

Causes of hyperthyroidism
• Excess exogenous thyroid hormone
• Diffuse toxic goiter (Graves' disease)
• Hyperfunctioning adenoma (toxic nodule)
• Toxic multinodular goiter
• Painless thyroiditis
• Subacute thyroiditis
• Thyroid stimulating hormone (TSH)–secreting adenoma
• Human chorionic gonadotrophin (hCG)–secreting tumours

Fig. 11.5 Causes of hyperthyroidism (from Page et al., 2002).

Management of thyroid dysfunction
Hyperthyroidism and antithyroid drugs
Thioamides
Methimazole and propylthiouracil (PTU) are examples of thioamides. The thioamides are the first-line drugs for treatment of hyperthyroidism.

Mechanism of action: The thioamides cause inhibition of thyroid peroxidase with a consequent reduction in thyroid hormone synthesis and storage (see Fig. 11.2). The effects of PTU may take several weeks to manifest, as there are stores of T_3 and T_4. PTU also inhibits the peripheral deiodination of T_4 to T_3.

Route of administration: Oral.

Indications: The thioamides are used for hyperthyroidism.

Contraindications: The thioamides should not be given to people with a large goiter. PTU should be given at a reduced dose in patients with renal impairment.

Adverse effects: Nausea and headache; allergic reactions, including rashes; hypothyroidism; and, rarely, hepatotoxicity, bone marrow suppression, and alopecia.

Therapeutic regimen: Methimazole is given at 30–40 mg daily until the patient is euthyroid (4–12 weeks later), then the dose is progressively reduced to a maintenance level of 5–15 mg daily. Treatment is usually given for 18 months. PTU is given at 200–400 mg daily until the patient is euthyroid; then the dose is progressively reduced to a maintenance level of 50–150 mg daily. PTU is safer in pregnant women.

Anion inhibitors
Iodine, iodide, and potassium perchlorate are examples of anion inhibitors.

189

Potassium perchlorate inhibits the uptake of iodine by the thyroid (see Fig. 11.2), but it is no longer used because of the risk of aplastic anemia.

Iodide is the most rapidly acting treatment against thyrotoxicosis, and it is given in thyrotoxic crisis ("thyroid storm").

Mechanism of action: Iodine and iodide cause inhibition of conversion of T_4 to T_3, or organification, and of hormone secretion. They also reduce the size and vascularity of the gland, which is evident after 10–14 days.

Route of administration: Oral.

Indications: Thyrotoxicosis and preoperatively.

Contraindications: Iodine and iodide should not be given to breastfeeding women, as they cause goiter in infants.

Adverse effects: Iodine and iodide can cause hypersensitivity reactions, including rashes, headache, lacrimation, conjunctivitis, laryngitis, and bronchitis. With long-term treatment, depression, insomnia, and impotence can occur.

Therapeutic regimen: Iodine and iodide are given 10–14 days before partial thyroidectomy, with either carbimazole or PTU. They should not be given long term, as iodine becomes less effective.

Beta-adrenoceptor antagonists

Propranolol and atenolol are examples of β-adrenoceptor antagonists. They are used to attenuate the symptoms of increased thyroid hormone levels and the effect of increased numbers of adrenoceptors caused by thyroid hormone.

Mechanism of action: β-adrenoceptor antagonists reduce tachycardia, the BMR, nervousness, and tremor.

Route of administration: Oral.

Indications: Thyrotoxic crisis and preoperatively.

Contraindications: β-adrenoceptor antagonists should not be given to people with asthma.

Adverse effects: The side effects of β-adrenoceptor antagonists are given in Chapter 7.

Radioiodine

The use of radioactive iodine to treat hyperthyroidism is not classically considered pharmacology, although the reader should be aware of its place in the management of thyroid disorders and is advised to consult a general medical textbook.

Hypothyroidism and thyroid replacement therapy
Levothyroxine

Thyroxine is given as thyroxine sodium in maintenance therapy. It has a half-life of 6 days and a peak onset of 9 days.

Mechanism of action: Thyroxine is converted to T_3 *in vivo.*

Route of administration: Oral.

Indications: Hypothyroidism.

Contraindications: Thyroxine should not be given to people with thyrotoxicosis, and it should be used with caution in those who have cardiovascular disease.

Adverse effects: Arrhythmias, tachycardia, anginal pain, cramps, headache, restlessness, sweating, and weight loss.

Therapeutic regimen: The starting dose of thyroxine should be no greater than 100 µg daily (reduce in elderly or those with cardiovascular disease) and increased by 25–50 µg every 4 weeks until a dose of 100–200 µg is reached.

Liothyronine (l-triiodothyronine sodium)

As liothyronine is bound only slightly by thyroid-binding globulin, it has a more rapid onset of effects and a shorter duration of action than levothyroxine.

Mechanism of action: Liothyronine is rapidly metabolized *in vivo* to T_3. It has a half-life of 2–5 days and a peak onset of 1–2 days.

Route of administration: Oral, intravenous.

Indications: Liothyronine is given for severe hypothyroidism where a rapid effect is needed.

Contraindications: Liothyronine should not be given to people with cardiovascular disorders.

Adverse effects: Arrhythmias, tachycardia, anginal pain, cramps, headache, restlessness, sweating, and weight loss.

Therapeutic regimen: The dosage of liothyronine should be gradually increased as with thyroxine (20 µg liothyronine is equivalent to 100 µg thyroxine). Intravenous liothyronine is the drug of choice in the emergency treatment of myxedema (hypothyroid) coma.

Endocrine pancreas

Control of plasma glucose

Blood glucose levels are maintained at a concentration of about 5 mmol/L and usually do not exceed 8 mmol/L. A plasma glucose concentration of

2.2 mmol/L or less may result in hypoglycemic coma and death due to a lack of energy reaching the brain. A plasma glucose concentration of more than 10 mmol/L exceeds the renal threshold for glucose, which means that glucose will be present in the urine. Osmotic diuresis then occurs.

The islets of Langerhans, located in the pancreas, contain glucose receptors, and they secrete the hormones glucagon and insulin. These hormones are short-term regulators of plasma glucose levels with opposite effects. In addition, their release can be influenced by gastrointestinal hormones and autonomic nerves.

Glucose receptors are also found in the ventromedial nucleus and lateral areas of the hypothalamus. These are able to regulate appetite and feeding, and they also indirectly stimulate the release of a variety of hormones, including adrenaline, growth hormone, and cortisol, all of which affect glucose metabolism.

The hormones involved in blood glucose regulation target the liver, skeletal muscle, and adipose tissue.

Insulin

Insulin is a 51-amino-acid-residue peptide made up of an α- and a β-chain linked by disulfide bonds. It has a half-life of 3–5 minutes, and it is metabolized to a large extent by the liver (40–50%), but also by the kidneys and muscles.

In response to high blood glucose levels (as occurs after a meal), as well as to glucosamine, amino acids, fatty acids, ketone bodies, and sulfonylureas (see below), the β-cells of the endocrine pancreas secrete insulin along with a C peptide.

Insulin release is mediated by ATP-dependent potassium channels, located in the membrane of the β-cells. These close in response to elevated cytoplasmic ATP and decreased cytoplasmic ADP levels, resulting in depolarization of the membrane. This triggers calcium entry into the cell through voltage-dependent calcium channels, and subsequent insulin release (Fig. 11.6).

Insulin release is inhibited by low blood glucose levels, growth hormone, glucagon, cortisol, and sympathetic nervous system activation.

The insulin receptor consists of two α- and two β-subunits linked by disulfide bonds. Insulin binds to the extracellular α-subunits, resulting in the internalization of the receptor and its subsequent breakdown.

The β-subunits display tyrosine kinase activity upon the binding of insulin to the receptor. Autophosphorylation of the β-subunits ensues, resulting in the phosphorylation of phospholipase C with subsequent liberation of diacylglycerol (DAG) and inositol triphosphate (IP_3).

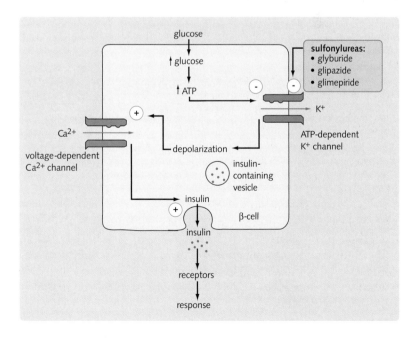

Fig. 11.6 Mechanism of insulin secretion from pancreatic β-cells.

The effects of insulin are summarized in Fig. 11.7.

Diabetes mellitus

Diabetes mellitus involves an inability to regulate plasma glucose within the normal range. It is characterized by an absolute or relative insulin deficiency, leading to hyperglycemia, glycosuria (glucose in the urine), polyuria (production of large volumes of dilute urine) associated with cellular potassium depletion, and polydipsia (intense thirst).

There are two forms of diabetes mellitus: insulin-dependent and non-insulin-dependent. The differences between the two forms are summarized in Fig. 11.8.

The long-term consequences of both types of diabetes are similar, and they include increased risk of cardiovascular and cerebrovascular events, peripheral and autonomic neuropathy, nephropathy, and retinopathy.

Insulin-dependent diabetes mellitus (type 1)

In insulin-dependent diabetes mellitus (IDDM), pancreatic β-cells are destroyed by an autoimmune T-cell attack. This leads to a complete inability to secrete insulin, and ketoacidosis is a problem. Some untreated IDDM patients have a plasma glucose concentration of up to 100 mmol/L due to insulin deficiency. In this situation, lipolysis is increased, as is the production of ketone bodies from fatty acids. This leads to ketonuria and metabolic acidosis; body fluids become hypertonic, resulting in cellular dehydration, and eventually in hyperosmolar coma.

IDDM is most often apparent at a young age.

Non-insulin–dependent diabetes mellitus (type 2)

In non-insulin–dependent diabetes mellitus (NIDDM), insulin is often secreted because on average 50% of the β-cells remain active, although there is also peripheral resistance to insulin. Unlike IDDM, this is relatively common in all populations enjoying an affluent lifestyle. The prevalence of NIDDM increases with age and the degree of obesity.

Ketosis is not a feature of NIDDM, as ketone production is suppressed by the small amounts of insulin produced by the pancreas. Hyperosmolar nonketotic coma is the NIDDM equivalent to ketoacidosis, and it can be fatal if untreated, although it responds rapidly to fluids and insulin.

Effects of insulin on fuel homeostasis	
Carbohydrates	Increase glucose transport Increase glycogen synthesis Increase glycolysis Inhibit gluconeogenesis
Fats	Increase lipoprotein lipase activity Increase fat storage in adipocytes Inhibit lipolysis (hormone-sensitive lipase) Increase hepatic lipoprotein synthesis Inhibits fatty acid oxidation
Proteins	Increase protein synthesis Increase amino acid transport

Fig. 11.7 Metabolic effects of insulin on fuel homeostasis (from Page et al., 2002).

Features of insulin-depedent and non-insulin–dependent diabetes mellitus	
Insulin-dependent diabetes mellitus (IDDM)	**Non-insulin-dependent diabetes mellitus (NIDDM)**
0.5% prevalance in adults	0.5% prevalance in adults
Juvenile onset (<30 years)	Maturity onset (>30 years)
Absoulte lack of insulin	Relative lack of, or excess, insulin
Not associated with obesity	Often associated with obesity
Insulin therapy	Oral agents (sulphonylureas) usually suffice
Ketoacidosis frequent	Ketoacidosis uncommon
Linked to the presence of islet cell antibody and genetic markers (HLA antigens)	No known autoimmune origin

Fig. 11.8 Features of insulin-dependent and non-insulin–dependent diabetes mellitus.

Secondary diabetes mellitus

Not to be confused with NIDDM, secondary diabetes mellitus accounts for less than 2% of all new cases of diabetes, and it is most commonly due to pancreatic disease (pancreatitis, carcinoma, cystic fibrosis), endocrine disease (Cushing's syndrome, acromegaly), or drug-induced (thiazide diuretics or corticosteroid therapy).

Management of diabetes mellitus
Insulin

The aim of exogenous insulin preparations is to mimic basal levels of endogenous insulin and meal-induced increases in insulin.

Insulin preparations can be human (recombinant), porcine, or bovine in origin, and they are available as short-, intermediate-, and long-acting preparations (Fig. 11.9).

Short-acting insulins are soluble. These preparations most resemble endogenous insulin, and they can be given intravenously in the hospital. The rapid-acting insulins aspart and lispro have recently been introduced, which have a faster onset and shorter duration of action than the traditional short-acting insulin.

Intermediate- and long-acting insulins are not as soluble as the short-acting preparations. Their solubility is decreased by precipitating the insulin with zinc or protamine (a basic protein), which prolongs their release into the bloodstream.

The intermediate- and long-acting preparations include:
- Isophane (NPH) insulin.
- Lente insulin.
- Insulin zinc suspension (ultralente).
- Insulin glargine.

Mechanism of action: Insulin preparations mimic endogenous insulin.

Route of administration: Insulin must always be given parenterally (intravenously, intramuscularly, or subcutaneously), as it is a peptide and, therefore, destroyed in the gastrointestinal tract. Short-acting insulin is given intravenously in emergencies, but administration of the insulin preparations in maintenance treatment is usually subcutaneous.

Indications: IDDM and NIDDM uncontrolled by other means.

Adverse effects: Local reactions and, in overdose, hypoglycemia. Protamine can cause allergic reactions. Rarely, there may be immune resistance.

Therapeutic regimen: The following regimens are recommended, according to the patient:
- Short-acting insulin 3 times daily (before breakfast, lunch, and dinner) and intermediate-acting insulin at bedtime.
- Short-acting insulin and intermediate-acting insulin mixture twice daily before meals.
- Short-acting insulin and intermediate-acting insulin mixture before breakfast, short-acting insulin before dinner, and intermediate-acting insulin before bedtime.
- Short-acting insulin and intermediate-acting insulin mixture before breakfast is adequate for some NIDDM patients needing insulin.

Therapeutic notes: Preparations are now available that contain mixtures of short- and intermediate- and long-acting insulins, allowing patients to inject themselves only once each time they administer their insulin.

Oral hypoglycemics

The oral hypoglycemics are administered orally, and, like insulin, they act to lower plasma glucose. The sulfonylureas and the biguanides are the main drugs used from this class, but newer drugs are also now available.

Insulin preparations (subcutaneous)			
Insulin preparation	Action	Peak activity (h)	Duration (h)
Rapid-acting insulin	Very rapid	0–2	3–4
Short-acting insulin	Rapid	1–3	3–7
Isophane insulin	Intermediate	2–12	12–22
Insulin zinc suspension	Prolonged	4–24	24–28

Fig. 11.9 Insulin preparations.

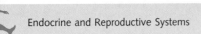

Sulfonylureas

Glyburide, glipizide, and glimepiride are examples of currently prescribed sulfonylureas.

Mechanism of action: Sulfonylureas block ATP-dependent potassium channels in the membrane of the pancreatic β-cells, causing depolarization, calcium influx, and insulin release.

Route of administration: Oral.

Indications: Sulfonylureas are given for diabetes mellitus, in patients with residual β-cell activity.

Contraindications: Breastfeeding women or people with ketoacidosis. Long-acting sulfonylureas (chlorpropamide) should be avoided in the elderly and in those with renal and hepatic insufficiency, as these drugs can induce hypoglycemia.

Adverse effects: Weight gain; sensitivity reactions, including rashes; gastrointestinal disturbances; headache; and hypoglycemia.

Therapeutic regimen: Glyburide is given at 5–20 mg/day (once or in divided doses); glipizide is given at 10–20 mg/day (once or in divided doses); and glimepiride is given at 1–4 mg once daily.

Biguanides

Metformin is the only drug in this class.

Mechanism of action: Metformin increases the peripheral utilization of glucose by increasing uptake and decreasing gluconeogenesis. To work, metformin requires the presence of endogenous insulin; therefore, patients must have some functioning β-cells.

Route of administration: Oral.

Indications: NIDDM where dieting and sulfonylureas have proved ineffective.

Contraindications: Metformin should not be given to patients with hepatic or renal impairment (owing to the risk of lactic acidosis) or heart failure.

Adverse effects: Anorexia, headache, nausea and vomiting, diarrhea, lactic acidosis, and decreased vitamin B$_{12}$ absorption.

Therapeutic regimen: Metformin is given at 500 mg two or three times daily. It can be used alone or with sulfonylureas. Metformin should be taken with or after food.

Other antidiabetics
Alpha-glucosidase inhibitors

Acarbose and miglitol are the available drugs in this class.

Mechanism of action: These drugs act to inhibit intestinal α-glucosidases and delay the absorption of starch and sucrose.

Route of administration: Oral.

Indications: Diabetes mellitus inadequately controlled by diet alone or in combination with other oral hypoglycemics.

Contraindications: Pregnancy, breastfeeding, bowel disease.

Adverse effects: Flatulence, diarrhea.

Therapeutic notes: Like metformin, these drugs are particularly useful in the obese diabetic patient.

Thiazolidinediones

Rosiglitazone and pioglitazone belong to the thiazolidinediones.

Mechanism of action: These agents are believed to reduce peripheral insulin resistance, leading to a reduction in plasma glucose.

Route of administration: Oral.

Indications: Uncontrolled NIDDM.

Contraindications: Hepatic impairment, history of heart failure.

Adverse effects: Gastrointestinal disturbance, fluid retention, weight gain. Potentially, liver failure.

Therapeutic notes: The thiazolidinediones should be prescribed only by a physician experienced in treating NIDDM, and they are currently licensed only for use in combination with either a sulfonylurea or metformin.

Diet and fluid replacement
Dietary control

Dietary control is important for both IDDM and NIDDM.

The diet should aim to derive its energy from the following constituents, in the following amounts:

- 50% carbohydrate (slowly absorbed forms).
- 35% fat.
- 15% protein.

This regimen aims to reduce total fat intake, increase protein intake, and increase the intake of high fiber foods, which slow the rate of absorption from the gut.

Simple sugars, as found in sweet drinks and cakes, should be avoided.

Meals should be small and regular, thus avoiding large swings in blood glucose levels.

Rehydration therapy

In the acute diabetic patient, the fluid deficit can be as high as 7–8 L. Rehydration therapy is essential in order to regain fluid and electrolyte balance, and this takes precedence over the administration of insulin.

The management of the acute diabetic patient is essential to know. Not only is this a very common exam question, you will also encounter it on the wards.

Untreated diabetic patients suffer from hyperkalemia, as potassium requires insulin to enter cells. As soon as insulin is administered, however, potassium follows glucose into cells, and hypokalemia becomes the danger. The rehydration fluid should, therefore, contain potassium, and plasma potassium concentration should be measured hourly.

Diabetic patients are also at risk of metabolic acidosis due to excessive ketone production. If the acidosis is severe (pH < 7.0), bicarbonate can be administered intravenously, although evidence to support this is weak.

Hypoglycemia

Hypoglycemia is an uncommon presentation in the untreated diabetic patient, although very common in those taking insulin and sulfonylureas.

The symptoms of hypoglycemia are driven by the sympathetic nervous system and include:

- Sweating.
- Tremor.
- Anxiety.
- Altered consciousness.

The history may reveal that the patient has not eaten as scheduled, has not exercised, or has taken too much insulin.

Management depends upon the consciousness of the patient. If the patient is alert, glucose can be given orally as a syrup or as simple sugar. If consciousness is altered, oral administration of glucose is dangerous, and there is a risk of the patient aspirating. In this situation, glucose should be administered intravenously, or glucagon can be given by intramuscular or intravenous injection.

Glucose (dextrose monohydrate)

Glucose is administered parenterally as dextrose monohydrate.

Mechanism of action: Dextrose mimics endogenous glucose, and it is utilized by cells.

Route of administration: Intravenous.

Indications: Hypoglycemia, as part of rehydration therapy.

Contraindications: Hyperglycemia.

Adverse effects: Venous irritation and thrombophlebitis. Hypokalemia may occur.

Therapeutic notes: Glucose is also available in numerous oral preparations, although the patient must be alert and conscious before these are administered, as aspiration can occur.

Glucagon

Glucagon is a polypeptide hormone, normally secreted by the pancreatic α-cells.

Mechanism of action: Glucagon acts on the liver to convert glycogen to glucose and to synthesize glucose from noncarbohydrate precursors (gluconeogenesis). The overall effect is to raise plasma glucose levels.

Route of administration: Parenteral.

Indications: Insulin-induced hypoglycemia.

Contraindications: Pheochromocytoma.

Adverse effects: Nausea, vomiting, diarrhea, and hypokalemia.

Therapeutic notes: Unlike intravenous glucose, glucagon can be administered easily by nonmedical personnel, and it can be carried by the patient as a prefilled syringe-pen.

 In an acute hyperglycemic attack, it is essential that fluids and soluble insulin be given intravenously to rehydrate the patient rapidly and decrease blood sugar levels.

Adrenal cortex

The adrenal cortex secretes several steroid hormones into the bloodstream. These are categorized by their actions into two main classes—mineralocorticoids and glucocorticoids.

Of the mineralocorticoids, aldosterone is the main endogenous hormone, synthesized in the zona glomerulosa. It affects water and electrolyte balance, and it possesses salt-retaining activity.

Of the glucocorticoids, hydrocortisone (cortisol) and cortisone are the main endogenous hormones, synthesized in the zona fasciculata and zona reticularis. These affect carbohydrate, fat, and protein metabolism, and they suppress inflammatory and immune responses. Cortisol and cortisone also possess some mineralocorticoid activity.

Small quantities of some sex steroids, mainly androgens, are also produced by the adrenal cortex.

Adrenal corticosteroids
Synthesis and release
Adrenal corticosteroids are not preformed; they are synthesized when required from cholesterol.

Glucocorticoids
The release of cortisol is controlled by negative feedback upon the hypothalamic–pituitary–adrenal axis (Fig. 11.10). There is a diurnal pattern of activity with an early morning peak in cortisol release.

A variety of sensorineural inputs regulate the release of corticotrophin-releasing factor (CRF) in the hypothalamus; examples include physiologic and psychological "stress," injury, and infection.

CRF, a 41-amino-acid-residue polypeptide, reaches the anterior pituitary in the hypothalamo-hypophysial portal system, where it stimulates the release of adrenocorticotropic hormone (ACTH).

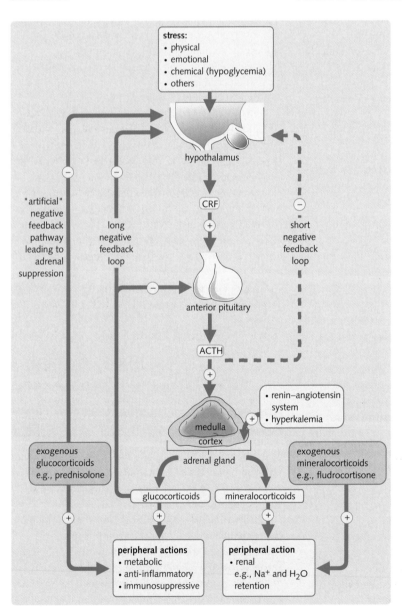

Fig. 11.10 Hypothalamic–pituitary–adrenal axis; control of adrenal corticosteroid synthesis and secretion (ACTH, adrenocorticotropin hormone; CRF, corticotropin-releasing factor).

ACTH is formed from a larger molecule, pro-opiomelanocortin, and it is released into the circulation, where it stimulates the synthesis and release of cortisol from the adrenal cortex.

Natural and artificial glucocorticoids circulating in the blood exert a negative feedback effect on the production of both CRH and ACTH.

Mineralocorticoids

Aldosterone release is also partially controlled by ACTH, but other factors, especially the renin–angiotensin system (RAS) and plasma potassium levels, are more important.

Mechanism of action of corticosteroids

Endogenous and synthetic corticosteroids act in a similar way (Fig. 11.11). The hormone or drug circulates to peripheral tissues, where it enters cells (steroids are lipid-soluble) and binds to cytosolic corticosteroid receptors (CR). After hormone binding, these receptors are translocated to the nucleus, where they interact with DNA, leading to the transcription of corticosteroid-responsive genes (CRGs).

The products of these CRGs lead to diverse effects on the target tissues (Fig. 11.12). The actions of corticosteroids are divided into effects on inorganic metabolism (mineralocorticoid effects) and effects on organic metabolism (glucocorticoid effects).

Therapeutic use of corticosteroids

Corticosteroids have wide-ranging and powerful effects on human physiology. There are two main areas where these properties are taken advantage of in the therapeutic use of corticosteroids—physiologic replacement therapy of corticosteroid deficiency, and anti-inflammatory therapy and immunosuppression (Chapters 4 and 11).

Exogenous corticosteroids

Both naturally occurring and a number of synthetic corticosteroids are available for clinical use. These vary in their potency, half-life, and the balance between glucocorticoid versus mineralocorticoid activity (Fig. 11.13).

Mechanism of action: Exogenous corticosteroids imitate endogenous corticosteroids.

Indications: The therapeutic use of corticosteroids falls into the two main categories of physiological replacement therapy, and anti-inflammatory therapy and immunosuppression.

Corticosteroid replacement therapy is necessary when endogenous hormones are deficient, as happens in:

- Primary adrenocortical destruction (Addison's disease).
- Secondary adrenocortical failure due to deficient ACTH from the pituitary or after adrenalectomy.
- Suppression of the hypothalamic–pituitary–adrenal axis due to prolonged glucocorticoid therapy.

As all the actions of natural corticosteroids are required, a glucocorticoid with mineralocorticoid activity (cortisol) or separate glucocorticoid and mineralocorticoid are given.

The anti-inflammatory and immunosuppressive effects of glucocorticoids are used to treat a wide variety of conditions (Fig. 11.14). In these cases, synthetic glucocorticoids with little mineralocorticoid activity are used (Chapters 4 and 11).

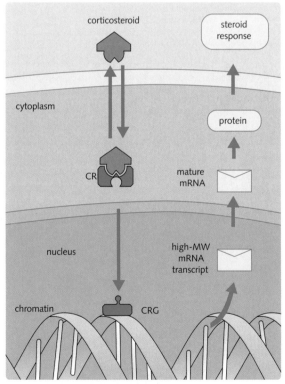

Fig. 11.11 Mechanism of action of corticosteroids at the cellular level (CR, corticosteroid receptor; CRG, corticosteroid response gene; MW, molecular weight). (Redrawn from Page et al., 2002.)

Major effects of the corticosteroids	
Glucocorticoids	
Immunological	• Decreased production of T and B lymphocytes and macrophages, involution of lymphoid tissue • Decreased function of T and B lymphocytes, and reduced responsiveness to cytokines • Inhibition of complement system
Anti-inflammatory	• Profound generalized inhibitory effects on inflammatory response • Reduced production of acute inflammatory mediators, especially the eicosanoids (prostaglandins, leukotrienes, etc.), owing to production of lipocortin, an enzyme that inhibits phospholipase A_2, thus blocking the formation of arachidonic acid and its metabolites-see Chapter 4 • Reduced numbers and activity of circulating immunocompetent cells, neutrophils, and macrophages • Decreased activity of macrophages and fibroblasts involved in the chronic stages of inflammation, leading to decreased inflammation and decreased healing
Carbohydrate metabolism	• Increased gluconeogenesis, decreased cellular uptake and utilization of glucose, increased storage of glycogen in the liver (hyperglycemic actions)
Fat metabolism	• Redistribution of lipid from steroid-sensitive stores (limbs) to steroid-resistant stores (face, neck, trunk)
Protein metabolosm	• Increased catabolism, decresed anabolism, leading to protein degradation
Cardiovascular	• Increased sensitivity of vascular system to catecholamines, reduced capillary permeability leading to raised blood pressure
Central nervous system	• High levels can cause mood changes (euphoria/depression) or psychotic states, perhaps due to electrolyte changes
Anterior hypothalamus and pituitary	• Negative feedback effect of CRF and ACTH with the result that endogenous secretion of glucocorticoids is reduced and may remain so after prolonged glucocorticoid therapy ("adrenal suppresssion")
Mineralocorticoids	
Kidney	• Increases permeability of the apical membrane of cells in the distal renal tubule to sodium • Stimulates the Na^+/K^+ ATPase pump leading to reabsorption of Na^+ and loss of K^+ in the urine • Water is passively reabsorbed owing to sodium retention; thus extracellular fluid and blood volume are increased (raising blood pressure).

Fig. 11.12 Major effects of corticosteroids (ACTH, adrenocorticotropin hormone; CRF, corticotropin-releasing factor).

Contraindications: Exogenous corticosteroids should not be given to people with systemic infection, unless specific antimicrobial therapy is being given.

Route of administration: Replacement therapy is given orally twice a day at physiologic doses to try to mimic, as closely as possible, the level and rhythm of natural corticosteroid secretion.

When used to suppress inflammatory and immune responses, corticosteroids may be given orally or intravenously, but, depending on the condition, the topical administration of glucocorticoids is preferred, if feasible, as it can deliver high concentrations to the target site while minimizing systemic absorption and adverse effects (see Fig. 11.14).

At high doses, even topically administered glucocorticoids can achieve systemic penetration.

Adverse effects: Overdosage or prolonged use of corticosteroids may exaggerate some of their normal physiological actions (see earlier), leading to mineralocorticoid and glucocorticoid side effects. Many of these effects are similar to those seen in Cushing's syndrome, a condition caused by excess secretion of endogenous corticosteroids (Fig. 11.15).

The metabolic side effects of glucocorticoids include:

- Central obesity and a "moon" face, as fat is redistributed.
- Hyperglycemia, which may lead to clinical diabetes mellitus, due to disturbed carbohydrate metabolism.
- Osteoporosis, due to catabolism of protein matrix in bone.
- Loss of skin structure, with purple striae and easy bruising, due to altered protein metabolism.

- Muscle weakness and wasting, due to protein catabolism.
- Suppression of growth in children.

Corticosteroid therapy suppresses endogenous secretion of adrenal hormones via negative feedback on the hypothalamic–pituitary–adrenal axis.

Adrenal atrophy can persist for years after withdrawal from prolonged corticosteroid therapy. Replacement corticosteroid therapy is needed to compensate for the lack of sufficient adrenocortical response in times of stress (e.g., illness, surgery).

Steroid therapy must be withdrawn slowly after long-term treatment, as sudden withdrawal can lead to an acute adrenal insufficiency crisis.

With glucocorticoid therapy, the modification of inflammatory and immune reactions leads to an increased susceptibility to infections. This can progress unnoticed because of the suppression of normal indicators of infection, such as inflammation.

Increased susceptibility occurs to normally pathogenic and opportunistic bacterial, viral, and fungal organisms. Reactivation of latent infections (e.g., tuberculosis, herpes viruses) can occur.

The effects are most serious when corticosteroids are being used systemically, although topical use can exacerbate superficial skin infections, and inhaled corticosteroids can encourage oropharyngeal thrush, etc.

The other effects of glucocorticoids include mood change (euphoria and, rarely, psychosis), peptic ulceration due to inhibition of gastrointestinal

Corticosteroids used therapeutically		
Glucocorticoids		Mineralocorticoids
"Natural hormones"	Synthetic	Synthetic
Hydrocortisone (cortisol)	Prednisolone Betamethasone Dexamethasone Beclometasone Triamcinolone	Fludrocortisone

Fig. 11.13 Examples of therapeutically used corticosteroids.

Conditions in which corticosteroids are used for their anti-inflammatory and immunosuppressive effects		
Systemic uses	Topical uses	
Acute inflammatory conditions (e.g., anaphylaxis, status asthmaticus, fibrosing alveolitis, angionecrotic edema)	Asthma	Aerosol
Chronic inglammatory conditions (e.g., rheumatoid arthritis, inflammatory bowel disease, systemic lupus erythematosus, glomerulonephritis)	Allergic rhinitis	Nasal spray
Neoplastic disease myelomas, lymphomas, lymphatic leukemias	Eczema	Ointment or cream
Miscellaneous organ transplantation	Inflammatory bowel disease	Foam enema

Fig. 11.14 Examples of conditions in which corticosteroids are used for their anti-inflammatory and immunosuppressive effects.

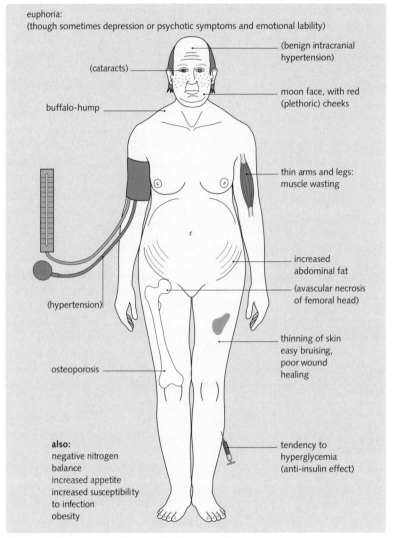

euphoria:
(though sometimes depression or psychotic symptoms and emotional lability)

(benign intracranial hypertension)

(cataracts)

moon face, with red (plethoric) cheeks

buffalo-hump

thin arms and legs: muscle wasting

increased abdominal fat

(avascular necrosis of femoral head)

(hypertension)

thinning of skin easy bruising, poor wound healing

osteoporosis

also:
negative nitrogen balance
increased appetite
increased susceptibility to infection
obesity

tendency to hyperglycemia (anti-insulin effect)

Fig. 11.15 Effects of prolonged corticosteroid use—the Cushingoid appearance.

prostaglandin synthesis, and eye problems such as cataracts and exacerbation of glaucoma.

Fluid retention, hypokalemia, and hypertension can all be side effects of any corticosteroids that possess significant mineralocorticoid activity.

Therapeutic notes on specific steroid agents
Glucocorticoids
Hydrocortisone (cortisol):
- Is administered orally for adrenal replacement therapy, and possesses mineralocorticoid activity.
- Is administered intravenously in status asthmaticus and anaphylactic shock.
- Is applied topically for eczema, inflammatory bowel conditions, etc.

Prednisolone:
- Is predominantly glucocorticoid in activity.
- Is the oral drug most widely used in allergic and inflammatory diseases.

Methylprednisolone:
- Is derived from prednisolone, with high glucocorticoid activity.
- Is administered orally, and indicated in inflammatory and allergic disorders.

Betamethasone and dexamethasone:
- Have very high glucocorticoid activity with insignificant mineralocorticoid activity.
- Are very potent drugs used orally and by injection to suppress inflammatory and allergic disorders

and to reduce cerebral edema. They do not possess salt- or water-retaining actions.

Beclomethasone:
- Is the dipropionate ester of betamethasone.
- Is a very potent drug with no mineralocorticoid activity that is useful topically, as it is poorly absorbed through membranes and skin.
- Is used as an aerosol in asthma, and as a cream and ointment in eczema to provide high local anti-inflammatory effects with minimal systemic penetration.

Triamcinolone:
- Is a moderately potent drug used in severe asthma.
- Is also administered by intra-articular injection for rheumatoid arthritis.

Mineralocorticoids
Fludrocortisone:
- Has such high mineralocorticoid activity that glucocorticoid activity is insignificant.
- Is administered orally, in combination with a glucocorticoid, in replacement therapy.

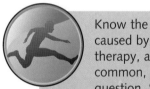

Know the adverse effects caused by corticosteroid therapy, as they are numerous, common, and a popular exam question. Some of the adverse effects caused by corticosteroids are logical exaggerations of their normal physiologic actions; others are more unexpected and must, therefore, be learned individually.

Reproductive system

Hormonal control of the reproductive system
Physiology of the female reproductive tract
The female gonads, or ovaries, are responsible for oogenesis and the secretion of the steroid sex hormones, namely estrogens (mainly estradiol) and progesterone.

The production of the female sex hormones is controlled by the hypothalamic–pituitary–ovarian axis (Fig. 11.16).

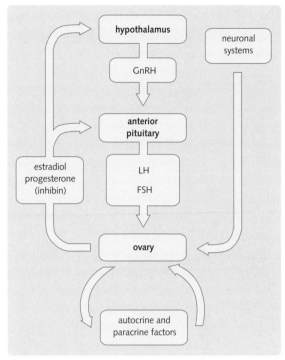

Fig. 11.16 Hypothalamic–pituitary–ovarian axis (GnRH, gonadotrophin-releasing hormone; LH, luteinizing hormone; FSH, follicle-stimulating hormone). (Redrawn from Page et al., 2002.)

Gonadotropin-releasing hormone (GnRH) is secreted by the hypothalamus and stimulates the pulsatile secretion of the gonadotropins, follicle-stimulating hormone (FSH), and luteinizing hormone (LH) by the anterior pituitary. In turn, these act upon the ovaries to stimulate the release of estradiol, progesterone, and other ovarian hormones.

The ovarian hormones are able to exert a negative feedback on the hypothalamus and/or the pituitary. Some of these are selective in their inhibition; for example, inhibin selectively inhibits FSH release from the pituitary; activin selectively stimulates FSH release from the pituitary, and gonadotrophin-surge-attenuating factor selectively inhibits LH secretion from the pituitary.

Menstrual cycle
The menstrual cycle is divided into a follicular phase (days 1–14) and a luteal phase (days 14–28).
The cycle proceeds as follows (numbers refer to Fig. 11.17):
1. Day 1 is the first day of menstruation, which involves the shedding of the uterine

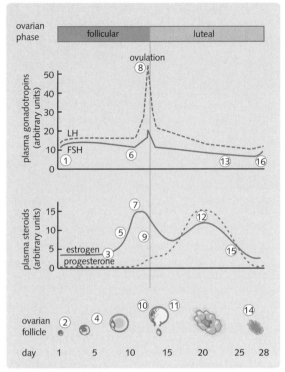

Fig. 11.17 The menstrual cycle (see text for details of numbered stages) (FSH, follicle-stimulating hormone; LH, luteinizing hormone).

8. An LH surge occurs. This results in a decrease in estrogen secretion, an increase in progesterone secretion by the granulosa cells, and the resumption of meiosis in the egg.
9. Estrogen levels decline after ovulation.
10. The first meiotic division is completed.
11. On day 14, ovulation, the release of the ovum occurs. This is approximately 18 hours after the LH surge.
12. The granulosa cells are transformed into the corpus luteum, which secretes both estrogen and progesterone in large quantities.
13. There is a rise in the levels of estrogen and progesterone. As a result, FSH and LH secretion is suppressed, and their levels fall.
14. If fertilization does not take place, the corpus luteum degenerates after about 10 days.
15. Estrogen and progesterone levels fall; menstruation is imminent.
16. FSH and LH secretion increase once more, and the 28-day cycle begins again.

Physiology of the male reproductive tract

The male gonads, or testes, are responsible for spermatogenesis and the secretion of the steroid sex hormone testosterone.

Spermatogenesis takes place in the lumen of the seminiferous tubules of the testis.

The production of the male sex hormones is controlled by the hypothalamic–pituitary axis (Fig. 11.18).

The Sertoli cells are connected to one another by tight junctions, and they extend from the basement membrane of the seminiferous tubules into the lumen. Under the influence of FSH, these synthesize testosterone receptors and inhibin.

The Leydig cells are found in the connective tissue between the tubules. Under the influence of LH, these synthesize testosterone. Testosterone acts locally to increase sperm production, and also peripherally on the testosterone-sensitive tissues of the body.

Testosterone and inhibin are able to exert negative feedback control over the anterior pituitary, the former decreasing LH secretion and the latter decreasing FSH secretion. In addition, testosterone and inhibin act on the hypothalamus to decrease GnRH secretion.

endometrium. Plasma estrogen levels are low; therefore, little negative feedback occurs. As a result, the secretion of LH and FSH begins to increase.
2. Ten to twenty-five preantral follicles start to enlarge and secrete estrogen.
3. FSH stimulates the granulosa cells to secrete estrogen, the levels of which rise.
4. About 1 week into the cycle, one of the follicles becomes dominant, and the others undergo atresia. The dominant follicle secretes increasingly larger amounts of estrogen.
5. Plasma estrogen levels rise significantly as a result of increased sensitivity of the granulosa cells to FSH.
6. Elevated estrogen levels provide negative feedback, and FSH secretion decreases.
7. Plasma estrogen levels are now so high (> 200 pg/mL) that they exert a positive feedback on gonadotropin secretion. This occurs for about 2 days, during which FSH stimulates the appearance of LH receptors on the granulosa cells.

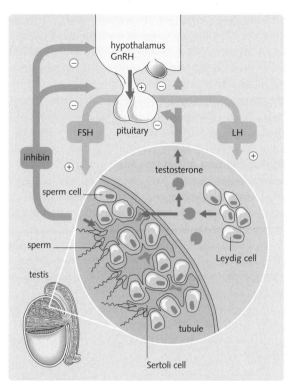

Fig. 11.18 Hormonal control of Sertoli, Leydig, and sperm cell function (FSH, follicle-stimulating hormone; GnRH, gonadotrophin-releasing hormone; LH, luteinizing hormone). (Redrawn from Page et al., 2002.)

Drugs that affect the reproductive system

Oral contraceptive drugs (OCDs)

Combined oral contraceptive pill

The combined oral contraceptive pill (COCP) contains both an estrogen (usually ethinylestradiol, 20–50 μg) and a progestogen (an analog of progesterone).

COCPs provide a highly effective form of contraception. Their efficacy is reduced by some broad-spectrum antibiotics, which reduce enterohepatic recirculation of estrogen by killing gut flora.

Mechanism of action: The levels of steroids mimic the luteal phase of the menstrual cycle and suppress, via negative feedback effects, the secretion of gonadotropins. As a result, follicular selection and maturation, the estrogen surge, the LH surge, and consequently ovulation, do not take place.

Route of administration: Oral.

Indications: Contraception and menstrual symptoms.

Contraindications: Pregnancy, breastfeeding, or a history of heart disease or hypertension, hyperlipidemia or any prothrombotic coagulation abnormality, diabetes mellitus, migraine, breast or genital tract carcinoma, or liver disease.

Adverse effects: Nausea, vomiting and headache, weight gain, breast tenderness, impaired liver function, impaired glucose tolerance in diabetic women, "spotting" (slight bleeding at the start of the menstrual cycle), thrombosis and hypertension, a slightly increased risk of cervical cancer, and possibly an increased risk of breast cancer.

Therapeutic regimen: COCPs are taken for 21 days (starting on the first day of the menstrual cycle) at about the same time each day, with a 7-day break to induce a withdrawal bleed. If the delay in taking the pill is greater than 12 hours, the contraceptive effect may be lost.

Progesterone-only pill (minipill)

The minipill consists of low-dose progestogen; ovulation still takes place, and menstruation is normal. The minipill is not as effective as the COCP.

Mechanism of action: The minipill causes thickening of cervical mucus, thus preventing sperm penetration. It also causes suppression of gonadotropin secretion and occasionally ovulation, but the latter effect does not occur in the majority of women.

Route of administration: Oral.

Indications: Contraception. It is more suitable for heavy smokers and patients with hypertension or heart disease, diabetes mellitus, and migraine, or patients who have other contraindications for estrogen therapy.

Contraindications: Pregnancy, arterial disease, liver disease, or breast or genital tract carcinoma.

Adverse effects: Menstrual irregularities, nausea, vomiting and headache, weight gain, and breast tenderness.

Therapeutic regimen: The minipill is taken as one tablet daily, at the same time, starting on day 1 of the menstrual cycle and then continuously. If the delay in taking the pill is greater than 3 hours, the contraceptive effect may be lost.

Other contraceptive regimens

Depo-progesterone

Examples of depo-progesterone drugs include medroxyprogesterone acetate and the

Many female patients forget to mention the oral contraceptive pill when they list their medications, so be sure to ask specifically because of the numerous important drug interactions to consider.

norgestrel-releasing implant. These provide contraception that is long term.

Mechanism of action: Depo-progesterone causes thickening of cervical mucus. It also causes suppression of gonadotropin secretion and occasionally ovulation, but the latter effect does not occur in the majority of women.

Route of administration: Medroxyprogesterone acetate is administered intramuscularly. The norgestrel-releasing implant system relies on a hormone rod placed subdermally.

Indications: Contraception.

Contraindications: Pregnancy, arterial disease, liver disease, or breast or genital tract carcinoma.

Adverse effects: Menstrual irregularities, nausea, vomiting and headache, weight gain, and breast tenderness.

Therapeutic notes: Medroxyprogesterone acetate provides protection for about 12 weeks. The norgestrel-implant system provides protection for 3 years.

Postcoital ("morning-after") pill

The postcoital or "morning-after" pill provides a form of emergency contraception.

Mechanism of action: High doses of a progestin alone or a progestogen with an estrogen prevent implantation of the fertilized egg. This is 75% effective. Contractions of the smooth muscle are induced, and these accelerate the movement of the fertilized egg into the unprepared uterine endometrium.

Route of administration: Oral.

Indications: The morning-after pill is used for emergency contraception after unprotected intercourse.

Contraindications: Preparations containing estrogens should not be used in patients who have contraindications to estrogens (see above).

Adverse effects: Nausea and vomiting, headache, dizziness, and menstrual irregularities.

Therapeutic regimen: The morning-after pill regimen depends upon the type of pill being taken, but commonly it consist of one or two tablets within 72 hours of intercourse and one or two subsequent tablets 12 hours later.

Possible contraceptives for males

Male contraceptive drugs remain purely experimental.

Estrogens and antiestrogens
Estrogen agonists

The adverse symptoms of the menopause can be attributed to decreased levels of estrogen that occur as the ovaries being to fail.

Evidence suggests that estrogen given in low doses to menopausal women will reduce postmenopausal osteoporosis, vaginal atrophy, and the incidence of stroke and myocardial infarction.

A progestogen is coadministered with estrogen in order to inhibit estrogen-stimulated endometrial growth and thus reduce the risk of uterine cancer and fibroids.

Examples of estrogen agonists include estradiol and estriol.

Mechanism of action: Estrogen agonists mimic premenopausal endogenous estrogen levels.

Route of administration: Oral or by transdermal patches, gels, or subcutaneous implants.

Indications: Estrogen agonists are used alone for hormone replacement therapy (HRT) in menopausal women who have undergone a hysterectomy and in conjunction with a progestin if the patient has a uterus.

Contraindications: Pregnancy, estrogen-dependent cancer, active or previous thromboembolic disease.

Adverse effects: Increased risk of endometrial cancer and, possibly, an increased risk of breast cancer after many years of treatment.

Therapeutic regimen: Estrogen agonists are given for several years, starting in the perimenopausal period.

Estrogen antagonists

Examples of estrogen antagonists include tamoxifen, clomiphene, and toremifene.

Mechanism of action: Antiestrogens act at estrogen receptors in estrogen-sensitive tissues, such as the breast, bone, and endometrium, and also give feedback to the pituitary, antagonizing endogenous estrogen.

Route of administration: Tamoxifen is administered orally or by intravenous or subcutaneous injection, while clomiphene is administered orally.

Indications: Estrogen antagonists are used to treat female infertility and breast cancer.

Contraindications: Hepatic disease, ovarian cysts, or endometrial carcinoma.

Adverse effects: Multiple pregnancies and hot flushes. Withdrawal causes visual disturbances and ovarian hyperstimulation.

Progestins and antiprogestins
Progestogen agonists
Examples of progestin agonists include progesterone, medroxyprogesterone, dimethyl Histerone, hydroxyprogesterone, and norethindrone.

Mechanism of action: Progestin agonists mimic endogenous progesterone.

Route of administration: Oral or by transdermal patches, gels, or subcutaneous implants.

Indications: Progestin agonists are given for premenstrual symptoms, severe dysmenorrhea, menorrhagia, endometriosis, contraception, and as part of HRT.

Contraindications: Pregnancy or women with arterial disease, liver disease, or breast or genitaltract carcinoma.

Adverse effects: Menstrual irregularities, nausea and vomiting, headache, weight gain, and breast tenderness.

Progestin antagonists
Mifepristone is an example of a progestin antagonist.

Mechanism of action: Progestin antagonists bind to progesterone receptors, but they exert no effect. They sensitize the uterus to prostaglandins; therefore, they can be used in combination with prostaglandins in the termination of early pregnancy.

Route of administration: Oral.

Indications: Progestin antagonists are used in the termination of pregnancy.

Contraindications: Progestin antagonists should not be given to pregnant women (64 days' gestation or more), to women with adrenal failure or hemorrhagic disorders, to women on anticoagulant or long-term corticosteroid treatment, or to smokers aged 35 years and over.

Adverse effects: Vaginal bleeding, faintness, and nausea and vomiting.

Androgens and antiandrogens
Androgen agonists
Testosterone and methyltestosterone are examples of androgen agonists.

Mechanism of action: Androgen agonists mimic endogenous androgens.

Route of administration: Orally, intramuscularly, or by implant or cutaneous patch.

Indications: Androgen agonists are given as androgen-replacement therapy in castrated men, for pituitary or testicular disease causing hypogonadism, and for breast cancer.

Contraindications: Androgen agonists should not be given to men with breast or prostate cancer, to people with hypercalcemia, or to women who are pregnant or breastfeeding.

Adverse effects: Sodium retention causing edema, hypercalcemia, suppression of spermatogenesis, virilism in women, and premature closure of epiphyses in prepubertal boys. The incidence of prostate abnormalities and prostate cancer is also increased.

Androgen antagonists
Cyproterone is an androgen antagonist that is a progesterone derivative. Both estrogens and progestins have antiandrogenic properties.

Mechanism of action: Androgen antagonists are partial agonists at androgen receptors, and they act on the hypothalamus to reduce the synthesis of gonadotropins. They inhibit spermatogenesis, causing reversible infertility, but they are not contraceptives.

Route of administration: Oral.

Indications: Androgen antagonists are used for male hypersexuality and sexual deviation, prostate cancer, acne, female hirsutism, and precocious puberty.

Contraindications: Androgen antagonists should not be given to people with hepatic disease or severe diabetes or to those aged 18 and under, as their bones are not fully matured.

Adverse effects: Fatigue and lethargy, and hepatotoxicity.

Therapeutic notes: Finasteride is technically an antiandrogen, although it inhibits the enzyme 5α-reductase, which metabolizes testosterone, to the more potent androgen dihydrotestosterone. Finasteride is indicated in benign prostatic hyperplasia and is administered orally.

Flutamide, bicalutamide, and nilutamide are androgen-receptor antagonists used to treat prostate cancer.

Like breast cancer in women, prostate cancer in men is most often hormone dependent. Exogenous androgens can promote and antiandrogens suppress tumor growth.

Anabolic steroids

Nandrolone and stanozolol are examples of anabolic steroids.

Mechanism of action: Anabolic steroids are androgenic; they stimulate protein synthesis and promote wound and fracture healing.

Route of administration: Nandrolone is administered by deep intramuscular injection, and stanozolol is given orally.

Indications: Anabolic steroids can be used for osteoporosis in postmenopausal women, aplastic anemias, and chronic biliary obstruction.

Contraindications: Hepatic impairment, men with prostate or breast cancer, or pregnant women.

Adverse effects: Acne, sodium retention causing edema, virilization in women, amenorrhea, inhibition of spermatogenesis, and liver tumors.

Gonadotropin-releasing hormone agonists and antagonists

Agonists

Goserelin, leuprolide, and nafarelin are examples of GnRH agonists.

Mechanism of action: GnRH agonists are given intermittently and mimic endogenous GnRH. Continuous use desensitizes the GnRH receptors on the gonadotrophs and inhibits gonadotropin synthesis.

Route of administration: Nafarelin is administered intranasally; goserelin and leuprolide are administered by subcutaneous injection.

Indications: GnRH agonists are used for ovulation induction in those with GnRH deficiency as well as for endometriosis, precocious puberty, sex-hormone–dependent cancers, and prostate cancer.

Adverse effects: Menopause-like symptoms, including hot flushes, palpitations, decreased libido due to hypoestrogenism, and breakthrough bleeding.

Therapeutic regimen: Pulsatile administration of GnRH agonists is every 90 minutes for a few minutes. The treatment must not exceed 6 months, and it should not be repeated.

Antagonists

Danazol and mifepristone can suppress GnRH actions.

Mechanism of action: These drugs inhibit the release of GnRH and the gonadotropins. They bind to the sex-steroid receptors, displaying androgenic, antiestrogenic, and antiprogestin effects.

Route of administration: Oral.

Indications: GnRH antagonists are given for endometriosis, menstrual disorders (including menorrhagia), cystic breast disease, and gynecomastia.

Contraindications: Pregnancy; hepatic, renal, or cardiac impairment; or vascular disease.

Adverse effects: Nausea and vomiting, weight gain, and androgenic effects such as acne and hirsutism.

Therapeutic notes: Cetrorelix and ganirelix are luteinizing hormone-releasing hormone antagonists, inhibiting the release of the gonadotropins. They are administered parenterally, and they are used to treat infertility in specialist centers.

Oxytocic drugs

The oxytocic drugs include oxytocin, ergonovine, prostaglandins E and F (e.g., misoprostol [PGE_1 analog] and dinoprostone [PGE_2 analog]), and carboprost (15-methyl PGF_{2a}). All cause uterine contractions.

Oxytocin is a posterior pituitary hormone that acts on uterine muscle to induce powerful contractions. It does this directly and also indirectly by stimulating the muscle to synthesize prostaglandins.

In addition, prostaglandins ripen and soften the cervix, further aiding the expulsion of a uterine mass.

Mechanism of action: Oxytocin acts on oxytocin receptors. The mechanism for ergonovine is not well understood, but it may be via partial agonist action at α-adrenoceptors or 5-hydroxytryptamine receptors. The prostaglandins act at prostaglandin receptors.

Route of administration: Misoprostol and dinoprostone are administered by vaginal pessary; dinoprostone can also be administered extra-amniotically; oxytocin is administered by slow intravenous infusion, and oxytocin and ergonovine together are injected intramuscularly. Prostaglandins can be administered by intravenous infusion.

Indications: Prostaglandins are used to induce abortion. Oxytocin and dinoprostone are used for the induction of labor while oxytocin, ergonovine, and carboprost (in those unresponsive to oxytocin and ergometrine) are used for the management of the third stage of labor, and for prevention and treatment of postpartum hemorrhage.

Contraindications: Oxytocic drugs should not be given to women with vascular diseases; ergonovine should not be used to induce labor.

Adverse effects: Nausea and vomiting, vaginal bleeding, and uterine pain. Oxytocin can cause hypotension and tachycardia.

Bone and calcium

Bone and calcium physiology
Bone is a tissue comprised mainly of calcium, phosphates, and a protein meshwork, in addition to the components of the bone marrow.

Bone functions to provide support, and it enables us to carry out various physiological processes, such as respiration and movement. Bone is also an active tissue and crucial in the homeostasis of calcium and phosphate.

Serum calcium is ultimately controlled by the peptide, parathyroid hormone (PTH) derived from the parathyroid glands. PTH maintains serum calcium by acting on the kidney to reabsorb calcium from the tubular filtrate, and to stimulate the activation of vitamin D. PTH also acts directly on bone, mobilizing calcium. Activated vitamin D (1,25-dihydroxycholecalciferol) promotes absorption of calcium from the gut. PTH is secreted in response to low serum calcium.

Calcitonin, from the thyroid gland, inhibits calcium mobilization from bone and decreases reabsorption from the renal tubules.

Disorders of bone and calcium
Osteoporosis is an overall loss of bone mass, and it commonly occurs in women after the menopause, when estrogens fall and bone mobilization slowly increases. Other common causes of osteoporosis include thyrotoxicosis and excessive glucocorticoids (exogenous or endogenous).

Osteodystrophy occurs in renal failure and is driven by secondary hyperparathyroidism.

Rickets (vitamin D deficiency) is now rare in the west, although the adult variant, osteomalacia, is not uncommon.

Hypercalcemia is a medical emergency, and it is most often due to malignancy.

Rehydration therapy is as important in hypercalcemia as it is in ketoacidosis (hyperglycemia), because fluid will be lost in the urine due to osmotic diuresis.

Drugs used in bone and calcium disorders
Bisphosphonates
Alendronate, risedronate, and disodium pamidronate are bisphosphonates.

Mechanism of action: Bisphosphonates inhibit and potentially destroy osteoclasts, which are responsible for mobilizing calcium from bone.

Route of administration: Oral, parenteral.

Indications: Prevention of postmenopausal osteoporosis and corticosteroid-induced osteoporosis, and management of hypercalcemia of malignancy.

Contraindications: Renal impairment, hypocalcemia.

Adverse effects: Nausea, esophageal reactions (with oral preparations), hypocalcemia.

Calcium salts
Calcium gluconate and calcium lactate are calcium salts.

Mechanism of action: Calcium supplementation replaces calcium deficiencies.

Route of administration: Oral, intravenous.

Indications: Hypocalcemia, calcium deficiency, osteoporosis.

Contraindications: Hypercalcemia.

Adverse effects: Mild gastrointestinal disturbance, bradycardia, arrhythmias.

Therapeutic notes: If calcium is given parenterally, serum calcium should be repeatedly monitored.

Vitamin D
Vitamin D can be administered in its inactive form as ergocalciferol or in its active form as calcitriol.

Mechanism of action: Vitamin D acts on the gut to absorb calcium from the diet.

Route of administration: Oral, parenteral.

Indications: Vitamin D deficiency, hypocalcemia secondary to hypoparathyroidism, renal failure, and postmenopausal osteoporosis.

Contraindications: Hypercalcemia.

Adverse effects: Symptoms of overdosage include anorexia, lassitude, nausea and vomiting, weight loss, and hypercalcemia.

Therapeutic notes: Serum calcium should be monitored closely once vitamin D therapy has started and if symptoms of hypercalcemia appear.

Calcitonin

Mechanism of action: Calcitonin binds specific receptors on osteoclasts, inhibiting their mobilization of bone, and acts on the kidney to limit calcium reabsorption from the proximal tubules.

Route of administration: Subcutaneous or intramuscular.

Indications: Hypercalcemia, Paget's disease of bone, bone pain in neoplastic disease.

Contraindications: Caution with history of allergy or renal impairment.

Adverse effects: Nausea, vomiting, flushing, diarrhea, tingling of hands.

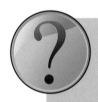

- How are the thyroid hormones produced? How is the process controlled?
- What are the physiologic functions of the thyroid hormones?
- What is the difference between hypothyroidism and hyperthyroidism?
- What are the classes of drugs used to treat hyperthyroidism and hypothyroidism? What are their mechanism of action and potential side effects?
- How are plasma glucose levels controlled?
- What are the differences between type 1 and type 2 diabetes mellitus?
- What are the actions of insulin? What are the various insulin preparations, their route of administration, and potential adverse effects?
- What other classes of drugs can be used to treat diabetes mellitus? How do these drugs act?
- What is the immediate management of the acute diabetic patient presenting with ketoacidosis?
- What are the clinical features of hypoglycemia? What drugs are used in such a situation?
- What are the different types of endogenous steroids produced by the adrenal glands? How do their actions differ?
- How are endogenous steroid levels regulated in the human body?
- What are the physiologic and cellular effects of steroids?
- By what route are exogenous steroids administered to patients? What are the common side effects of prolonged steroid therapy?
- What are the common sex hormones and regulatory hormones, and their main actions?
- What are the principles of the female reproductive cycle?
- What are the agents currently used as contraceptives, their mechanism of action, and their potential adverse effects?
- What other drugs, aside from those mentioned, affect reproductive function? What is the mode of action of each?
- What are the roles and sites of synthesis for vitamin D and parathyroid hormone?
- What are the drugs used to treat metabolic bone disease, their mechanism of action, and potential adverse effects?

12. Eyes and Skin

Eyes

Anatomy and physiology

The eyeball is a 25-mm sphere made up of two fluid-filled compartments (the aqueous humor and the vitreous humor) separated by a translucent lens, all encased within four layers of supporting tissue (Fig. 12.1). These four layers consist of:

- The cornea and sclera.
- The uveal tract, comprising the iris, ciliary body, and choroid.
- The pigment epithelium.
- The retina (neural tissue containing photoreceptors).

Light entering the eye is focused by the lens onto the retina, and the signal reaches the brain via the optic nerve.

Control of pupil size
Light
Light levels affect the pupil in two ways (Fig. 12.2):
- High light levels cause pupil constriction, termed miosis.
- Low light levels cause pupil dilation, termed mydriasis.

Autonomic control
The pupils are innervated by the autonomic nervous system, such that:
- Parasympathetic stimulation causes miosis.
- Sympathetic stimulation causes mydriasis.

The dilator pupillae (radial smooth muscle of the iris) is innervated by the sympathetic system, which causes contraction when norepinephrine activates α_1-adrenoceptors. The constrictor pupillae (sphincter smooth muscle of the iris) is innervated by the

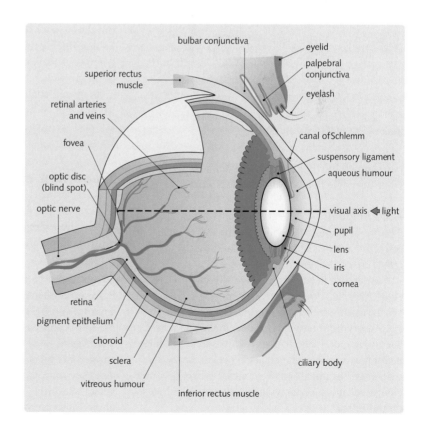

Fig. 12.1 Anatomy of the eye (redrawn from Page et al., 2002).

209

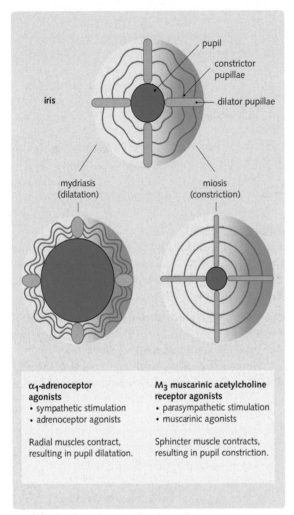

α₁-adrenoceptor agonists
- sympathetic stimulation
- adrenoceptor agonists

α_1-adrenoceptor agonists
- sympathetic stimulation
- adrenoceptor agonists

Radial muscles contract, resulting in pupil dilatation.

M_3 muscarinic acetylcholine receptor agonists
- parasympathetic stimulation
- muscarinic agonists

Sphincter muscle contracts, resulting in pupil constriction.

Fig. 12.2 Mechanisms involved in controlling pupil size (redrawn from Page et al., 2002).

parasympathetic system, which causes contraction when acetylcholine activates M_3 receptors.

Accommodation

Accommodation is the ability of the eye to change its refractive power. This is determined by the curvature of the lens.

Suspensory ligaments connect the lens to the ciliary muscle. When the ciliary muscle contracts (parasympathetic M_3 receptor activation), the suspensory ligaments relax, resulting in the lens becoming more spherical so that it is able to focus near objects. When the ciliary muscle relaxes, the suspensory ligaments tighten, and the lens becomes elongated and thin, allowing far objects to be focused on the retina.

Production of aqueous humor

Aqueous humor fills the anterior chamber of the eyeball. It is continuously produced at a rate of 3 mL/day by a special vascular tissue associated with the ciliary body (Fig. 12.3).

The ciliary epithelial cells contain carbonic anhydrase and an ATPase, which transport bicarbonate and sodium.

The aqueous humor flows through the pupil and into the anterior aqueous chamber. Draining fluid leaves the aqueous chamber via the trabecular meshwork and the canal of Schlemm within the surface of the sclera before entering the episcleral veins.

Glaucoma

Glaucoma can be defined as a disorder in which the intraocular pressure (IOP) is raised. This may result in structural changes within the eye, such as cupping of the optic disc, as well as visual field deficits and potentially blindness.

There are two types of glaucoma: open-angle and closed-angle.

Open-angle glaucoma is the most common type of glaucoma and may be congenital. It is caused by pathology of the trabecular meshwork that reduces the drainage of the aqueous humor into the canal of Schlemm. Treatment involves either reducing the amount of aqueous humor produced or increasing its drainage.

In closed-angle glaucoma, the angle between the iris and the cornea is very small, and this results in forward ballooning of the iris against the back of the cornea.

Treatment of open-angle glaucoma

Most drugs used to treat eye disease can be given topically in the form of drops and ointments. To enable these drugs to penetrate the cornea, they must be lipophilic or uncharged.

Drugs used to inhibit aqueous production
Beta-adrenoceptor antagonists

Timolol and betaxolol are examples of β-adrenoceptor antagonists used in glaucoma.

Mechanism of action: Beta-adrenoceptor antagonists block β_2-receptors on the ciliary body, and they may also block β-receptors on ciliary blood vessels, resulting in vasoconstriction (they are almost universally referred to as "beta blockers" in clinical

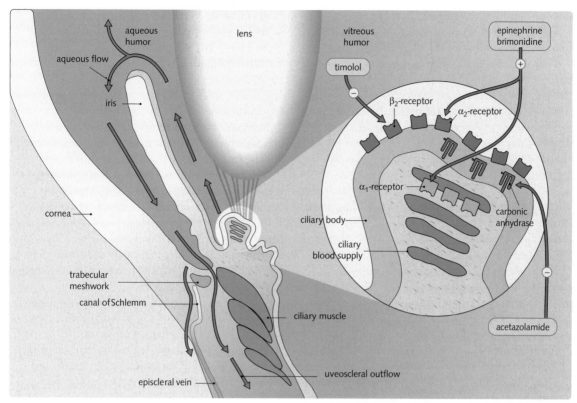

Fig. 12.3 Production and drainage of the aqueous humor (redrawn from Page et al., 2002).

practice) (see Fig. 12.3) and reduced aqueous production.

Route of administration: Topical.

Indications: Open-angle glaucoma. β-adrenoceptor antagonists are also used in cardiovascular disease (Chapter 7).

Contraindications: Beta-adrenoceptor antagonists should not be given to patients with asthma, bradycardia, heart block, or heart failure.

Adverse effects: Systemic side effects include bronchospasm in asthmatic patients, and potentially bradycardia owing to their nonselective action on β-receptors. Other side effects include transitory dry eyes and allergic blepharoconjunctivitis.

Sympathomimetics (adrenoceptor agonists)

Epinephrine, dipivefrin, and brimonidine are commonly used sympathomimetics.

Mechanism of action: Agonist at α-adrenoceptors is thought to be the principal means by which these agents reduce aqueous production from the ciliary body. Adrenaline may also increase drainage of aqueous via the trabecular meshwork (see Fig. 12.3).

Route of administration: Topical.

Indications: Open-angle glaucoma. Sympathomimetics are also used in the management of cardiac and anaphylactic emergencies (Chapter 7) and in reversible airways disease (Chapter 8).

Contraindications: Closed-angle glaucoma, hypertension, and heart disease.

Adverse effects: Pain and redness of the eye.

Therapeutic notes: Epinephrine is not very lipophilic; therefore, it does not penetrate the cornea effectively. This can be overcome by administering dipivefrin hydrochloride, a prodrug that crosses the cornea and that is metabolized to epinephrine once inside the eye.

Carbonic anhydrase inhibitors

Acetazolamide and dorzolamide are carbonic anhydrase inhibitors (CAIs).

Mechanism of action: CAIs inhibit the enzyme carbonic anhydrase, which catalyses the conversion of carbon dioxide and water to carbonic acid, which dissociates into bicarbonate and H^+. Bicarbonate is required by the cells of the ciliary body, and

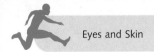

under-production of bicarbonate limits aqueous secretion (see Fig. 12.3). CAIs given systemically have a weak diuretic effect (Chapter 9).

Route of administration: Oral, topical, intravenous.

Indications: Open-angle glaucoma.

Contraindications: Hypokalemia, hyponatremia, renal impairment. These effects can be reduced if the drug is given in a slow-release form.

Adverse effects: Irritation of the eye, nausea, vomiting, diarrhea, diuresis.

Drugs used to increase the drainage of aqueous humor

Miotics—muscarinic agonists

Pilocarpine is a muscarinic agonist.

Mechanism of action: Pilocarpine causes contraction of the constrictor pupillae muscles of the iris, constricting the pupil and allowing aqueous to drain from the anterior chamber into the trabecular meshwork (see Fig. 12.3).

Route of administration: Topical.

Indications: Open-angle glaucoma.

Contraindications: Acute iritis, anterior uveitis.

Adverse effects: Eye irritation, headache and brow ache, blurred vision, hypersalivation. May exacerbate asthma.

The prostaglandin analog latanoprost is a novel treatment for open-angle glaucoma, and it promotes outflow of aqueous from the anterior chamber. This topically applied drug is indicated in open-angle glaucoma that is resistant to conventional treatment; it may result in a brown pigmentation of the iris.

Glaucoma has a prevalence of approximately 1% in people aged over 40 years.

Treatment of closed-angle glaucoma

Drugs to treat closed-angle glaucoma are used in emergencies as a temporary measure to lower IOP.

Pilocarpine and a carbonic anhydrase inhibitor are often first-line treatments. Mannitol and glycerol have been administered systemically to reduce IOP in more serious cases.

YAG (yttrium-aluminium-garnet) laser surgery provides a permanent cure for closed-angle glaucoma.

A hole is made in the iris (iridectomy) to allow increased flow of aqueous humor.

Examining the eye

Mydriatic drugs dilate the pupil (i.e., cause mydriasis), while cycloplegic drugs cause paralysis of the ciliary muscle (i.e., cycloplegia).

Mydriatic and cycloplegic drugs are used in ophthalmoscopy to allow a better view of the interior of the eye.

Mydriasis and cycloplegia reduce the drainage of the aqueous humor; therefore, they should be avoided in patients with closed-angle glaucoma.

Muscarinic antagonists

The most effective mydriatics are the muscarinic antagonists. These block the parasympathetic control of the iris sphincter muscle.

The type of muscarinic antagonist chosen will depend on the length of the procedure and on whether or not cycloplegia is required.

The most commonly used muscarinic antagonists, their duration of action, and their mydriatic and cycloplegic effects are summarized in Fig. 12.4.

Alpha-adrenoceptor agonists

Alpha-adrenoceptor agonists can cause mydriasis by stimulating the sympathetic control of the iris dilator muscle. However, the sympathetic system does not control the ciliary muscle; therefore, these drugs do not produce cycloplegia.

The α-agonist most commonly used to produce mydriasis is phenylephrine.

Muscarinic agonists and α-antagonists

A muscarinic agonist such as pilocarpine or an α-antagonist such as dapiprazole may be used to reverse mydriasis at the end of an ophthalmic examination. This is not usually necessary.

Skin

Anatomy and physiology

The skin is the largest organ in the body, making up on average 16% of the total body weight and covering an area of approximately 1.8m^2 (Fig. 12.5).

Functions of the skin

The skin has several functions. These include:

Effects of commonly used muscarinic antagonists			
Drug	Duration (h)	Mydriatic effect	Cycloplegic effect
Tropicamide	1 – 3	++	++
Cyclopentolate	12 – 24	+++	+++
Atropine	168 – 240	+++	+++

Fig. 12.4 Mydriatic and cycloplegic effects of the commonly used muscarinic antagonists.

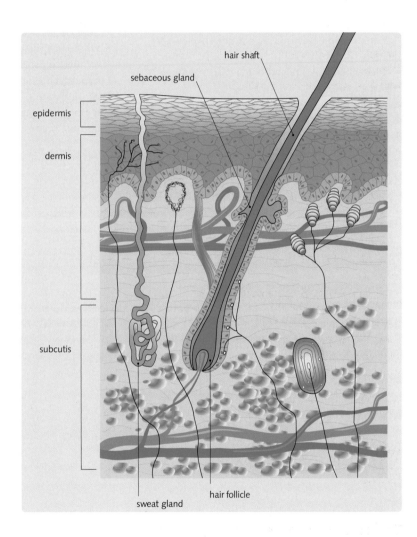

Fig. 12.5 Anatomy of the skin.

- Protection—the skin provides a barrier against chemical, mechanical, and thermal stresses; ultraviolet light; dehydration; heat loss; and microorganisms.
- Thermoregulation—hair and subcutaneous fat provide the body with insulation, whereas the sweat glands and increased dermal blood flow allow heat loss.
- Sensation—the skin contains receptors for touch, pressure, temperature, and pain.
- Metabolism—synthesis of vitamin D takes place in the epidermis, and adipose tissue

213

provides a store of energy in the form of triglycerides.

Skin disorders

The most common skin diseases are eczema, acne, psoriasis, skin cancer, viral warts, and urticaria.

Eczema (dermatitis)

Eczema is an inflammatory disease of the skin, defined by the presence of epidermal intercellular edema or spongiosis.

Eczema can be caused by a number of factors, such as:

- Exogenous irritants and contact allergens.
- Infections.
- Atopy.
- Drugs.
- Certain environmental conditions such as low humidity and ultraviolet light.

Drugs used to treat eczema are summarized in Fig. 12.6.

Acne

Acne affects the pilosebaceous unit and occurs where these are numerous, such as on the face, back, and chest.

Acne is characterized by the presence of keratin plugs in the sebaceous duct openings, known as comedones. Other signs of acne of worsening degrees of severity include inflammatory papules, pustules, nodules, cysts, and scars.

Acne is stimulated by androgens, which is why it is related to puberty, and why the antiandrogen cyproterone is often used in females with acne (Chapter 11).

The drugs used to treat acne are summarized in Fig. 12.7.

Psoriasis

Psoriasis is a genetic skin disorder that manifests under certain conditions including stress, infection, damage from ultraviolet light, or trauma.

In psoriasis, the turnover rate of skin is eight times that of normal skin (7 instead of 56 days).

Psoriasis is characterized by:

- Thickened skin plaques.
- Superficial scales.
- Dilated capillaries in the dermis (these might act to initiate psoriasis or as nourishment for hyperproliferating skin).
- An infiltrate of inflammatory cells, especially lymphocytes and neutrophils, in the epidermis and dermis, respectively.

Drugs used to treat psoriasis are summarized in Fig. 12.8.

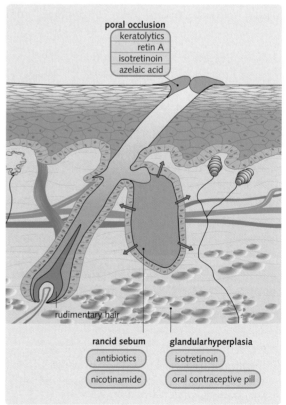

Fig. 12.7 Characteristics of acne and its drug treatment (redrawn from Page et al., 2002).

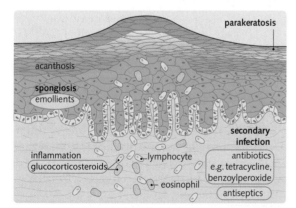

Fig. 12.6 Characteristics of eczema and its drug treatment (redrawn from Page et al., 2002).

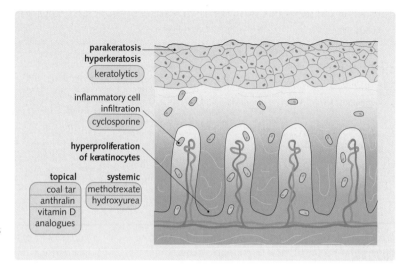

Fig. 12.8 Characteristics of psoriasis and its drug treatment (redrawn from Page et al., 2002).

Treatment of skin disorders

Much is made of the potentially serious effects of steroid therapy, but their usefulness in treating many dermatologic conditions should not be ignored. Use steroids with care—but use them!

Corticosteroids

Examples of corticosteroids include clobetasol propionate, betamethasone, clobetasone butyrate, and hydrocortisone (Fig. 12.9).

Mechanism of action: Corticosteroids suppress components of the inflammatory reaction (see Chapter 11 and Fig. 12.6).

Route of administration: Topically, orally, intradermally or intravenously in severe disease.

Indications: Corticosteroids are used for the relief of symptoms due to inflammatory conditions of the skin other than those due to infection (e.g., in eczema).

Contraindications: Rosacea or untreated skin infections.

Adverse effects: Most likely to occur with prolonged, or high dose therapy. Local—spread or worsening of infection, thinning of the skin, impaired wound healing, irreversible striae atrophicae. Systemic—immunosuppression, peptic ulceration, osteoporosis, hypertension, cataracts.

Therapeutic notes: Withdrawal of corticosteroids after high doses or prolonged use should be gradual (Chapter 11).

Anthralin

Anthralin is the most potent topical drug for the treatment of psoriasis.

Mechanism of action: Anthralin modifies keratinization, but the mechanism is unclear (see Fig. 12.8).

Route of administration: Topical.

Contraindications: Anthralin should not be given to people with hypersensitivity or acute and pustular psoriasis.

Adverse effects: Local skin irritation, staining of skin and hair.

Vitamin D analogs

Calcipotriene is a vitamin D analog derivative.

Vitamin D analogs are keratolytics, although they are also used in vitamin D deficiency related to gastrointestinal/biliary disease and renal failure (Chapter 9).

Mechanism of action: The exact mechanism of action is still unclear, but several effects of vitamin D analogs have been observed. These include inhibition of epidermal proliferation and induction of terminal keratinocyte differentiation (Fig. 12.8).

The anti-inflammatory properties of vitamin D analogs include inhibition of T-cell proliferation and of cytokine release, decreased capacity of monocytes to stimulate T-cell proliferation and to stimulate

Potency of some topical steroids		
Group	**Approved name**	**Proprietary name**
I (very potent)	Clobetasol propionate	Temovate®
II (potent)	Betamethasone valerate 0.1% Beclomethasone dipropionate Hydrocortisone 17-butyrate	Valisone® Diprolene® Westcort®
III (moderately potent)	Hydrocortisone butyrate	Locoid®
IV (mild)	Hydrocortisone 1% Hydrocortisone 2%	Various Various

Fig. 12.9 Potency of some topical steroids.

lymphokine release from T cells, and inhibition of neutrophil accumulation in psoriatic skin.

Route of administration: Topical.

Indications: Psoriasis.

Contraindications: Vitamin D analogs should not be given to people with disorders of calcium metabolism. They should not be used on the face, as irritation may occur.

Adverse effects: Side effects of vitamin D analogs include local irritation and dermatitis. High doses may affect calcium homoeostasis.

Tar preparations

Coal tar, made up of about 10,000 components, is a keratolytic that is more potent than salicylic acid. It also has anti-inflammatory and antipruritic properties.

Mechanism of action: Coal tar modifies keratinization, but the mechanism is unclear (see Fig. 12.8).

Route of administration: Topical.

Indications: Psoriasis and occasionally eczema.

Contraindications: Coal tar should not be given to people with acute or pustular psoriasis or in the presence of an infection. It should not be used on the face, or on broken or inflamed skin.

Adverse effects: Skin irritation and acne-like eruptions, photosensitivity, and staining of the skin and hair.

Salicylates

Salicylic acid is keratolytic at a concentration of 3–6%.

Mechanism of action: Salicylic acid causes desquamation via the solubilization of cell-surface proteins that maintain the integrity of the stratum corneum.

Route of administration: Topical.

Indications: Hyperkeratosis, eczema, psoriasis (combined with coal tar or dithranol preparations), acne, wart, and callous eradication.

Contraindications: Sensitivity to the drug or broken or inflamed skin. High concentrations, such as those needed to treat warts, should not be given to people with diabetes mellitus or peripheral vascular disease, as ulceration may be induced.

Adverse effects: Side effects of salicylic acid include anaphylactic shock in those sensitive to the drug, skin irritation and excessive drying, and systemic effects if used over the long term.

Emollients

Emollients are used to soothe and hydrate the skin.

A simple preparation is aqueous cream, which is often as effective as more complex drugs.

Most creams are thin emollients, whereas a mixture of equal parts soft white paraffin and liquid paraffin is a thick emollient.

Camphor, menthol, and phenol preparations have antipruritic effects, whereas zinc- and titanium-based emollients have mild astringent (contracting) effects.

Mechanism of action: Emollients hydrate the skin and reduce transepidermal water loss.

Route of administration: Topical. Many emollients can be added to bath water.

Indications: Emollients are used for the long-term treatment of dry scaling disorders.

Contraindications: None.

Adverse effects: Some ingredients, such as lanolin or antibacterials, may induce an allergic reaction.

Therapeutic notes: The use of emollients lessens the need for topical steroids, thereby limiting potential side effects.

216

Other drugs used in skin disease		
Drug	**Indication**	**Mechanism of action**
Benzoyl peroxide	Acne vulgaris	Antibacterial/keratolytic
Retinoids (vitamin A derivatives)	Psoriasis/acne	Keratolytic/cyto-inhibitory
Psoralen	Psoriasis	Mutates DNA/cytotoxic
Methortrexate	Psoriasis	Cytotoxic
Cyclosporine	Psoriasis	Immunosuppressant
Antibacterial, antiviral, antifungal	Skin infections/warts	Antimicrobial
Antiparasite preparations	Skin/hair infestations	Parasite toxins

Fig. 12.10 Other drugs used in skin disease, their indications, and mechanism of action (from *Mosby's Color Atlas and Text of Dermatology*, by Graham-Brown et al., Mosby, 1998).

Other drugs used in skin disease

Many other drugs are employed in the management of skin disease. Some of the more common drugs are summarized in Fig. 12.10.

Preparations of drugs for use on skin

Drugs applied to the skin are delivered by a variety of vehicles such as ointments, creams, pastes, powders, aerosols, gels, lotions, and tinctures.

Factors affecting the choice of vehicle include:
- The solubility of the active drug.
- The ability of the drug to penetrate the skin.
- The stability of the drug–vehicle complex.

- The ability of the vehicle to delay evaporation, this being greatest for ointments and least for tinctures.

Factors that affect the absorption of the drug include:
- Body site, in that absorption is greatest from the scrotum and vulva, high from the scalp and face, and lowest from the palms and soles.
- Skin hydration, as occlusive dressings can increase the absorption of a drug tenfold, for example.
- Skin condition, because damage caused by burns and inflammation increases absorption.
- The concentration gradient across the skin (the greater this is, the greater the rate of absorption).

- How is pupil size controlled?
- How is aqueous humor produced and drained from the eye?
- What are the differences between open-angle and closed-angle glaucoma?
- What are the different classes of drugs used to treat glaucoma? For each class, list an example, mechanism of action, route of administration, and major adverse effects.
- In which situation are mydriatic and cycloplegic drugs used?
- What are the common skin disorders and their treatments?
- What are the different classes of drugs used to treat skin disease? For each class, list examples, mechanism of action, route of administration, indications, and major adverse effects.
- Which factors affect the choice of vehicles for drugs used on the skin?
- Which skin diseases may benefit from the use of antibiotic therapy?
- Which factors affect the absorption of drugs used on the skin?

Index

Page numbers for figures are indicated in bold type.

A

Absorption, of drugs, 11–2
ACE inhibitors. *See* Angiotensin-converting
    enzyme inhibitors
Acetaminophen
  for headaches, 68
  poisoning, 14–5, **61**
Acetic acid, **61**
Acetylcysteine, **163**
Acetylsalicylic acid. *See* Aspirin
Acne, 214
Acyclovir, 44
Adenosine, for cardiac treatment, 136
Adenylyl cyclase/cyclic AMP system, 6–7
Adrenal cortex, **195–201**
  description of, **195–6**
  treatment of, **196–201**
Adrenal corticosteroids
  for endocrine therapy, 28
  mechanism of, **197, 198**
  synthesis and release of, **196–7**
  therapeutic use of, **197–200**
Adrenal medulla, **82**
Adrenoceptor agonists, **211**
Adrenoceptors, 82–3, **82**
Affective disorders, 99–103, **100, 101**
  bipolar, 99, 103
  description of, 99
  monoamine theory of depression,
     99–100, **100**
  treatment of, 100–3, **100, 101**
  unipolar, 99–103, **100, 101**
Agonists, 9
Albuterol, 159
Aldosterone, in adrenal cortex, **197**
Alkylating agents, **24**, 26
Allergic disorders, **163–5**
  description of, **163, 164**
  drug therapy of, **163–4, 165**
Allopurinol, **63**
Allylamines, 48–9, **48**
Alpha-adrenoceptor agonists, 212
Alpha-adrenoceptor antagonists, 173

Alpha-blockers. *See* Alpha-adrenoceptor
    antagonists
Alpha-glucosidase inhibitors, 194
Alprostadil, 174
Alzheimer's disease. *See* Dementia
Amantadin, 42–4, **42**
Amebiasis, 52
Amikacin, 37
Aminoglycosides
  description of, **34–5**, 37, **38**
  as NMJ drug, **79**
para-Aminophenols, **61**
4-Aminoquinolines, 51
8-Aminoquinolines, 52
Aminosalicylates, 184
Amoxicillin, 33
Amphetamines
  description of, 120
  in norepinephrine release, **84**
Ampicillin, 33
Amsacrine, 28
Anabolic steroids, 206
Anal disorders, 185
Analeptic drugs, 162
Androgens, 205
Androgens antagonists. *See* Antiandrogens
Anemia
  description of, 153
  treatment of, 153–4
Angina pectoris, 132
Angiotensin-converting enzyme inhibitors
    (ACE inhibitors), **139, 140–1**
Anion inhibitors, 189–90, **189**
Antacids, **178**
Antagonists
  competitive, 9–10
  description of, 9–10
  noncompetitive, 10
Anthelminthic drugs, 53–5
Anthralin, **215**
Antiandrogens
  in reproductive system, 205
  for urinary retention treatment, 173

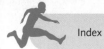

Antianginal drugs, 136–8
  beta-adrenoreceptor blocker as, 137, **138**
  calcium-channel blockers as, 137–8, **138**
  organic nitrates as, 136–7, **138**
Antiarrhythmic drugs
  adenosine as, 136
  classifications, 134–6
    epinephrine as, 136
Antibacterial drugs, 31–41
  antimycobacterial, 40–1, **41**
    antileprosy therapy, **41**
    antituberculosis therapy, 40
  cell-wall synthesis inhibition
      by, **32**, 33–6
    aztreonam, 36
    carbapanems, 36
    cephalosporin, 34–6, **34**
    glycopeptides, 34–5, **34–6,** 36
    penicillin, **32,** 33–4, **34–5**
  choices of, **34–5**
  concepts of, **31,** 31–3
  miscellaneous, 39–40
    bacitracin, **34–5,** 39
    metronidazole, **34–5,** 39
    nitrofurantoin, **34–5,** 39
    polymyxins, **32, 34–5,** 40
  nucleic acid inhibition by, **32,** 36–7
    antifolates, **32, 34–5,** 36–7
    quinolones/fluoroquinolones, **32, 34–5,** 37
  protein synthesis inhibition by, 37–9
    aminoglycosides, **34–5,** 37, **38**
    chloramphenicol, **34–5, 38,** 38–9
    clindamycin, 39
    macrolides/ketolides, **34–5,** 39
    tetracyclines, **34–5,** 37–8, **38**
Antibiotics, classification of, **32**
  definition of, **31–2**
  prescribing, 33
  resistance to, 32–3, **32**
Anticholinergic agents
  description of, 94
  for reversible airways
      disease, 159
Anticholinesterases
  description of, 80–1, **81**
  in parasympathetic nervous
      system, **87**
Anticoagulants, **149, 150–1**
Antidepressants
  as anxiolytic/hypnotic, 99
  atypical, **100,** 103

Antidepressants *(Continued)*
  carbamazepine, 103
  for headaches, **68**
  lithium, 103
  MAOIs, **100, 101,** 102–3
  for neuralgic pain, 69
  SNRIs, **100, 101,** 102
  SSRIs, **100, 101,** 102
  tricyclic, **100, 101,** 101–2
Antidiabetics, 194
Antidiarrheal drugs, 182–3
Antiemetic drugs
  for headaches, **68**
  for nausea, vertigo, and
      vomiting, 108, **179,** 179–80
Antiepileptics, **109–11,** 109–13
  compounds, **111,** 111–3
  mechanisms of, **109–11**
  for neuralgic pain, 69
Antiestrogens. *See* Estrogen
    antagonists
Antifibrinolytic agents, 153
Antifolates, **32, 34–5,** 36–7, 52
Antifungal drugs, **47,** 47–9
  fungal infection, **47**
  imidazoles, **47–8**
  miscellaneous, **48,** 48–9
  polyene macrolides, **47, 48**
  trazoles, **48**
Antihistamines
  for allergic disorders, **164–5**
  as anxiolytic/hypnotic, 99
Antihypertensive drugs, 143
Anti-inflammatory drugs, **57–61**
  NSAIDs, **57–61**
  for reversible airways disease, 161
Antimetabolites, **24,** 26, 27
Antimicrobial drugs, 183
Antimuscarinics
  for intestinal motility, **181**
  for urinary incontinence
      treatment, 173
Antimycobacterial drugs, 40–1, **41**
    antileprosy therapy, **41**
    antituberculosis therapy, 40
Anti-obesity drugs, 184–5
Antiplatelet agents, **151,** 151–2
Antiprogestins, 205
Antiprotozoal drugs, 49–53
    malaria, 49–52
    other infections, 52–3

Antiprotozoal drugs (Continued)
  for protozoal infection, 49, **50**
Antispasmodics, 181–2, **181**
Antithyroid drugs, **189**, 189–90
Antitussives, 162–3
Antiviral drugs, 41–6
  description of, **41–2**
  host cell attachment and penetration
      inhibition, **42**, 42–4
    amantadin/arimantidine, **42**, 42–4
    immunoglobulins, **43**, 43–4
    neuraminidase inhibitors, 43
  immunomodulators, 46
  nucleic acid replication inhibition, 44–5, **45**
    acyclovir and related drugs, 44
    ganciclovir, 44
    nonnucleoside reverse transcriptase
        inhibitors, **45**
    nucleoside analog reverse transcriptase
        inhibitors, 44–5, **45**
    ribavirin, 44
  post-translation event inhibition, **45**, 45–6
  viral infection, **41**
Anxiety, 95–9, **96–7**
Anxiolytics
  barbiturates, 98
  benzodiazepine, **96–7**
  description of, 95
  miscellaneous agents, 99
  nonbenzodiazepine, **97**
  serotonergic receptor blocking, 98
Aprotinin, 153
Aqueous humor
  drugs influencing, **210**, 210–2, **211**
  production of, **210, 211**
Arachidonic acid metabolites, 57, **58**
Arimantidine, **42**, 42–4
Arrhythmias, **131**
Asparaginase, **24**, 28
Aspirin, 57–8, **58, 59, 60**
  as antiplatelet agent, **151–2**
  drug absorption and, 12
Asthma, 157–9
  pathogenesis of, 157–9
  types of, 157
Atenolol
  for cardiac treatment, **135**, 137
  for hyperthyroidism, 190
Autonomic ganglia, **81–2**
  ganglion-blocking drugs, **82**
  ganglion-stimulating drugs, **81–2**

Autonomic nervous system, **81**, 81–8, **82, 84–8**
  autonomic ganglia, **81–2**
  concepts of, **81, 89**
  parasympathetic nervous
      system, **86–8**
  sympathetic nervous system, **82**, 82–6, **86**
Azathioprine
  as immunosuppressant, 62, 71
  for inflammatory bowel disease, 184
Azithromycin, 39
Aztreonam, 36

B
Bacitracin, **34–5**, 39
Bacterial infection
  description of, **31**
  drug choices for, **31–41, 34–5**
Barbiturates
  as antiepileptic drug, 113
  as hypnotic/anxiolytic drug, 98
BDZs. See Benzodiazepines
Benzimidazoles, **54**
Benzocaine, 162
Benzodiazepines (BDZs), 122
  as antiepileptic drug, 113
  as hypnotic/anxiolytic drug, 95–7, **96, 97**
Beta-adrenoceptor agonists
  for hyperthyroidism, 190
  for reversible airways disease, 159
Beta-adrenoceptor antagonists
  as antianginal drugs, 137, **138**
  as anxiolytic drug, 98
  for glaucoma, **210–1**
Betamethasone, 200–1
Betaxolol, **210–1**
Biguanides, 194
Bipolar affective disorder (BPAD), 99, 103
Bismuth, **178**
Bisphosphonates, 207
Bleeding disorders, **149–50**
Bleomycin, 26
β-Blockers. See Beta-adrenoceptor antagonists
Blood, 153–4
  anemia, 153–4
  myeloproliferative disorders, 154
Bone, 207–8
  disorders of, 207
  drugs for, 207–8
  physiology of, 207
Botulinum toxin, **79**
BPAD. See Bipolar affective disorder

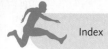

Bran, 182
Bronchodilators, 159–61
    anticholinergics, 159
    beta-adrenoceptor agonists, 159
    leukotriene receptor antagonists, 161
    xanthines, 159–61
Budesonide, 184
Buprenorphine, **66, 67**
Butyrophenones, 106

C
CAIs. *See* Carbonic anhydrase inhibitors
Calcitonin, 208
Calcium salts, 207
cAMP. *See* Cyclic adenosine
        monophosphate
Cancer, 23–9
    chemotherapy, 23–9
        cytotoxic therapy, 23–8
        endocrine therapy, 28
        future of, 29
        immunotherapy, 28–9
    description of, 23
Cannabinoids, 123
Cannabis, 123
Capreomycin, 40
Carbachol, 81
Carbamazepine
    as antiepileptic drug, **111,** 112
    in BPAD, 103
Carbapanems, 36
Carbonic anhydrase inhibitors (CAIs), **211,** 211–2
Cardiac glycosides, **130,** 132–3, **138**
Cardiovascular system, 127–55
    blood, 153–4
    circulation, 138–48
    fluid replacement, 154
    heart, 127–138
Carrier molecules, **4**
Catechol-*O*-methyl transferase (COMT)
    inhibitors of, 94
    in sympathetic nervous system, **84**
Celecoxib, **61**
Central nervous system, 91–125
    affective disorders, 99–103, **100, 101**
    anxiety and sleep disorders, 95–9, **96, 97**
    dementia, 95
    depressants of, 121–2
    drug misuse, 118–24
    epilepsy, 108–13
    general anesthetics, 113–8

Central nervous system (*Continued*)
    nausea and vertigo, 108
    parkinsonism, **91,** 91–4, **92**
    psychotic disorders, 104–8, **105–7**
    stimulants of, 120–1
Cephalosporin, 34–6, **34**
Chelates, **178**
Chemotherapy, 23–9
    cytotoxic therapy, 23–8
    definition of, **31**
    endocrine therapy, 28
    future of, 29
    immunotherapy, 28–9
CHF. *See* Congestive heart failure
Chlorambucil, 26
Chloramphenicol, **34–5, 38,** 38–9
Chloroquine, 51
Cholera, 6
Cholestyramine, 185
Cholinesterase, inhibitors of, 95
Chronic obstructive pulmonary disease
        (COPD), 159
Ciprofloxacin, 37
Circulatory system, 138–48
    hemostasis and thrombosis, 148–53
    hypertension in, **139,** 139–43
        description of, 139
        treatment of, **139,** 139–43
    lipoprotein circulation and atherosclerosis
        in, 145–8
        description of, 145
        hyperlipidemias, 145–6, **146**
        treatment of, **146,** 146–8
    pheochromocytoma in, 143
    vascular tone control, **138,** 138–9, 140
    vasoconstrictors and shock in, 143–5
        description of, 143–4
        management of, 144–5
Clarithromycin, 39
Clindamycin, 39
Clofazimine, **41**
Clopidogrel, 152
Clotting factors, **150**
Cocaine, 120
COCP. *See* Combined oral contraceptive pill
Codeine, **66, 68**
Colchicine, **63**
Combined oral contraceptive pill
        (COCP), 203
Compliance, 10–1
COMT. *See* Catechol-*O*-methyl transferase

Congestive heart failure (CHF), **130–1**
Contraceptive regimens, **203**, 203–4
COPD. *See* Chronic obstructive pulmonary disease
Corticosteroids
    for circulatory treatment, 145
    exogenous, **197–200**
    as immunosuppressant, 62
    for skin treatment, **214, 215, 216**
Cortisol, **196–7, 200**
Cyclic adenosine monophosphate (cAMP)
    in arrhythmias, **131**
    G-proteins and, 83
    phosphodiesterase and, 134
    in sympathetic nervous system, 83, **84**
Cyclophosphamide, 26
Cycloserine, 40
Cyclosporine, 62, 69–71
Cyproterone, 205
Cytarabine, 27
Cytokines, 29
Cytotoxic antibiotics, 26
Cytotoxic chemotherapy, 23–8
    agents of, **25–8**
        alkylating, 26
        antimetabolites, 27
        cytotoxic antibiotics, 26
        miscellaneous agents, 27–8
        mitotic inhibitors, 27
    mechanisms of action, 23, **24, 25**
    resistance to, **25**
    selectivity, 23–5, **24–5**

D
Dactinomycin, 26
DAG. *See* Diacylglycerol
Danazol, 206
Dapsone, **41**, 51
Decongestants in, **163**
Dementia, 95
Depo-progesterone, 203–4, **203**
Depression, monoamine theory of, 99–100, **100**
Desmopressin, **150**
Dextropropoxyphene, **66, 68**
Diabetes mellitus, **192**, 192–5
    description of, **192–3**
    management of, 193–5
Diacylglycerol (DAG)
    G-proteins and, 7
    in parasympathetic nervous system, **86**
    in sympathetic nervous system, 83

Diethylcarbamizine, **54**, 55
Diethylstilbestrol, 28
Dihydrocodeine, **66, 68**
Diltiazem, 136–7
Dinoprostone, 206–7
Diphenhydramine, **164**
Dipyridamole, 152
Disease-modifying antirheumatic drugs (DMARDs), **61**, 61–2
    antimalarials, **61**, 62
    Gold salts, **61**, 62
    immunosuppresants, **61**, 62
    Penicillamine, **61**, 62
    sulfasalazine, **61**, 62
Distal tubule
    diuretics for, 171–2
    in nephron, **170**
Diuretic drugs
    for cardiac treatment, 134, **138**
    for hypertension treatment, 139, 142–3
    NSAIDs interaction with, 18
DMARDs. *See* Disease-modifying antirheumatic drugs
DNA-linked receptors, 8
Dopamine
    antagonists, **179**, 179–80
    for circulatory treatment, 144
    drugs to increase, **92**, 92–4
Doxapram, 162
Doxorubicin, 26
Doxycycline, 37
Drug(s)
    absorption of, 11–2
    administration routes of, 11
        enteral, 11
        local anasthetics, **75–6**
        parenteral, 11
        topical, 11
    adverse effects of, 18–9
    agonists, 9
    antagonists, 9–10
    definition of, 3
    dependence on, 118
    development of, 19–20
    distribution in body of, 12–3
    excretion of, 15
        gastrointestinal, 15
        renal, 15
    interactions of, 17–8
    kinetics of, 15–6
    mechanism of, 3

Drug(s) *(Continued)*
  metabolism of, 13–5
  names and classification of, 3
  patient compliance with, 10–1
  patient history of, 19
  potency of, 10
  receptors and, 8–10
  tolerance of, 118
  withdrawal from, 119
Drug misuse, 118–24
  concepts of, 118–9
  drugs of, 119–23
    cannabinoids, 123
    central depressants, 121–2
    central stimulants, 120–1
    opioid analgesics, 122
    psychotomimetic drugs, 123
  legal aspects of, 119

E
Ecstasy. *See* Methylenedioxymethamphetamine
Eczema, **214**
Edema, 171–2
  causes of, 171
  treatment of, 171–2
    loop diuretics, **169,** 171
    osmotic diuretics, 172
    potassium-sparing diuretics,
      170, 172
    thiazide diuretics, 171–2
Eicosanoids. *See* Arachidonic acid
      metabolites
Endocrine chemotherapy, 28
Endocrine pancreas, 190–5, **191–2**
  diabetes mellitus, **192,** 192–5
  hypoglycemia, 195
  insulin release from, **191–2**
  plasma glucose control by, 190–1, **191**
Endocrine system
  adrenal cortex, 195–201, **196–201**
  endocrine pancreas, 190–5, **191–2**
  thyroid gland, **187,** 187–90
Enflurane, 117
Enzymes, **4**
Ephedrine
  for circulatory treatment, 144
  in norepinephrine release, **84**
Epilepsy, 108–13, **109–11**
  causes of, **109**
  description of, 108–9, **109**
  treatment of, 109–13, **109–11**

Epinephrine
  for allergic disorders, **164**
  for cardiac treatment, 136
  for circulatory treatment, 144
  in sympathetic nervous system, 83, **85**
Erectile dysfunction, 173–4
Erythromycin, 39
Erythropoietin, 153–4
Estrogen antagonists, 204–5
Estrogens
  for endocrine therapy, 28
  in reproductive system, **201–2,** 204, 205
Ethambutol, 40
Ethanol, 121–2
Etomidate, **115**
Excretion, of drugs, 15
Eyes, **209–11,** 209–12
  anatomy and physiology, **209–10**
  aqueous humor production, **210, 211**
  examination of, 212
  glaucoma, **210, 211,** 210–2

F
Fecal softeners, 182
Fenemates, **61**
Fibrates, **146,** 147
Fibrinolytic agents, 152
Flucytosine, 49
Fludrocortisone, 201
Fluoroquinolones
  in antituberculosis therapy, 40
  description of, **32, 34–5,** 37
Fluorouracil, 27
Flutamide, 28
Folate, 153
Fungal infection
  concepts of, **47**
  drugs for, **47,** 47–9

G
Gallbladder, 185
Gamma-aminobutyric acid (GABA),
      receptors of, 95–6, **96**
Ganciclovir, 44
Gastroesophageal reflux disease, 176, **178**
Gastrointestinal system, 175–86
  gallbladder, 185
  intestines, 180–5
  nausea and vomiting, 179–80, **179**
  pancreas, 185
  stomach, **175,** 175–9, **179**

General anesthetics, 113–8, **114–5**
  agents of, **114, 115,** 114–8
    inhalation, 116–8
    intravenous, 115–6, **115**
  concepts of, 113–4, **117**
  neuromuscular blockers in, 118
Gentamicin, 37
Giardiasis, 52
Glaucoma, **210, 211,** 210–2
  description of, **210**
  treatment of, **210, 211,** 210–2
Glucagon, 195
Glucocorticoids, **58, 61**
  in adrenal cortex, **196–7, 199**
  for allergic disorders, **164**
  as immunosuppression drugs, 71
  for inflammatory bowel disease, 184
  for reversible airways disease, 161
  side effects of, **199–200**
  therapeutic notes on, **200–1**
Glucose, 195
Glycopeptides, **34–5,** 36
Glycoprotein inhibitors, 152
Gonadotropin-releasing hormones, 206
Gout
  description of, 62–3, **63**
  drugs for, 62–3, **63**
G-proteins, **5**
  cAMP and, 83
  receptors and, **5,** 6
  targets for, **5–8**
    ion channels, **5–6**
    second messengers, 6–8
Griseofulvin, 49
Guanylyl cyclase system, 7–8

H
H$_1$ receptor antagonists, **179**
Half-life, of drug, 16
Hallucinogens. *See* Psychotomimetic drugs
Halothane, 117
Headache, **68–9**
  migraine, **68**
Heart, 127–38
  anatomy and physiology of, **127–9,** 127–30
    autonomic control in, **129**
    cardiac contractility in, **129–30**
    functioning of, **127, 128**
    nodal and nonnodal cells, **128–9**
  dysfunction of, 130–8
    abnormal impulse conduction, 132

Heart *(Continued)*
  dysfunction of *(Continued)*
    abnormal impulse generation, **131–2**
    angina pectoris, 132
    arrhythmias, **131**
    CHF, **130–1**
  treatment for, 132–8, **138**
    antianginal drugs, 136–8
    antiarrhythmic drugs, 134–6
    cardiac glycosides, **130,** 132–3, **138**
    diuretics, 134, **138**
    phosphodiesterase inhibitors, **130,** 134, **138**
Helicobacter pylori, eradication for stomach disease, **178–9**
Helminthic infection
  concepts of, 53
  drugs for, 53–5
Hemicholinium, **78**
Hemostasis, 148–53
  anticoagulants in, **149, 150–1**
  antifibrinolytic agents in, 153
  antiplatelet agents in, **151,** 151–2
  bleeding disorders of, **149–50**
  fibrinolytic agents in, 152
  principles of, 148–9, **149**
Heparins, **150–1**
Heroin, 122
Hirudins, **150–1**
Histamine H$_2$ receptor antagonists, 176–7
Histamines
  in allergic disorders, **163**
  description of, **164, 165**
HIV. *See* Human immunodeficiency virus
Human immunodeficiency virus (HIV), drug therapy, **42,** 44–6
Hydralazine, **139,** 142
Hydrocortisone. *See* Cortisol
Hydrolysis, of drugs, 13
Hydroxyprogesterone, 205
Hydroxyurea, **24,** 26, 27–8
Hyperlipidemias, 145–6
Hypertension, **139,** 139–43
  description of, **139**
  treatment of, **139,** 139–43
    antihypertensive drugs, 143
    diuretic drugs, **139,** 142–3
    hydralazine, **139,** 142
    minoxidil, **139,** 142
    sodium nitroprusside, **139,** 142
    vasolidators, **139, 140–1**

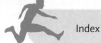

Hyperthyroidism, **188–9,** 188–90
  description of, **188, 189**
  management of, **188, 189,** 189–90
Hypnotics
  barbiturates, 98
  benzodiazepine, **96–7**
  description of, 95
  miscellaneous agents, 99
  nonbenzodiazepine, **97**
  serotonergic receptor blocking, 98
Hypoglycemia, 195
Hypothyroidism, **188, 189,** 190
  description of, **188, 189**
  management of, 190

I

Ibuprofen. *See* Propionic acid
IFNs. *See* Interferons
Imidazoles, **47–8**
Immunoglobulins, 43–4
Immunomodulators, 46
Immunosuppression, 69–71
  description of, 69
  drugs for, 69–71
    azathioprine, 71
    cyclosporin, 69–71
    glucocorticoids, 71
Immunotherapy, for cancer, 28–9
Indomethacin. *See* Acetic acid
Infectious diseases, 31–56
  anthelminthic drugs, 53–5
    benzimidazoles, **54**
    diethylcarbamizine, **54,** 55
    ivermectin, **54,** 55
    niclosamide, 53, **54**
    piperazine, **54**
    praziquantel, 53–4, **54**
  antibacterial drugs, 31–41
  antifungal drugs, **47–9**
  antiprotozoal drugs, 49–53
  antiviral drugs, 41–6, **41**
Inflammation, 57–63, **58–61**
  anti-inflammatory drugs, 57–61, **58–61**
    glucocorticoids, **58, 61**
    NSAIDs, 57–61, **58–61**
  arachidonic acid metabolites, 57, **58**
  description of, 57
  DMARDs, **61,** 61–2
  gout drugs, 62–3, **63**
Inflammatory bowel disease, 183–4
  description of, 183

Inflammatory bowel disease (*Continued*)
  treatment of, 184
Inhalers, 161–2
Inositol (1,4,5) triphosphate (IP$_3$)
  G-proteins and, 7
  in parasympathetic nervous
    system, **86**
  in sympathetic nervous
    system, 83, **84**
Insulin
  description of, **191,** 191–2
  for diabetes management, **193**
Interferons (IFNs), 43, 46
Intestines, 180–5
  anal disorders, **185**
  inflammatory bowel disease, 183–4
  motility of, 180, **181**
    antidiarrheal drugs, **181,** 182–3
    antispasmodics, **181,** 181–2
    control of, 180
    stimulants for, 180
  obesity, 184–5
Iodine, **189,** 189–190
Ion channels, 3–4, **4**
  as G-proteins targets, **5–6**
  receptors and, **4–5**
IP$_3$. *See* Inositol (1,4,5) triphosphate
Iron, 153
Isoflurane, 117–8
Isoniazid, 40
Ivermectin, **54,** 55

K
Ketamine, 116
Ketolides, **34–5,** 39
Kidney system, **167,** 167–71
  drug excretion, 18
  nephrons of, **167,** 167–71
  principle functions of, **167**
Kinetics
  of drugs, 15–6
  first-order, 16
  zero-order, 15–6

L
Laxatives, 182
Leishmaniasis, 52–3
Leukotriene receptor
    antagonists, 161
Levamisole, 29
Levothyroxine, 190

Lidocaine, **135**
Lincosamide, 39
Liothyronine, 190
Lithium, 103
Liver, drug metabolism and, 13, 18
Local anesthetics, 74–6, **76, 77**
  routes of administration, **75–6**
Loop of Henle
  diuretics for, **169,** 171
  in nephron, **169**

M
Macrolides
  in antituberculosis therapy, 40
  description of, **34–5,** 39
Malaria, 49–52
  description of, 49–51
  drugs for, 51–2
MAO. *See* Monoamine oxygenase
MAOIs. *See* Monoamine oxidase inhibitors
Mast-cell stabilizers, 161
Medroxyprogesterone, 205
Medroxyprogesterone acetate, **203,** 203–4
Mefloquine, 51
Melphalan, 26
Menstrual cycle, **201–2**
Menthol vapor, 162
Meperidine, **66, 67**
Mercaptopurine, 27
Metabolism, of drugs, 13–5
  acetaminophen poisoning, 14–5
  factors influencing, 14
  hydrolysis of, 13
  oxidation of, 13
  phase 1, 13
  phase 2, 14
  reduction of, 13
  sites of, 13
Methimazole, **189**
Methotrexate
  as antimetabolite, 27
  for inflammatory bowel disease, 184
Methylcellulose
  as anti-obesity drugs, 185
  for intestinal motility, **182,** 182–3
Methylenedioxymethamphetamine, 120–1
Methylprednisolone, **200**
Methyltestosterone, 205
Metoprolol, **135,** 137
Metronidazole
  description of, **34–5,** 36, 39

Metronidazole *(Continued)*
  for inflammatory bowel disease, 184
  use of, 52–3
Mifepristone, 205, 206
Migraine, **68**
Mineral oil, 182
Mineralocorticoids
  in adrenal cortex, **197, 199**
  side effects of, **199–200**
Minipill, **203**
Minocycline, 37
Minoxidil, **139,** 142
Miotics, **211,** 212
Misoprostol
  in reproductive system, 206–7
  for stomach acid-related
      disease, **177–8**
Mitotane, **24,** 28
Mitotic inhibitors, **24,** 26, 27
Monoamine oxidase inhibitors (MAOIs)
  for affective disorder treatment, 100,
      101, 102–3
  in sympathetic nervous system, 84
Monoamine oxygenase (MAO)
  inhibitors of, 94
  in sympathetic nervous system, 83–5
MOPP therapy, **25**
"Morning-after" pill. *See* Postcoital pill
Morphine
  drug absorption and, 12
  as opioid, **66–7**
Mucolytics, **163**
Muscarinic agonists, **211,** 212
Muscarinic antagonists, 87–8
  for glaucoma, 212, **213**
Myeloproliferative disorders, 154

N
Nafarelin, 206
Nalbuphine, **66, 68**
Naloxone, **68**
Naltrexone, **68**
Nandrolone, 206
Nausea, **179,** 179–80
  description of, **179**
  treatment of, **179,** 179–80
Nebulizers, 161–2
Nephrons, **167,** 167–71, **168**
  blood supply to, **167**
  glomerular filtration in, **167**
  tubular function in, **168,** 168–71

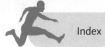

Nerve conduction
    description of, **73**, 73–4, **75**
    size of nerve fiber, 74
    sodium channel, 74
Nervous system
    autonomic, **81, 82, 86–8,** 81–8
    central, 91–125
    nitrergic, **88**
    parasympathetic, **86–8**
    peripheral, 73–90, **75–90**
    sympathetic, **82–6**
Neuralgic pain, 69
Neuraminidase inhibitors, 43
Neuroleptic drugs
    adverse effects of, **106, 107,** 106–8
    compounds, **105, 106**
    description of, **105–6**
    malignant syndrome, 108
Neuromuscular blockers, 118
Neuromuscular junction (NMJ), **76–9,** 76–81
    drugs for, **78,** 78–81, **79, 81**
        anticholinesterases, **80–1**
        postsynaptic agents, **79–80**
        presynaptic agents, **78–9**
    nicAChR in, **76–7**
        physiology of, **76–7**
        targets of, **78, 79**
Niacin. *See* Nicotinic acid
nicAChR. *See* Nicotinic acetylcholine receptor
Niclosamide, 53, 54
Nicotine, 121
Nicotinic acetylcholine receptor (nicAChR)
    ganglionic v. NMJ, **81**
    in NMJ, **76–7**
Nicotinic acid (niacin), **146,** 147
Nitrergic nervous system, **88**
Nitric oxide
    in erectile dysfunction, 173
    G-proteins and, 8
    in nitrergic nervous system, 88
Nitrofurantoin, **34–5,** 39
Nitrous oxide, 117
NMJ. *See* Neuromuscular junction
Nonbenzodiazepine hypnotics, 97
Nonnucleoside reverse transcriptase
        inhibitors, **45**
Nonsteroidal anti-inflammatory drugs (NSAIDs)
    description of, 57–61, **58–61**
    diuretics interaction with, 18
    as gout drug, **63**
    for headaches, **68**

Norepinephrine
    for circulatory treatment, 144
    in sympathetic nervous system,
        83–5, **84–5**
Norethindrone, 205
NSAIDs. *See* Nonsteroidal anti-inflammatory
        drugs
Nucleoside analog reverse transcriptase
        inhibitors, 44–5

O
Obesity, 184–5
    description of, 184
    treatment of, 184–5
OCDs. *See* Oral contraceptive drugs
Opioid analgesics, 122
Opioid receptors, **65–6**
    analgesic drugs for, **66,** 66–8
    antagonists of, **68**
    endogenous opioids, **66**
    types of, **65–6**
Opioids, 162–3
Opium, **66**
Oral contraceptive drugs (OCDs), **203**
Oral hypoglycemics, **193,** 193–4
Oseltamivir, 43
Osteoporosis, 207
Oxicams, **61**
Oxidation, of drugs, 13
Oxygen, 161–2
Oxytocic drugs, 206–7

P
P450 cytochrome
    drug metabolism and, 13–4
    imidazole inhibition of, **48**
    phenytoin induction of, 111
    rifampin inducement of, 40
    triazole inhibition of, **48**
Pain, **63–8,** 63–9
    description of, **63–4**
    headache, **68,** 68–9
    neuralgic, 69
    opioid receptors, **65–6**
        analgesic drugs for, **66–8**
        antagonists of, **68**
        description of, **65–6**
    perception of, **64–5**
Pancreas, 185
Parasympathetic nervous system, **86–8**
    drugs acting on, **87–8, 89**

Parasympathetic nervous system *(Continued)*
  heart influence by, **129**
  receptors of, **86–7**
Parasympathomimetics, 173
Parkinsonism, **91–2,** 91–4
  description of, **91**
  etiology of, **91–2**
  pathogenesis in, **91**
  treatment of, **92,** 92–4
Penicillin
  description of, **32,** 33–4, **34–5**
  resistance to, **32**
Pentazocine, **66,** 68
Peptic ulceration, **175,** 175–6
  acid secretion and, 176, **177**
  description of, **175**
  protective factors against, **175**
Peripheral nervous system, **73, 79,**
      81–2, 84–8, 73–90
  autonomic nervous system, 81–8, **82, 84–8**
  concepts of, **73,** 73–6, **75, 76**
    local anesthetics, 74–6, **75, 76, 77**
    nerve conduction, **73,** 73–4, **75**
  nitrergic nervous system, **88**
  somatic nervous system, **76–9,** 76–81
Pertussis, 6
Pharmacodynamics
  definition of, 10
  drug interactions in, 17–8
Pharmacokinetics
  compliance, 10–1
  definition of, 10
  drug absorption, 11–2
  drug distribution, 12–3
  drug excretion, 15
  drug interactions in, 18
  drug metabolism, 13–5
  of local anesthetics, 74
  mathematical aspects of, 15–7
    kinetics, 15–6
    model independent approach, 17
    one-compartment model, 16–7
    two-compartment model, 17
  routes of administration, 11
Pharmacology
  definition of, 3, 10
  molecular basis of, 3–8, **4, 5**
    enzymes, **4**
    receptors, **4,** 4–8
    transport systems, 3–4, **4**
Phenothiazines, 106, **179**

Phenoxybenzamine, 143
Phenytoin
  as antiepileptic drug, 111–2
  for cardiac treatment, **135**
Pheochromocytoma, 143
Phosphodiesterase inhibitors
  for cardiac treatment, **130,** 134, **138**
  for erectile dysfunction
      treatment, 173–4
Phospholipase C/inositol phosphate system, 7
Pilocarpine, **211,** 212
Piperazine, **54**
Pneumocystis pneumonia, 53
Polmonary surfactants, 162
Polyene macrolides, **47, 48**
Polymyxins, **32, 34–5,** 40
Postcoital pill, 204
Potassium perchlorate, **189,** 189–90
Potency, of drugs, 10
PPI. *See* Proton pump inhibitors
Praziquantel, 53–4
Prednisolone
  in adrenal cortex, **200**
  for endocrine therapy, 28
  for inflammatory bowel
      disease, 184
Prednisone, 184
Primaquine, 51
Probenecid, **63**
Procarbazine, **24,** 26, 27
Progesterones
  for endocrine therapy, 28
  in reproductive system, **201–2,** 205
Progestin antagonists. *See* Antiprogestins
Progestins, 205
Proguanil, 51
Promethazine, **164**
Propanolol
  for cardiac treatment, **135,** 137
  for hyperthyroidism, 190
  salmeterol interaction with, 18
Prophylactic drugs, 161
Propionic acid, **60**
Propofol, **115**
Prostaglandin E, 174
Prostaglandins, 206–7
Protamine, **150**
Protease inhibitors, **45,** 45–6
Proton pump inhibitors (PPI), 176
Protozoal infection
  concepts of, 49, **50**

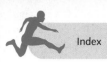

Protozoal infection (Continued)
  drugs for, 49–53
Proximal tubule
  diuretics for, 172
  in nephron, **168**
Pseudoephedrine, **163**
Psoriasis, **214, 215**
Psychotic disorders, 104–8, **105–7**
  concepts of, 104
  neuroleptic drugs for, **105–7**, 105–8
  schizophrenia, 104–5, **105**
Psychotomimetic drugs, 123
Psyllium, 182
Pyrazinamide, 40
Pyrazolones, 61
Pyrimethamine, 51

Q
Quinidine, 134
Quinine, 51
Quinoline-methanols, 51
Quinolones
  description of, **32, 34–5,** 37
  as DMARD, 61, 62

R
Radioiodine, 190
Receptors, **4**
  DNA-linked, 8
  drugs and, 8–10
  G-proteins and, **5,** 6
  ion channels and, **4–5**
  reserve of, 10
  tyrosine-kinase-linked, 8
Reduction, of drugs, 13
Reproductive system, **201–3,** 201–7
  drug influences on, **203,** 203–7
    anabolic steroids, 206
    contraceptives, **203,** 203–4
    hormones, 204–5
    oxytocic drugs, 206–7
  hormonal control of, **201–2**
    female reproductive tract, **201**
    male reproductive tract, **202, 203**
    menstrual cycle, **201–2**
Reproductive tract
  female, **201**
  male, **202, 203**
Resistance to antibiotics
  acquired, **32,** 32–3
  innate, **32**

Respiratory system, 157–65, **163–5**
  allergic disorders in, **163–5**
  antitussives in, 162–3, **163**
  decongestants in, **163**
  mucolytics in, **163**
  polmonary surfactants in, 162
  reversible airways disease, 157–62
    asthma, 157–9
    COPD, 159
    management of, 159–62, **163**
  stimulants in, 162
Reversible airways disease, management of, 159–62, **163**
  bronchodilators, **159–61**
  inhalers, nebulizers and oxygen for, **161–2**
  prophylactic and anti-inflammatory drugs, **161**
Ribavirin, 44
Rickets, 207
Rifampicin, **41**
Rifampin
  in antituberculosis therapy, 40
  description of, 36
Rituximab, 29

S
Salicylates, 57–8, **58,** 59
  for skin treatment, **216**
Salmeterol
  propanolol interaction with, 18
  for reversible airways disease, 159
Schizophrenia, 104–5, **105**
  symptoms and signs of, 104
  theories of, 104–5, **105**
Second messengers
  adenylyl cyclase/cyclic AMP system, 7
  as G-protein targets, 6–8
  guanylyl cyclase system, 7–8
  phospholipase C/inositol phosphate system, 7
Serotonergic receptors, 98
Serotonin agonists, **68,** 68–9
Serotonin receptor agonists, 180
Serotonin-norepinephrine reuptake inhibitors (SNRIs), **100, 101,** 102
Sildenafil, 173–4
Skin, 212–7, **213–7**
  anatomy and physiology of, 212–4, **213–4**
  disorders of, **214**
    acne, **214**

Skin *(Continued)*
  disorders of *(Continued)*
    eczema, **214**
    psoriasis, **214, 215**
    treatment of, **215–7**
      anthralin, **215**
      corticosteroids, **214, 215, 216**
      emollients, **216**
      other drugs, **217**
      salicylates, **216**
      tar preparations, **215, 216**
      vitamin D, **215–6**
Sleep disorders, 95–9
Smoking cessation, 123–4
SNRIs. *See* Serotonin-norepinephrine
    reuptake inhibitors
Sodium nitroprusside, **139,** 142
  G-proteins and, 8
Somatic nervous system, **76–9,** 76–81
Specific serotonin reuptake inhibitors
    (SSRIs), **100, 101,** 102
SSRIs. *See* Specific serotonin reuptake
    inhibitors
Stanozolol, 206
Statins, **146,** 146–7
Steroidal anti-inflammatory drugs. *See*
    Glucocorticoids
Stomach, **175,** 175–9
  acid-related disease, 176–9
    acid secretion reduction, 176–7, **177**
    antacids, 178
    Helicobacter pylori eradication, **178–9**
    mucosal strengtheners, **177–8**
    gastroesophageal reflux disease,
      176, **178**
    peptic ulceration of, **175,** 175–6
Stool modifiers, 183
Streptokinase, 152
Streptomycin
  as aminoglycoside, 37
  in antituberculosis therapy, 40
  as NMJ drug, **79**
Succinylcholine, 80
Sulfinpyrazone, **63**
Sulfonamides, 51
  as antifolate, 36
Sulfones, 36
Sulfonylureas, 194
Sympathetic nervous system, **82, 84–6,** 82–6
  adrenal medulla, **82**
  adrenoceptors, **82,** 82–3

Sympathetic nervous system *(Continued)*
  drugs acting on, 83–6, **84–6**
  heart influence by, **129**
Sympathomimetics. *See* Adrenoceptor agonists

T
Tamoxifen, 28
Telithromycin, 39
Terbutaline, 159
Testosterone, 202, 205
Tetracycline(s)
  description of, **34–5,** 37–8
  resistance, **32**
Theophylline, 159–61
Thiazide diuretics, **171,** 171–2
Thiazolidinediones, 194
Thioamides, **189**
Thiopental, **115**
Thioxanthenes, **106**
Thrombosis, **149**
Thyroid gland, **187,** 187–90
  dysfunction of, **188,** 188–90
    hyperthyroidism, **188,** 188–90
    hypothyroidism, **188, 189,** 190
  function of, **187, 188, 189**
Thyroid replacement therapy, 190
Thyroxine. *See* Levothyroxine
Timolol, **210–1**
Tinidazole, 39
Tissue-type plasminogen activators
    (t-PAs), 152
t-PAs. *See* Tissue-type plasminogen
    activators
Tranexamic acid, 153
Transport systems, 3–4, **4**
  carrier molecules, **4**
  ion channels, 3–4, **4**
Trastuzumab, 29
Trazoles, **48**
Triamcinolone, **201**
Trichomonas vaginitis, 52
Trimethoprim
  as antifolate, 36
  resistance to, **32**
Trypanosomiasis, 52
Tyrosine-kinase-linked receptors, 8

U
Uricosurics, **63**
Urinary incontinence, 173
Urinary retention, 172–3

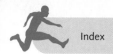

Urinary system, 172–4
  erectile dysfunction in, 173–4
  urinary incontinence in, 173
  urinary retention in, 172–3
Ursodeoxycholic acid, 185

V
Vaccines, 29
Vancomycin
  as glycopeptide, 36
  resistance to, **32**
Vasopressin, 144–5
Verapamil, 136–7
Vinblastine, 27
Vincristine, 27
Vinorelbine, 27
Viral infection
  concepts of, **41**
  drugs for, **41**–6
Vitamin B$_{12}$, 153

Vitamin D
  for bone treatment, 207–8
  for skin treatment, **215–6**
Vitamin K, **150**
Vitamin K antagonists, **150–1**
Vomiting, **179,** 179–80
  description of, **179**
  treatment of, **179,** 179–80

W
Warfarin, **150–1**

X
Xanthines, 159–61

Z
Zanamivir, 43
Zolpidem, **97,** 97–8